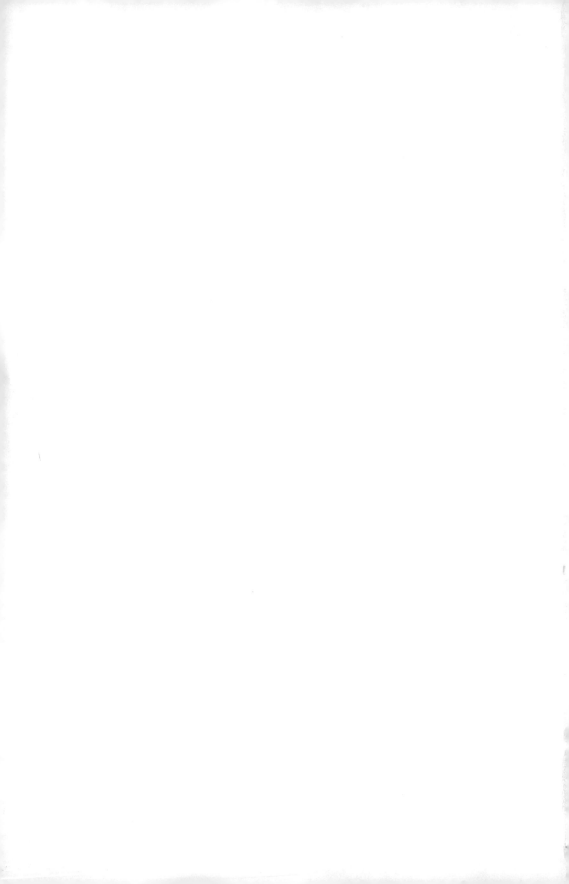

THE PSYCHOTHERAPIST'S GUIDE TO PSYCHOPHARMACOLOGY

Second Edition

MICHAEL J. GITLIN, M.D.

THE FREE PRESS
NEW YORK   LONDON   TORONTO   SYDNEY   SINGAPORE

THE FREE PRESS
A Division of Simon & Schuster Inc.
1230 Avenue of the Americas
New York, NY 10020

THE FREE PRESS and colophon are trademarks
of Simon & Schuster Inc.

Designed by Michael Mendelsohn of MM Design 2000, Inc.

Manufactured in the United States of America

10 9 8 7 6 5 4 3 2 1

Library of Congress Cataloging-in-Publication Data

Gitlin, Michael J.
     The psychotherapist's guide to psychopharmacology / Michael J. Gitlin.—2nd ed.
     p.   cm.
     Includes bibliographical references and index.
     ISBN 0-684-82737-9 (hc)
     1. Mental illness—Chemotherapy.   2. Psychotropic drugs.
3. Psychopharmacology.   I. Title.
     [DNLM: 1. Mental Disorders—drug therapy.   2. Psychotropic Drugs—
therapeutic use.   3. Psychotropic Drugs—pharmacology.   WM 402
G536p 1996]
RC483.G55   1996
616.89'18—dc20
DNLM/DLC
for Library of Congress   95-43353
                                                                      CIP

To Jeanie,
with love and admiration,
for what you have given me, taught me, and shared with me

Contents

SECTION FOUR

SECTION FIVE

List of Illustrations and Tables

Preface

WHEN THE FIRST EDITION of this book was published, its stated goal was to bridge the gap between those who prescribe medications—psychiatrists—and those who do not—nonphysician therapists and some psychoanalyst physicians. With six years' difference between editions, the need for that bridge has, if anything, increased. Pharmacotherapy has become a progressively dominant option in treating psychiatric/psychological disorders. At the same time, the split-treatment model (discussed in detail in chapter 14), in which one professional (typically a nonphysician therapist) provides psychotherapy while another (either a psychiatrist or an internist) prescribes the medication, has become more prevalent over the last few years. Therefore, those practitioners in closest touch with many patients taking psychotropic medications need even greater access to the kind of information that would allow them to be knowledgeable participants in the treatment.

Unfortunately, sources of information that would fill that need are still scarce. Psychopharmacology textbooks continue to be published on a regular basis. Virtually all of them, however, also continue to be written for professionals who already have some experience in prescribing medications. For therapists who have neither training nor experience in the medical model, these textbooks can be alienating in their use of technical language and assumption of basic knowledge of biological aspects of psychiatry.

As with the first edition, the purpose of this book is to bridge this gap, to provide a source of information about the medical aspects of modern psychiatry to therapists who cannot or do not often prescribe psychotropic medications. In the six years since the first edition was published, psychopharmacology has continued its rather rapid evolution. Some areas, such as the use of ECT and pharmacological options for generalized anxiety disorder, have been refined but not substantially changed. In so many other areas, however, the types of clinical thinking that were appropriate in the 1980s are simply outdated now. For many of these changes, the predominant factor has been the availability of new medications that have revolutionized the treatment of some disorders—such as powerfully serotonergic antidepressants for depressive disorders and obsessive compulsive disorder, and atypical neuroleptics for psychotic disorders. In other clinical situations, the changes over such a short period of time are secondary to greater recognition of the expanding spectrum of pharmacologically responsive disorders. Given this evolution, the purpose of this second edition is to keep up with these changes and to provide interested readers with the requisite information to stay current and knowledgeable. Anticipating that psychopharmacology will continue to evolve and hoping to retard a too-rapid obsolescence of this edition, some medications that are likely to be released in the next few years are described within the text.

The intended audience of the book is the same as previously: clinical psychologists, social workers, marriage and family counselors, clinical nurse therapists, and those psychiatrists whose knowledge of psychopharmacology is not extensive. Some family practitioners or internists may also find it useful. As before, I have attempted to utilize nontechnical language and to define technical terms when they are introduced.

It seems useless to describe medication treatments for disorders that may not in all cases be familiar to readers. Therefore a significant portion of the book is devoted to describing disorders for which medications are prescribed. With rare exception, I have drawn on the *Diagnostic and Statistical Manual,* Fourth Edition (American Psychiatric Association, 1994a), or DSM-IV as it is called, for this purpose. (See chapter 1 for a more detailed discussion of the DSMs.) As I point out repeatedly in the text, by no means does this imply a wholesale acceptance of these criteria. Neither DSM-IV nor any other manual or textbook can be considered the revealed truth. In many places in the text, I have noted my disagreements with DSM-IV. Although the DSM-IV diagnostic criteria vary in how well they describe discrete clinical syndromes, they at least give us a starting point for diagnosis. With the increasing emphasis on outcome studies to justify health care costs, the demand for clearly defined diagnoses will only increase in the near future. DSM-IV provides these definitions.

The format of the book is unchanged from the previous edition, allowing the reader to approach psychopharmacology in two ways: focusing on a psychiatric disorder and the medications used in its treatment, or on the medication itself and the disorders for which it is useful. The book is divided into five sections:

Chapter 1 explores concepts of diagnosis and treatment effects.

Chapter 2 provides an overview of brain function. It describes how cells within the brain communicate with each other, how these mechanisms may go awry in some major psychiatric disorders, and how medications may work biochemically. A new section on neuroimaging studies has been added for this edition. Although the information in this chapter is not directly relevant to the clinical focus of the book, it does provide a background for those interested and, more importantly, it introduces certain terms and concepts regarding medications that are referred to in later chapters.

Chapters 3 through 8 are devoted to the disorders and clinical situations for which medications are currently prescribed. For each disorder, the following issues are addressed: how the diagnosis is made (including, for the major disorders, a list of pertinent questions to ask); the possible genetic components; the natural history of the disorder. Differential diagnosis, that is, of disorders, both medical and psychiatric, that are often confused with the disorder in question, is also treated. The second half of each chapter discusses medication treatment. Here the emphasis is on how decisions on medication can and should be made, with less attention to technical aspects of treatment, such as doses and side effects.

Chapters 9 through 13 focus on the medications themselves: the disorders for which they might be prescribed, their likely mechanisms of action, the names of the different medications, how they are prescribed, the doses used, and the major side effects that might be seen.

Finally, chapter 14 discusses psychotherapy/psychopharmacology interactions: theoretical considerations, how to evaluate and select a pharmacotherapist in your area, and ways in which two professionals, one of whom prescribes medications and the other of whom provides psychotherapy, can best work together.

Case histories are presented throughout the book. These may illustrate types of disorders not easily recognized or complex situations that are most easily explicated by a specific case, or they may be typical vignettes involving medications. All case histories are real ones, altered to preserve anonymity but with the essential features intact.

Because this book is intended as a clinical guide and not as an exhaustive review, references are provided only intermittently. References are generally given for classic or unique studies, little known findings, the most recent study of its type, or for recent reviews of a topic. For those interested in more extensive reading, suggestions are provided at the end of the book.

Tables that list all medications of a class give both the trade names and generic names. However, within the text, in order to avoid advertising a specific product of a pharmaceutical firm, medications are called by their generic names with trade names only occasionally given in parentheses. The appendix lists all medications referred to in the book alphabetically by generic names, trade names, and medication class. Dosage ranges should be considered as approximate; occasionally patients may respond to smaller doses than expected while other patients will need higher doses than are generally recommended.

The following linguistic conventions are used: (1) Because the concern is with the more severe psychiatric/psychological problems for which the medical model can be applied relatively easily (except for personality disorders), the people we treat will be described as patients, not clients. The use of this term simply acknowledges that the types of problems described for which medications might be prescribed are different from, for instance, marital conflict. (2) The professional prescribing medication will be described as the psychopharmacologist, pharmacotherapist, or consultant, these terms being used interchangeably. The term "therapist" is used for any mental health professional who is treating the patient using some form of talking therapy. This would include clinical psychologists, social workers, marriage and family counselors, clinical nurse therapists, and psychiatrists.

Acknowledgments

T HE SIMPLE EXISTENCE of a second edition of a book implies at least a reasonable response to the first edition. I appreciate the positive responses received from those of you who read the first edition. Just as much, however, I am grateful to those of you who took the time to tell me or write me with suggestions on how to improve the book. Some of those changes have been incorporated in this edition.

In large part, teaching skills, whether verbal or written, derive from the demands, requests, and requirements of good students. In this regard, I have continued to reap the benefits of working with the exceptionally bright and inquisitive residents, psychology interns, and medical students at the UCLA psychiatry residency program, the psychology internship program at the hospital, and the UCLA Medical School. In the two settings in which I teach the most—the Affective Disorders Clinic (an outpatient clinic specializing in evaluating and treating mood disorders) and the inpatient units at the UCLA Neuropsychiatric Hospital where I am an attending physician—the residents, interns, and students have (appropriately) demanded clear explanations of psychiatric diagnosis and psychopharmacology. I am indebted to all of these students for forcing me to hone my teaching skills and for providing such intoxicating intellectual stimulation. Following my previous working relationship with Dr. Kay Jamison, my ongoing work with Drs. Connie Hammen and Keith Nuechterlein and their students has continued to provide me with the close interface with medical psychology that enhances my sensitivity for collaborative work. I am indebted to Migdalia (Micky) Richardson for her help in gathering endless references and typing the tables in this book, and for her continual good cheer and endless resourcefulness. Although he recently left UCLA for the University of New Mexico, my internalized image of Dr. Joel Yager continues to sustain a vision of patient care, teaching, writing, and intellectual joy as attainable goals in academic medicine, even at the present time.

For this edition, David Feinberg, MD, Barry Guze, MD, and Vicki Hendrick, MD read new sections of the book in their areas of expertise and provided thoughtful critiques. Charles Reynolds, PharmD, was always available for the latest update on the availability of medications. Susan Arellano of The Free Press quietly but consistently queried me over the last few years as to when a new edition would be appropriate. Her message was clear and her encouragement helpful.

Given the multiple demands of professional and personal life, it is difficult to carve out the time needed to write a book, even with less time devoted to sleep and more efficiency in the tasks of life. Some of the time invested in writing this edition was taken from Josh, Katie, and Rebecca, my three children who were patient and loving as always. My deepest gratitude, however, goes to my wife, Jean Gitlin, PhD, a clinical psychologist who, much to my amazement, encouraged this second edition because of her conviction of its value. Consistent with her being the best therapist I know and the wisest and most loving person in my life, she was far more patient with me than I might have been in the reverse situation.

SECTION

ONE

1

Diagnosis and Treatment: Basic Principles

I N THE LAST THIRTY YEARS, we in the mental health field have witnessed a veritable explosion of new information that has shifted the emphasis from the more psychoanalytically based models and treatments that dominated psychiatry and psychology for the preceding thirty years to descriptive and biological ones. The new approach is based on a number of assumptions, three of which are relevant to this book. The first is that psychiatric disorders can be reliably classified according to diagnostic methods used in medicine before the introduction of laboratory tests. The second is that pharmacological treatments—medications—are effective in treating a variety of psychiatric disorders. The third is that the efficacy of psychiatric therapies can be evaluated by empirical studies. Not surprisingly, the bulk of these treatment studies have involved medications. In this chapter, these three assumptions—that psychopathology can be usefully described by symptom-based terms, that medications effectively treat psychiatric disorders, and that scientific methods can be applied to evaluate treatments—will be discussed. The goals of medication treatment, some general principles of psychopharmacological treatment, and criteria for the selection of appropriate patients for psychopharmacological evaluation will then be presented.

DESCRIPTIVE PSYCHIATRY AND DSM-IV

Although the introduction of a descriptive, diagnosis-based approach to psychopathology was a radical shift from the etiologically based language of psychoanalysis, it was far from new. During the late nineteenth and early twentieth centuries, descriptive approaches dominated European psychiatry and resulted in the first diagnostic distinction between manic-depressive illness and schizophrenia (then called dementia praecox) on the basis of their differing clinical pictures. However, the descriptive approach fell into disfavor in this country for many decades, resurfacing only with the emergence of the *Diagnostic and Sta-*

tistical Manual of Mental Disorders, Third Edition (DSM-III) in 1980, the revised edition (DSM-III-R) in 1987, and DSM-IV in 1994. The goal of DSM-IV, as for any other diagnostic classification scheme is "to provide a helpful guide to clinical practice, . . . to improve communication among clinicians and researchers . . . , for improving the collection of clinical information and as an educational tool for teaching psychopathology" (DSM-IV, p. xv). By defining disorders consistently, both clinicians and researchers may better agree on what is meant by terms such as depression, thereby allowing better prediction of important clinical variables such as prognosis and treatment response.

Because the first half of this book is organized according to the DSM's classifications, it is worth reviewing their essential components.

The most important question in the descriptive approach used by DSM-IV is "what," in contrast to the centrality of "why" in psychoanalysis. It attempts (with only varying degrees of success) to be atheoretical with regard to etiology. Thus, when a 37-year-old man goes through a period of depressed mood with alterations in sleep, appetite, energy, and concentrating ability, the reason *why* is irrelevant for making the diagnosis of depression. Whether this patient's depression is best understood by his poor introject of a maternal object, depressogenic assumptions (using a cognitive framework), or by an alteration in the regulation of norepinephrine or serotonin in certain parts of the brain does not alter the diagnosis.

Among the objections to the descriptive approach is that patients are pigeonholed into diagnostic boxes and not understood for the unique constellation of intrapsychic, historical, and environmental variables that set each one apart from others. This objection is valid *if* clinicians view the patient's identity as synonymous with his diagnosis. Is the patient viewed as a person with manic-depressive disorder or is he a manic-depressive? The difference is far from semantic. Although the descriptive approach can be misused to objectify and distance patients, that is neither its purpose nor its proper use. DSM-IV classifies disorders, not individuals.

The second essential feature of the DSMs is their multiaxial approach. Patients are rated along five axes simultaneously, each of which utilizes different types of information. Psychiatric disorders are listed on Axes I and II while Axes III, IV, and V describe associated medical conditions, psychosocial and environmental stressors, and level of functioning. Axis I disorders comprise all clinical syndromes except for personality disorders and developmental disorders arising in childhood, which are listed on Axis II. Thus, Axis II disorders are, in general, more stable and long lasting. When a clinician describes a patient as having an Axis I disorder, he is referring to the presence of a symptom-based disorder, such as depression, phobias, or schizophrenia. Describing an adult patient as having an Axis II disorder is equivalent to saying he has a personality disorder. Among the goals of separating Axis I from Axis II is to encourage clinicians to conceptualize coexistent disorders. Instead of deciding whether the patient suffers from major depression *or* narcissistic personality disorder, the clinician can diagnose both disorders. This approach makes evaluation more difficult, but also more accurate. In this way, either/or formulations can be replaced by richer, more complex models.

It is in the evaluation and diagnosis of personality disorders that the descriptive approach of DSM-IV is most problematic. Inherently, personality features are difficult to describe using the language of symptoms and signs. As an example, criteria used to diagnose personality disorders such as lack of empathy or persistent identity disturbance simply do not fit well into a classification system that is defined as atheoretical and descriptive. Compounding the problem of classifying personality disorders in the DSMs is the use of a categorical system in which patients either meet criteria for a diagnosis (a category) or they don't. Another type of diagnostic system describes patients along a number of dimensions without specific cutoffs demarcating normal from abnormal (or having a disorder vs. not having it). It is especially in the diagnosis and description of personality disorders that a dimensional system has the strongest and most persuasive proponents—and that the categorical system has the most difficulties (see chapter 7 for more details about dimensional approaches to personality).

It is rather easy to criticize, with merit, the entire DSM system. Three different manuals—DSM-III, III-R, and IV—have been published over the short span of fourteen years, an insufficient time to gather enough new data to warrant many of the diagnostic definitions and changes in the new editions (Zimmerman, 1990). Disorders are defined and undefined in successive DSM editions without obvious justification. As an example, a manic episode precipitated by an antidepressant was diagnosed as bipolar disorder in DSM-III-R. In DSM-IV, that same episode would be called substance-induced mood disorder and specifically prohibited from contributing to a diagnosis of bipolar disorder, despite a lack of published data supporting or refuting either definition in the last six years. Furthermore, it continues to be difficult to use DSM-IV to describe patients with milder disorders, such as those with low self-esteem or heightened rejection sensitivity without significant depressive symptoms.

Additionally, the DSMs have done a better job at defining disorders reliably (can three clinicians agree that a certain patient has these specific symptoms and therefore meets specified criteria for a diagnosis?) than in demonstrating validity (do these diagnostic criteria have practical value with regard to prognosis, family history, treatment responsiveness, and so on?). Since for clinicians reliability is far less important than validity, the utility of the diagnostic system is not always apparent.

Despite these valid criticisms, the DSMs have accomplished a great deal and fill a vital need for mental health professionals. They have forced us to become more precise in our terminology, fostering both clearer thinking and clearer communication between ourselves and with those governing the finances of health care. Each succeeding DSM edition has been increasingly based on data and changes have often been made in response to feedback from the clinical community. If mental health professionals are to be taken seriously in our chaotic, rapidly changing system of health care (whatever its ultimate form), it is mandatory that we have clear definitions of disorders—even if those definitions change somewhat over time—and that we be able to perform the large-scale studies demonstrating both the prevalence and morbidity of these disorders. The DSMs foster these goals in ways that other systems might not.

Another major stumbling block for the acceptance of the descriptive approach as used in DSM-IV has been an understandable concern that this new model would replace and discount all other ways of understanding psychopathology. Descriptive models, however, should *never* preclude other ways of understanding psychological phenomena. For any clinical disorder, for any individual patient, different models will each have advantages and disadvantages in explaining the psychopathology. The clinical phenomenon of acute mania may be best viewed using the descriptive model, while adjustment disorders or narcissistic personalities will be better understood by an interpersonal or psychoanalytic perspective. A patient with a mild to moderate depression triggered by a loss, however, might be best understood using both descriptive and psychological concepts, with each model clarifying only a piece of the puzzle. It would be redundant and disruptive to point out continually in this text that other ways of understanding patients are helpful and, at times, mandatory. The use of multiple conceptual models should be considered a basic prerequisite for the full understanding of patients.

PHARMACOTHERAPY AND ITS IMPLICATIONS
FOR OTHER THERAPIES

The second assumption of the medical model in psychiatry, that some psychiatric disorders are effectively treated by medications, has been established through the astonishing amount of research over the last forty years devoted to the discovery, development, and documentation of psychopharmacologically active drugs. Initially used for severe depressions and psychotic disorders, medications have now been demonstrated to be useful for at least some patients with a wide variety of disorders. The simple existence of two editions of this book is testimony to the extent to which medications have been established as a treatment modality for psychiatric disorders. Despite the dramatic effect of medications in reducing or preventing psychopathology, however, their limitations have tempered some of the early, unrealistic hopes of the more biologically oriented clinicians. In a variety of disorders, medications are profoundly effective, yet still leave untouched some core aspects of the disorder which must be treated with other modalities. These limitations are most obvious in schizophrenia (see chapter 5), but are apparent also in panic disorder, bipolar disorder, and others.

Since 1987, with the release of fluoxetine (Prozac) as the first of the powerfully serotonergic antidepressants with fewer side effects than the older antidepressants, an increasing number of individuals with relatively mild psychiatric disorders and difficulties have taken one of these new medications. As an example, through early 1995, approximately 16 million patients had taken fluoxetine alone (Dista, 1995). The rapid proliferation of these medications in psychiatric treatment has led many therapists and interested laypeople to be concerned that prescribed drugs would soon become the quick fix for all problems, that a patient suffering distress would be given a medication to feel better at the risk of ignoring psychological and psychosocial factors. ("I just want to be more assertive with my girlfriend" or "I want to be bolder and more creative.") The explosion of media interest in these new medications has only exacerbated the problem, as exemplified by one *Newsweek* cover that pictured a Prozac capsule (labeled by its trade name and not its generic name) and by the controversy surrounding Peter Kramer's book *Listening to Prozac* (1993). (See chapters 3 and 7 for more detailed discussions of the serotonergic antidepressants for mild depressions and personality disorders.)

It is likely that some individuals have been prescribed one of the serotonergic antidepressants with little clinical justification. However, a great number of people with mild psychiatric disorders, many of whom have worked hard in psychotherapy but are still symptomatic, have greatly benefited from one of these newer medications. Moreover, in the treatment of the more serious psychiatric disorders, extraordinary numbers of patients continue to go untreated. In the most recent epidemiological study, only 42 percent of those with a psychiatric disorder had ever sought treatment for that disorder (Kessler et al., 1994). Of those with an active psychiatric disorder within the last year, less than 30 percent had received any type of treatment (Regier et al., 1993; Kessler et al., 1994). There is even evidence that only one quarter of chronically anxious patients use tranquilizers (Uhlenhuth, Balter, Mellinger, Cisin, and Clinthorne, 1983). Finally, of those patients with a severe mental illness as defined by psychosis or marked functional impairment, almost 40 percent sought no treatment within a one-year period (National Advisory Mental Health Council, 1993). Together, these studies suggest that, even now, we continue to be more of an undertreated than an overtreated society.

Another concern of psychotherapists about the advent of medications was their implication for the etiology of psychiatric disorders. There is a natural assumption that if medications are helpful, they must be correcting some biochemical abnormality which would then be viewed as the sole cause of the disorder. With the simplistic information promulgated in the press, patients come to their primary care physicians claiming that they know they have a serotonin deficiency and that they want a medication to fix this problem! Despite a remarkable amount of research over the last twenty-five years, however, there is still no definitive biological explanation for any psychiatric disorder (see chapter 2). Furthermore, even if a biological cause might be found for one or a number of disorders, it would not, by itself, imply the proper or effective methods of treatment. For example, coronary artery disease culminating in heart attacks has genetic and biological causes. Yet its course and outcome can be altered by life-style changes, such as diet, smoking, exercise, and the like. Similarly, even if depression or rejection sensitivity were shown to be caused by a specific neurotransmitter abnormality, this would have no necessary implication for the efficacy of psychotherapy in treating it.

In summary, just as descriptive models of psychopathology, as exemplified by DSM-IV, must be supplemented by other models to best understand our patients' problems, pharmacotherapy *never* precludes other methods of treatment. For some disorders, such as mild to moderate depression or obsessive compulsive disorder, there may be a variety of different, valid therapeutic approaches. As discussed in more detail in chapter 14, even with those disorders for which medications are the most effective treatments available, such as bipolar disorder, psychotherapy is likely to enhance the treatment and help patients in ways not measured in research studies. Moreover, since there is no evidence that, when utilized together, medication and psychotherapy interfere with the efficacy of each other, combination treatment should always be considered. Because this book focuses on pharmacological therapies, it will often not discuss the use of other valid treatments. Nonetheless, it should be assumed that other approaches do exist and may at times be preferable to medications for specific patients with certain disorders.

EVALUATING TREATMENTS: THE MEANING OF THE WORD EFFECTIVE

The application of scientific methods of evaluating treatment is the third important assumption inherent in the medical model approach to psychiatric disorders. An in-depth discussion of statistics is hardly necessary or relevant for this book. What is important, however, is a clarification of the use of the word "effective," since throughout the book statements will be made referring to a medication's effectiveness in treating a psychiatric disorder. At first glance, the meaning of the word "effective" seems clear—that the medication is useful in diminishing the manifestations of the disorder being treated. However, a number of questions about the use of this word must be addressed.

First and most important, how does this treatment compare to others? As already noted, the effectiveness of a medication does not bear on that of another type of treatment. For instance, the efficacy of certain antidepressants in diminishing the symptoms of obsessive compulsive disorder (see chapter 4) does not, in any way, negate the well-documented efficacy of behavior therapy for the same disorder. Similarly, the effectiveness of a medication does not bear on the potential value of other treatments administered simultaneously. In the treatment of schizophrenia, for instance, antipsychotics, although vital, are rarely sufficient for maximal response. A combination of medication with psychotherapy is likely to be the best treatment.

Another important question is that of assessment: how is effectiveness evaluated? During the twentieth century, and increasingly over the last thirty years, the hallmark of efficacy is that the medication has been shown to be effective in research studies using a double-blind, placebo-controlled design. In these studies, patients are randomly assigned to receive either the medication or an identical looking placebo. Patients and investigators are unaware of (i.e., blind to) the identity of the treatment actually received. In this way, the enthusiasm of the investigator as well as that of the patient ("I'm receiving a new pill that will make me all better") is similar for both the real medication and the placebo. If a drug is consistently associated with more improvement than a placebo in these studies, it is considered an effective treatment. For new drugs to be released in the United States, efficacy in double-blind studies (along with numerous other requirements) must be demonstrated.

A third important question is that of relativity: what is meant when one active treatment is described as more effective than another? As a generalization, this means that a larger percentage of patients responded (or improved to a greater degree) to one treatment compared to another. The magnitude of this difference may be relatively small (e.g., 60 percent vs. 50 percent) or large (70 percent vs. 30 percent). In both examples, however, *some* patients responded to the less effective treatment. (The inclusion of a placebo group would help evaluate whether the less effective treatment was superior to a placebo.) In a number of clinical situations, it is entirely appropriate to use the less effective treatment. If the more effective of two treatments has significantly more side effects, the less effective medication might be preferable. Furthermore, statements of comparative efficacy do not predict the response of an individual patient to either treatment since studies refer to groups, not individuals. Thus, a number of individual patients may respond better to the less effective treatment. The comparison statement simply states that a greater number of patients will respond to one medication than another.

Furthermore, even if a methodologically careful study demonstrates the effectiveness of a medication (compared to a placebo or to another drug), it should never be accepted as conclusive or proven. The recent history of medicine in general, and psychiatry specifically, is filled with carefully executed initial studies, the results of which are never replicated. There are a variety of explanations for this phenomenon, including subtle biases in the study design or selection of unusual patients (for instance, depressed patients seen at a university medical school may not be representative of the types of patients seen in the community and might respond to treatment differently). Despite the occasional story in the press, fraud is rarely responsible for contradictory findings in research. In general, any finding that is valid will be demonstrated in a number of different studies. Unfortunately, in their zeal for "hot" news, television and newspapers quote single studies as if they discovered the revealed truth. Patients who read these reports often look for this new magic. Therapists as well as psychopharmacologists need to help keep our patients from being swayed by these distortions.

A more recent consideration in clinical psychopharmacology distinguishes between efficacy and effectiveness, two terms that are typically used synonymously. For this distinction, efficacy refers to the percent of patients responding to a medication in a controlled study. Although controlled studies are vital for comparing treatments and for describing the percent of patients who respond under optimal conditions, patients in these studies tend to be highly motivated and physically healthy and typically do not suffer from any of a host of other concomitant psychiatric disorders common in the community. Thus, efficacy in controlled studies bears an uncertain relationship to the usefulness of a medication for the majority of more complicated patients seen in everyday clinical practice. The more clinically relevant variable is effectiveness, which takes into account ease of administration, side effects, and rates of noncompliance, and examines the utility of a medication for real patients who frequently suffer from multiple disorders, both psychiatric and medical. Using these definitions, it is effectiveness, not efficacy, that ultimately dictates which medications are prescribed in the community. As recently acknowledged (Klein, 1993b), almost no research studies have explored the types of practical questions confronted in everyday practice. Thus, from research studies we know very little on topics such as how quickly to raise the dose of a medication, what dose schedule should be used (once daily vs. twice daily), how to treat side effects, how long to keep patients on medications once they are better, and the optimal time to discontinue medications. By necessity, there is much accumulated experience and wisdom in these matters, but surprisingly little data. Therefore, much of what will be presented in the rest of the book will rely heavily on this wisdom, with the results of studies quoted when available.

Finally, the relationship between starting an individual patient on a medication (or any new treatment) and the resulting clinical response is not always as clear as it may seem. A patient's improvement may be due to one of three variables. First, the medication itself may have a pharmacological effect. Second, a placebo response may occur, defined here as improvement from any and all aspects of treatment that have no specific value for the condition being treated. Thus, a patient who is given a medication may improve because of increased hope, the magic of taking a pill administered by a societally sanctioned healer, or positive transference to a parental figure. This would be described as a placebo response insofar as the clinical change was unrelated to the pharmacological effects of the specific medication. A third variable is spontaneous remission. A variety of psychiatric disorders for which medications are prescribed are self-limited by nature, with or without treatment. As an example, major depressive disorder lasts an average of six to eight months. Thus, if a medication is started during the eighth month, it might be difficult to know whether the improvement seen was due to the treatment or the lifting of the depression that would have occurred anyway at that time.

GOALS OF PHARMACOTHERAPY

Pharmacological treatments can be considered to have more than one goal. Specifically, medications may be prescribed to (1) treat an acute disorder, (2) prevent a relapse soon after clinical improvement, or (3) prevent future episodes of the disorder. These three goals or phases are termed acute, continuation, and maintenance treatment.

Acute treatment is used to alleviate the symptoms of an actively occurring disorder. When most people think of treatment as necessary, they are referring to acute treatment. A depressed patient is given antidepressants to alleviate the active symptoms of the disorder; lithium is prescribed to diminish the symptoms of an acute manic episode.

The goal of continuation treatment is to prevent a relapse into the same episode for which treatment was begun. As an example, the depressed patient who is given an antidepressant may improve over four weeks. Once the symptoms of the disorder have remitted, acute treatment ends and continuation treatment begins. If the antidepressant is stopped at this point, when the patient has only recently become asymptomatic, the risk of relapse is high. The analogy in general medicine is the standard recommendation to continue antibiotics after the cough of a respiratory infection has stopped. The cough may remit after three to four days, but the antibiotics are typically prescribed for an additional seven to ten days as a continuation treatment. For psychiatric disorders, continuation treatment is typically extended for many months. Recommendations as to the length of continuation treatment are slightly different for each disorder. These will be covered in the chapters on the individual disorders. Unfortunately, there is an astonishing paucity of research regarding the appropriate length of continuation treatment. Thus, as with many of the practical issues noted above, the recommendations given will reflect clinical wisdom more than validated research findings.

Maintenance treatment is synonymous with preventive treatment. Because many psychiatric disorders occur in episodes throughout a person's lifetime, a decision can be made whether to treat each episode only when it arises (acute treatment), or to prevent recurrences by the ongoing, maintenance use of a medication. The two most common examples of medication maintenance treatment in psychiatry are lithium for bipolar disorder and antipsychotics for schizophrenia. In both disorders, there is an overwhelming likelihood of repeated recurrences. The decision to institute a psychopharmacological maintenance treatment is based on a judgment that takes into account such factors as the length of time between episodes, the severity and destructiveness of the episodes, the ease of treating acute episodes, the rapidity with which the episodes begin, patients' capacity for insight into the beginning of an episode (that is, can they recognize the warning signs so that acute treatment can begin quickly?), the potential toxicity of the treatment, and alternative preventive therapies. Thus, for each patient and for each disorder, somewhat different considerations apply. Maintenance treatment is discussed further in the chapters covering individual disorders.

SOME GENERAL ISSUES IN PSYCHOPHARMACOLOGICAL TREATMENT

A number of issues pertinent to all psychopharmacological treatments are relevant for any mental health professional seeing patients taking medications.

FDA Approval and PDR Doses

One series of concerns sometimes expressed by both patients and mental health professionals surrounds the regulation of medications by the Food and Drug Administration (FDA). New medications are approved by the FDA and then released based on their safety and efficacy for a specific disorder (or disorders) as demonstrated by rigorous double-blind studies. The medication is then described as being indicated or approved for the treatment of that disorder. This information is listed in the *Physicians' Desk Reference* (PDR), along with the dosage range that was tested during the research trials. The specific language and information given in the PDR is negotiated and ultimately approved by the

FDA. As such, the PDR should be considered as providing information for marketing purposes and medicolegal protection for the pharmaceutical firms. It specifies what pharmaceutical firms may claim for their products, and gives warnings and notes side effects in order to avoid a later charge of not informing physicians about their products.

Often, medications are prescribed for nonapproved uses—that is, for disorders or uses other than those evaluated and accepted by the FDA. Similarly, medications may be prescribed at doses higher than those recommended in the PDR or in the package insert given at pharmacies. This is acceptable and appropriate clinical practice (assuming the doses used are not dangerous and the rationale for the medication's use is reasonable). Neither the FDA indications nor the recommended maximal doses should be considered legally or ethically binding, nor are they necessarily based on the best scientific information.

To achieve an FDA indication requires enormous time and money. If a medication is already available and clinical studies and experience show that it is beneficial for a disorder other than the original indication, it is generally not worth the money for the pharmaceutical firm to submit an application to the FDA to obtain the additional indication. The most obvious example of this is the use of tricyclic antidepressants and imipramine (Tofranil) in particular for successfully treating panic disorder. Despite the ample evidence that these medications are effective antipanic medications and have been used for that purpose for over twenty years, they are not FDA indicated for panic disorder.

Similarly, dosage guidelines in the PDR and package inserts are conservative estimates, documented by studies submitted to the FDA by the pharmaceutical firm typically before the release of the medications. If clinicians and clinical researchers discover that higher doses of a certain medication are both safe and effective, it will generally not result in a change in the package insert which, like adding a new indication, is usually prohibitively expensive. Because of these limitations in the system, all psychiatrists—indeed, all physicians—routinely prescribe medications for nonapproved uses and intermittently at doses outside the package insert recommendations. Prescription must simply be consistent with sound medical judgment (although prescribing outside FDA indications and PDR dosage ranges may be factors used in a malpractice suit if a bad outcome ensues).

A far more difficult dilemma surrounds the use of FDA nonapproved medications—drugs that are unavailable in the United States but are available, for example, in Canada, Mexico, or Europe. Some of these medications have been prescribed for decades in other countries but their manufacturers never bothered to obtain FDA approval for release in the United States because of the extraordinary cost involved (currently estimated at many tens of millions of dollars). Clomipramine (Anafranil), the most well-documented treatment for obsessive compulsive disorder, was available in Europe for twenty years before its FDA approval in 1990. Only after epidemiological studies showed that obsessive compulsive disorder was common, and that therefore the potential market for the medication was large, was there a push for its release in this country. The FDA permits patients to carry nonapproved medications into the United States or to receive them by direct mail shipments, if they are for personal use (i.e., not for sale) and if the import is neither fraudulent nor dangerous (Kessler, 1989). Malpractice insurance companies are less consistently accepting of this practice and will at times refuse to cover physicians in their supervising the use of nonapproved medications. Thus, physicians who supervise use of nonapproved drugs find themselves in something of a limbo—the practice is legally acceptable but not consistently covered medicolegally. Because of this, only some psychiatrists are willing to participate in these prescribing practices.

Polypharmacy

In general, most psychopharmacological texts emphasize that polypharmacy—the use of multiple medications prescribed simultaneously—should be avoided whenever possible. With single agent treatment, interactions between drugs are avoided and side effects more easily understood. Yet, over time, the limitations of single treatments have become more apparent and the rationales for multiple medications increasingly persuasive. Polypharmacy can be very useful, but because it clearly introduces complications and some risks, it should only be undertaken thoughtfully and by a practitioner familiar with drug interactions.

The most common reasons for rational polypharmacy are listed in Table 1-1. An example of a patient with more than one disorder would be one with both panic disorder and depression who might require a benzodiazepine tranquilizer along with an antidepressant. The use of adjunctive treatments—second medications added to the first to augment effectiveness—has arisen with the awareness that single agent treatment does not result in sufficient improvement in many patients. The most common augmenting agents are those prescribed for treating depression, such as lithium or T_3 which, when added to an antide-

Table 1–1
Appropriate Reasons for Multiple Simultaneous Medications
(Rational Polypharmacy)

Treating patients with more than one disorder
The need for an adjunctive treatment
The need for combination treatment
Providing temporary symptomatic relief
Treating/minimizing side effects
Documented need for multiple medications in treating that specific disorder

pressant, enhance the antidepressant effect (see chapter 3 for details). Combination treatment is the prescription of two independently effective medications together, with the possibility that, when used concurrently, they will be more effective than either medication if prescribed alone. Examples are the use of two different mood stabilizers—such as lithium plus valproate —for difficult-to-manage bipolar disorder or a tricyclic antidepressant plus a serotonergic antidepressant for treating depression. Especially in the beginning of treatment, a medication may be temporarily prescribed as an aid for symptomatic relief along with the primary medication until the latter takes effect. For instance, a depressed patient with anxiety and insomnia might benefit from a brief prescription of a tranquilizer in the beginning of treatment until the antidepressant becomes effective (which may take a few weeks). In addition, increasing use is being made of second medications to treat the side effects of the primary medication. As an example, trazodone, a sedating antidepressant, is often properly and successfully prescribed to help combat the insomnia caused by the serotonergic antidepressants. Finally, a few disorders are well documented as being optimally treated with medications of two different types. The most well known example is psychotic depression which requires a combination of an antidepressant with an antipsychotic for effective treatment.

Despite these clear guidelines, all psychopharmacologists have had experiences with particularly difficult patients who end up being treated with multiple (up to seven or eight) simultaneous medications. Even though this may at times represent sloppy clinical practice, it may also represent the limitations of pharmacotherapy and the goal of minimizing side effects. As an example, a brittle bipolar depressed patient might be treated with two mood stabilizers (if neither one was sufficiently effective), an antidepressant, a hypnotic for sleep (if the antidepressant is effective but causes insomnia), a beta-blocker to reduce the tremors caused by the mood stabilizer, and a medication to counteract the sexual side effect of the effective antidepressant. This may look like psychopharmacology gone wild, but there is a clear rationale for each of these treatments and together they make the treatment both more effective and more tolerable. When multiple medications are prescribed, it is incumbent on the physician to regularly review the treatment regimen and to eliminate those medications that are no longer needed.

Practice Guidelines

Over the last two years, the American Psychiatric Association has published a series of practice guidelines for a variety of disorders such as eating disorders, major depression, bipolar disorder, and substance abuse. Future guidelines are planned for schizophrenia and other disorders. These documents contain consensus recommendations for suggested treatments (including medications) for specific indications, such as the proper role of antidepressants in bulimia nervosa or lab tests that should be checked during ongoing lithium use. The guidelines are not meant to define the standards of appropriate treatment to be followed in all cases, or specific treatment mandates for individual patients, but rather to provide overall direction (Zarin, Pincus, and McIntyre, 1993).

WHO SHOULD HAVE A MEDICATION CONSULTATION?

In deciding whether a psychotherapy patient should be referred for medication consultation, an initial problem is to elicit the relevant information needed to make the decision. Typically, the interviewing style in psychotherapy, in initial sessions and even more during the course of the therapy, is open-ended and nondirective. What is easily missed using that technique is the presence of symptoms that the patient is either unaware of or whose significance the patient does not grasp. In the past, the mental status examination, in which the patient's behavior in the interview setting was observed and systematically evaluated, was emphasized. To a great degree, this has been replaced by a heightened emphasis on obtaining an accurate history. With the current focus on longitudinal data (what symptoms are present and for how long?), it is less important (though not unimportant) to accurately describe the patient's affect in the interview or to distinguish between flight of ideas or loose associations than to find out how long the patient has been unable to concentrate or felt depressed. Thus, in evaluating patients for pharmacological consultation, the therapist may need to shift into a more directive style of questioning. The timing of these questions—whether in the first session or later—will depend, in great part, on the therapist's suspicion about the presence of a pharmacologically treatable disorder.

A series of clinical clues that are nonspecific with regard to diagnosis but that suggest the presence of the type of Axis I disorder for which medication might be appropriate are listed in Table 1-2. These items are broad-based and do not substitute for specific questions that are needed to diagnose specific disorders. Sample questions that will help diagnose specific disorders such as depression, bipolar disorder, a variety of anxiety disorders, or schizophrenia are given in the individual chapters.

Most important among the general items that should suggest a consultation is the ability to describe the patient's difficulties using the language of symptoms, such as insomnia or fatigue, as opposed to psychological feelings or interpersonal interactions. Marital conflict, as an example, can usually be described only using interactive terms. Axis I disorders, for which medications are most commonly prescribed, are defined by these types of symptoms. Therefore, the more the patient's problems or complaints focus on sensations or bodily feelings, the more a consultation should be considered. This is especially true when the symptoms involve cognitive capacities that have changed. Common examples include a new-onset memory disturbance or a diminution in concentrating ability. Psychotic symptoms, that is, those that involve a gross impairment in reality testing, comprise another group of important symptoms that usually require pharmacological intervention.

The presence of medical symptoms or disorders is another clue for

---

Table 1–2
**Clinical Characteristics That Should Suggest
a Psychopharmacological Consultation**

Psychiatric symptoms:
   Sleep or appetite disturbances, fatigue, panic attacks, ritualistic behavior
   Cognitive symptoms, such as poor memory, concentration difficulties, confusion
   Psychosis, such as delusions, hallucinations
Prominent physical symptoms or significant medical disorder
Significant suicidality
Family history of major psychiatric disorder
Marked mood lability, especially in response to environmental events, with (e.g.) rage
   or depressive symptoms
Nonresponse to psychotherapy

---

consultation. New or recent-onset medical symptoms, such as headaches, abdominal pain, or clumsiness may reflect a medical or a psychiatric disorder. If the patient has an ongoing medical problem that has not been recently reevaluated, or takes medication and has symptoms or physical complaints, an evaluation, either by a psychopharmacologist or an internist, should be done.

Patients who are significantly suicidal are also candidates for psychopharmacological consultation. The most important reason for this is that the majority of people who commit suicide suffer from types of Axis I disorders (the most common of which is depression) for which medications can often be helpful (Robins, 1986). Second, with the medicolegal climate as it currently exists, if a patient commits suicide without having been evaluated (but not necessarily treated) for medication, the therapist may be considered negligent and at higher risk for being sued.

As will be highlighted during the course of the book, the types of disorders for which medications are useful tend to run in families. It is usually impossible to tease apart early environmental variables from genetic ones, since the parent who may have transmitted the genetic vulnerability is usually the same one who raised the patient. Nonetheless, a patient who describes mood swings that are mild but whose mother and brother have clear-cut bipolar disorder is more likely to have a pharmacologically treatable disorder than is another patient with no history of mood disorders in the family.

Many patients generically described as moody or explosive have typically been conceptualized as having personality disturbances that were not amenable to pharmacotherapeutic treatment. Yet recent clinical experience suggests that many of these patients have pharmacologically responsive disorders or characteristics. (Chapter 7 discusses this issue in more detail.) Therefore, patients who are overly sensitive to rejection or get enraged in response to minor provocation, especially if they are not improving in their psychotherapy, should be considered for psychopharmacological consultation.

Finally, nonresponse to psychotherapy might also suggest a consultation. This often takes the form of patient and therapist acknowledging that the work of the therapy has gone well—a therapeutic alliance has been established, the patient has gained significant insight into the source and context of his problems—yet the depressed mood, or the chronic anxiety is unchanged. Certainly, an unsatisfactory response to psychotherapy does not by itself imply a pharmacologically treatable disorder, but it may be worth considering.

SECTION

TWO

2

Biological Basis of Psychopharmacology

U NDERSTANDING THE BRAIN and the intricate nuances of its function has been among the major goals of modern psychiatric research. The ultimate hope is that greater understanding will enhance our ability to accurately diagnose and more definitively treat those disorders characterized by brain dysfunction. Until now, however, virtually all the major advances in psychopharmacology—the discoveries of the first antipsychotics, antidepressants, antianxiety agents, and lithium—have depended far more on chance than on a detailed understanding of brain chemistry that then led to the synthesis of drugs capable of correcting known abnormalities. Recently, after almost thirty years of less than rapid progress in the development of innovative pharmacotherapies, the last decade has witnessed the emergence of genuinely new classes of effective medications. These new agents—selective serotonin reuptake inhibitors (SSRIs) for depression, azapirones for anxiety, atypical antipsychotics—work via novel mechanisms and are frequently associated with different clinical effects. New types of psychotropic agents not only enhance our understanding of how medications diminish psychiatric symptoms in general but also rekindle excitement in understanding the intricate workings of the brain and its dysfunctions.

In order to follow the evolving changes in the field, psychotherapists must understand some basic elements of brain biology. With greater understanding, familiarity, and comfort in this area, therapists can also help demystify the field for their patients who may be taking psychiatric medications. Additionally, as future research yields the fruits of new, more specific and effective biological treatments for the major psychiatric disorders, educated therapists will more easily be able to understand the significance of these discoveries and place them into a meaningful context for clinical practice.

In this chapter, we will examine the ways in which neurons (nerve cells) function, the way they communicate with each other, how medications exert their therapeutic effects, and the role of the most important brain chemicals (neurotransmitters) in the regulation of mood and thinking. After briefly reviewing the different neuroimaging techniques (e.g., brain scans) used in psychiatric research, the chapter will conclude with current hypotheses of the biology of the major psychiatric disorders for which medications are typically prescribed.

NEUROTRANSMISSION: HOW CELLS COMMUNICATE

In keeping with the variety of subtleties of its functions, the brain is the most sophisticated of our organs. Yet, like every other organ in the body, the brain is primarily (although not exclusively) composed of cells (called neurons in the nervous system) that interact with each other in rather predictable characteristic ways. The complexities are due to the extraordinary number of interconnections (estimated as greater than 100 trillion) that work in synchrony, creating the possibility of finely tuned, graded responses. For psychiatric and psychological functions, this translates into a wide repertoire of cognitive, affective, and behavioral capacities.

Within the brain messages are transmitted both electrically and chemically. Neurons are composed of three basic parts—the cell body, dendrites, and axons. The many dendrites of each neuron primarily receive information from other cells, while the axons, fewer in number, generally relay information to other cells. As shown in Figure 2–1, elec-

Figure 2–1   The Synapse

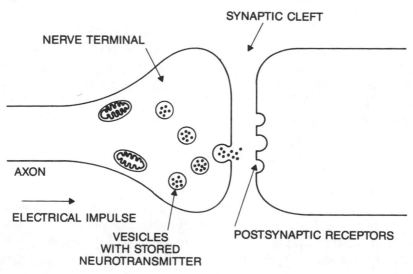

trical impulses travel through the cell to the axon, culminating at the nerve terminal. Since electrical impulses cannot bridge the physical gap between neurons, called the synapse (derived from the Greek word *synapto,* meaning "to join"), further propagation of the messages is dependent on chemical messengers, called neurotransmitters. When the electrical impulse reaches the nerve terminal on the presynaptic neuron, it causes the release of a neurotransmitter into the synaptic cleft. The neurotransmitter then diffuses across the synapse where it comes into contact with the postsynaptic neuron via an area on the surface of the neuron called a receptor site. These sites are specifically structured to bind with neurotransmitters. The binding of the neurotransmitter to the receptor leads to a variety of physiological responses (see below).

The brain utilizes a variety of neurotransmitters. Since new neurotransmitters are discovered regularly, their exact number will continue to change, but the list now numbers more than fifty (Hyman and Nestler, 1993). Although different parts of the brain utilize different neurotransmitters, they are all synthesized, stored, released, and inactivated by the same general mechanisms. Some are widely distributed, found over large areas of the brain. Others are found only in very specific parts, utilized in the regulation of just a few brain functions. As examples, glutamate, gamma-aminobutyric acid (GABA), and glycine are utilized by 75 to 90 percent of neurons as neurotransmitters. In contrast, the neurotransmitters that seem most involved in the regulation of mood, cognition, and sensory experiences (and therefore are the most likely to be disturbed in psychiatric disorders)—norepinephrine, serotonin, and dopamine—are each found in less than 2 percent of the synapses in the brain (Snyder, 1988). In these cases, it is helpful to think of neurotransmitter tracts, composed of groups of neurons all utilizing the same neurotransmitter.

Neurotransmitters can also be characterized as having predominantly excitatory (enhancing transmission of electrical impulses) or inhibitory properties. A good example of the latter is GABA, which is widely distributed but may have a very specific role to play in the regulation of anxiety and the mechanism of action of most effective tranquilizers (see chapter 11).

Neurotransmitters are synthesized within the neuron from precursors delivered to the cell from the outside. Enzymes within the neuron break down and alter these precursors, ultimately forming neurotransmitters, which are then stored in vesicles at the nerve terminals, ready for release into the synapse when an electrical impulse surges through the cell. Each vesicle contains from dozens to thousands of molecules of one type of neurotransmitter. In contrast to earlier thinking, it is now apparent that individual neurons frequently utilize more than one neurotransmitter (called colocalization). When multiple neurotransmitters are used together, the effects of one may modulate the effects of the other, thereby enhancing the fine tuning of the neurotransmission.

Soon after the neurotransmitter is released, it must be quickly inactivated in order for the postsynaptic neuron to be able to receive new messages. The most common methods for this inactivation are enzymatic degradation or reuptake. Enzymes on the cell surface break down or degrade some neurotransmitters into inactive components. In the process of reuptake, the neurotransmitter is transported back into the presynaptic neuron where it is repackaged into the vesicles—recycled, as it were.

A receptor is the lock for which the neurotransmitter is the key. Receptors are specific discrete countable protein structures located on the membrane (outside) of the cell. The neurotransmitter molecules bind to receptors specifically shaped to receive them. For any neurotransmitter, there may be subpopulations of receptors. These subpopulations are usually labeled by Greek letters and numbers such as alpha-one, alpha-two, beta-one, and so on. Each receptor subtype binds with slightly different affinity to a variety of neurotransmitters (or medications) and may be present in varying concentrations in the separate tracts utilizing that neurotransmitter. Because of this, the stimulation of each receptor subtype is associated with somewhat different effects. Moreover, any neuron may contain a variety of receptor subtypes for the same neurotransmitter. Over the last few years, many new receptor subtypes have been discovered. As an example, fourteen serotonin receptor subtypes have now been identified within seven types (Roth, 1994). More subreceptors for most if not all of the neurotransmitters are likely to be discovered in the near future. Additionally, receptors are found on both the pre- and postsynaptic neurons. The simultaneous existence of all these receptor types—some excitatory, others inhibitory, some presynaptic and others postsynaptic, with subpopulations for each neurotransmitter—as well as the multiple synapses that any one neuron may make with other neurons, reflect a system that is complex not only in the sheer volume of inputs but also in the competing nature of these inputs (see Figure 2–2). Finely tuned regulation and the need for maintaining sameness despite a variety of influences is vital for the brain to function correctly. The final effect, then, is a summation of the individual influences.

Implied in the discovery of subreceptors is the possibility of synthesizing more specific, "cleaner" drugs which, instead of enhancing

Figure 2–2   Receptor Sites

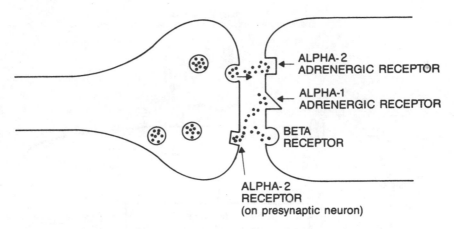

ALPHA-2
ADRENERGIC RECEPTOR

ALPHA-1
ADRENERGIC RECEPTOR

BETA
RECEPTOR

ALPHA-2
RECEPTOR
(on presynaptic neuron)

serotonin function, for instance, would selectively bind to the sero-
tonin-2A receptor. Theoretically, this would provide more specific
pharmacological effects, both in efficacy and in diminishing side effects
which are often due to a medication attaching to multiple receptors
other than the ones desired.

Once the neurotransmitter binds to the receptor, the message must
be passed to the interior of the cell in a process called signal transduction (Hyman and Nestler, 1993). Messages may be conveyed by either
changing electrical characteristics of the cell or by initiating some biochemical action within the cell or both. Those receptor systems that
directly alter electrical characteristics of the cell membrane utilize a
process called ligand-gated ion channels. (Neurotransmitters and drugs
are collectively referred to as ligands.) The majority of receptors, however, produce cellular effects by inducing certain chemical changes and
are called G protein-linked receptors.

G proteins, so named because they bind guanine nucleotides,
themselves translate the binding of neurotransmitters to receptors into
both electrical and biochemical effects within the cell (Gollub and
Hyman, 1995). The chemical effects of G proteins result from their activation of a group of other intracellular chemicals called second messengers (neurotransmitters being considered first messengers). Second
messengers, of which the most well known is cyclic AMP, in turn alter
the activity of certain enzymes that further translate the effect of the
neurotransmitter/receptor binding into cellular processes such as synthesizing neurotransmitters, further electrical changes, and so on. To
summarize then, as illustrated schematically in Figure 2–3, the binding

Figure 2–3   Signal Transduction: Relaying the Message

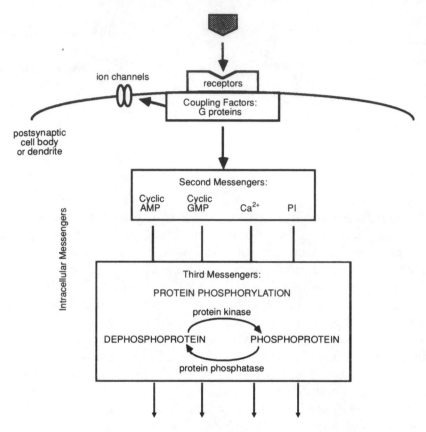

Multiple Physiological Responses

Adapted with permission from S. E. Hyman and E. J. Nestler, *The Molecular Foundations of Psychiatry*. Copyright 1993 American Psychiatric Press.

of the neurotransmitter to the receptor is simply the first step in an increasingly complex cascade of effects that alter the cell's functions.

HOW MEDICATIONS WORK

All medications discussed in this book work by affecting some aspect of the neurotransmitter/receptor system and/or by altering second messenger systems. The mechanisms of action of currently available medications are explainable by one or more of seven different effects on this system. These are shown schematically in Figure 2–4.

The simplest way that medications work is by directly binding to the receptor site (no. 1 in Figure 2–4). If the medication mimics the neurotransmitter by stimulating the receptor, it is described as being a receptor agonist. Morphine is a direct agonist for endorphin receptors, causing a diminution of pain as does the naturally occurring neuro-transmitter. Conversely, some medications, called receptor antagonists, bind to the receptor site but cause no response, thereby blocking the effect of the naturally occurring neurotransmitter. Conventional antipsy-chotics, which block postsynaptic dopamine receptors, are examples of this type of medication. A second method by which medications act is by causing the release of more neurotransmitter, thereby functionally increasing the effect of the system (no. 2). Stimulants, such as d-am-phetamine, work in part by stimulating the release of dopamine and norepinephrine. Further complicating the picture, some medications are partial agonists, causing some biological effect but less than the en-dogenous neurotransmitter.

Blocking the reuptake of neurotransmitters back into the presynap-tic neuron (no. 3) allows the chemicals more time in the synapse, en-hancing the possibility of stimulating the postsynaptic receptor. The effect is to increase the neurotransmission. Cyclic antidepressants and SSRIs work, in part, by blocking the reuptake of norepinephrine, sero-tonin, or both.

Two other ways (nos. 4 and 5) by which medications may work are

Figure 2–4   How Medications Work

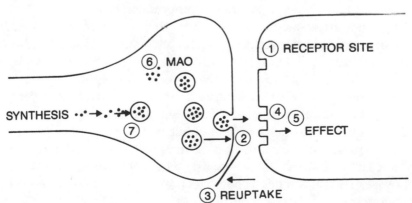

via their effects on receptor mechanisms. Antidepressants all cause changes in either the number of receptor sites (called down or up regulation for decrease or increase in the number respectively) or the sensitivity of receptors (i.e., altering the magnitude of response resulting from stimulation of the receptor). It is also possible to effect changes through the second messenger system. Lithium may exert its mood stabilizing effects by "dampening" the effects of one of these systems.

Altering the metabolism of a neurotransmitter will also change the amount available for release (no. 6). The class of antidepressants called monoamine oxidase (MAO) inhibitors exert their effects, in part, by diminishing the metabolism of a wide variety of neurotransmitters, all of which are metabolized by the enzyme MAO. Finally, the amount of neurotransmitter available could theoretically be altered by providing more or less of the precursor ingredients (no. 7). L-tryptophan is a naturally occurring amino acid that is metabolized into serotonin. Thus, ingesting large amounts of l-tryptophan might result in an increase in serotonin.

Focusing on one major biological effect of a medication and then correctly predicting its clinical effect, however, is rarely possible. One reason is that the brain's system of checks and balances works as much in response to outside influences as it does for the competing internal influences. Thus, taking a medication that blocks a neurotransmitter receptor—for example, taking an antipsychotic that blocks dopamine—will immediately cause an increase in dopamine release, as if the brain were trying to overcome the blockade by increasing the neurotransmitter blocked (Davis, Kahn, Ko, and Davidson, 1991). Similarly, taking an antidepressant that blocks the reuptake of norepinephrine, thereby functionally increasing the amount of available neurotransmitter, results in the decrease in the amount of norepinephrine released in another attempt to provide sameness or homeostasis.

Other than direct-acting agonists, how then can medications work at all if the system is designed to prevent changes? No single answer satisfies, but one possibility is that with more chronic influence such as taking a medication regularly over many weeks, the regulatory mechanisms themselves are altered. As an example, a presynaptic receptor (called an autoreceptor) generally decreases neurotransmission when stimulated. This would be the initial effect if, for example, an antidepressant increased the amount of norepinephrine or serotonin in the synaptic cleft (as it does). If the sensitivity of that autoreceptor diminished over weeks, it would respond less strongly to the presence of greater amounts of norepinephrine and serotonin caused by antidepressants, resulting in more of the neurotransmitter being available.

Another possible answer reflects the effects of medications on intracellular processes referred to above, such as G proteins and second messenger systems. Until very recently, virtually all research on the mechanisms of action of psychotropic medications focused on the neurotransmitter/receptor axis, ignoring the "downstream" effects of these drugs. Given that most psychotropic medications are effective over weeks and not hours to days, it seems probable that the mechanism of action of some medications may ultimately be better explained by these slower intracellular processes rather than by receptor activity.

Another difficulty that confuses our attempt to correlate the clinical effects of medications with biological changes in the brain is that all the older psychotropic agents and many of the newer ones have broad-based effects. As noted above, if medications were synthesized for the specific purpose we desired, they would bind to only one (or a few) specific receptor subtypes instead of binding to multiple receptors belonging to a variety of classes. Much of the current pharmacological research is predicated on this very concept—finding more biologically selective medications.

Our current pharmacopaeia, however, consists of medications that have one desired effect but also a host of other unwanted ones. In the case of conventional antipsychotics, dopamine blocking in the area controlling psychotic versus nonpsychotic thinking is wanted but the other biological effects, whether through dopamine blocking in other tracts or via interactions with other neurotransmitters, simply cause side effects. Thus, side effects can be considered to be due to the broad effects of medications and not central to their capacity to cause the desired clinical change.

NEUROTRANSMITTERS THAT HELP REGULATE MOOD AND BEHAVIOR

Dopamine, norepinephrine, and serotonin are the three neurotransmitters which seem most involved in the regulation of mood and thinking and for which there is evidence of disturbed functioning in major psychiatric disorders. (A fourth neurotransmitter, GABA, may be very important in the regulation of anxiety. Since much of what we know about the role of GABA in psychiatric disorders is linked to the mechanism of action of tranquilizers, it is discussed in chapter 11.)

Dopamine is derived from the amino acid tyrosine (available in health food stores), which is converted into dopa and then into dopamine. It is ultimately metabolized into homovanillic acid (HVA). Dopamine is utilized as a neurotransmitter in two tracts that are central to psychiatric disorders and their treatment. The more important of these pathways, called the mesocorticolimbic system, connects the midbrain to parts of the limbic system and the prefrontal cortex. These areas are involved in the regulation of a number of vital psychological functions related to thinking and moods, such as the ability to experience pleasure, reward systems, the selection of goal-directed behaviors, flexible decision making, and other cognitive processes (Le Moal, 1995). Evidence for the role of dopamine in some of these functions has been demonstrated in animals while for others, human evidence also exists. The other major dopamine pathway, called the nigrostriatal tract, helps regulate motor movements. Dopamine blockers, prescribed to decrease psychotic thinking, cause a number of motor side effects related to their effects in this area. A smaller dopamine pathway connects the hypothalamus to the pituitary gland and helps regulate certain aspects of endocrine (hormonal) function. Dopamine abnormalities are generally considered to be central in psychotic disorders, especially schizophrenia, and in disorders of attention such as attention deficit/hyperactivity disorder.

Like dopamine, norepinephrine is derived from tyrosine. The direct precursor of norepinephrine is dopamine, while its major metabolite in the central nervous system is initialed MHPG (3-methoxy-4-hydroxyphenylglycol). Together, norepinephrine and dopamine are described as catecholamines (referring to an aspect of their chemical structure). Catecholamines are inactivated both by reuptake into the nerve terminal and by enzymes such as monoamine oxidase (MAO). Because norepinephrine is also called noradrenaline, pathways utilizing this neurotransmitter are called noradrenergic or adrenergic. The single greatest concentration of norepinephrine in the brain is found in an area of the brainstem called the locus ceruleus. However, noradrenergic pathways and influences are found throughout the brain. Norepinephrine seems to be involved in the regulation of sleep-wake cycles, alertness, sustained attention, and biological responses to new stimuli (Robbins and Everitt, 1995). Anxiety, fear, and stress responses are also thought to be noradrenergically mediated. Not surprisingly, then, noradrenergic abnormalities are generally considered to be central in mood and anxiety disorders.

As noted above, l-tryptophan is a precursor amino acid which, after one intermediate step, is converted into serotonin, properly known as 5-hydroxytryptamine (or 5-HT). Serotonin's metabolic endproduct is 5-hydroxyindoleacetic acid (5-HIAA). Like the catecholamines, serotonin is inactivated both by reuptake and by enzymes such as MAO. The most important serotonergic tracts originate in the midline (raphe) of the brainstem with connections extending to most regions of the central nervous system. The range of psychobiological functions thought to be mediated in part by serotonin encompass many aspects of brain function including mood, anxiety, arousal, irritability/tranquility, cognition, appetite, sleep-wake cycles and so on (Dubovsky and Thomas, 1995). Given the diversity of these functions, another hypothesis about serotonin's function is that it serves to integrate a variety of more discrete functions, thereby explaining its wide-ranging roles. Because it is currently the most hotly researched neurotransmitter, serotonin has been implicated in the etiology of most psychiatric disorders, including mood disorders, anxiety disorders, and schizophrenia. The most consistent finding, however has been the link between low serotonergic function and impulsivity/aggression, regardless of the diagnosis (Coccaro and Siever, 1995).

Although the above discussion implies a relationship between specific neurotransmitters and isolated psychological/behavioral characteristics, it would be an error to take these generalizations too concretely. As alluded to above, neurons have extraordinary numbers of interconnections: dopaminergic neurons have important synapses with serotonergic neurons, norepinephrine and dopamine serve some overlapping functions, serotonergic neurons can alter adrenergic functions, and so on. Because of these diverse connections, no one neurotransmitter should ever be considered to control any complex behavior in isolation. Rather, most brain functions result from the multiple influences of a variety of different neurotransmitters, providing a system of extraordinary fine tuning.

NEUROIMAGING TECHNIQUES
IN PSYCHIATRIC DISORDERS

Replacing biochemical studies of neurotransmitters and receptors, neuroimaging techniques that provide visual images of the brain have become the powerful and exciting modality in biopsychiatric research. The potential clinical applications of neuroimaging include diagnosis and predicting course of disorder. Even more important, however, these techniques give extraordinary glimpses into both the structure and activity of the brain, providing unique, nondangerous methods of understanding brain function in both normal and abnormal states. With the capacity to quantify neurotransmitter tracts (e.g., providing estimates of the relative number of dopamine receptors in patients with a specific disorder or determining the percentage of dopamine receptors filled by a specific antipsychotic medication), neuroimaging techniques will also provide the next series of advances for biochemical studies.

Neuroimaging scans can be crudely divided into structural and functional types (Rauch and Renshaw, 1995). Structural techniques provide a window into the actual size and shape of various brain structures. The two most important structural techniques are computerized axial tomography (CT) and magnetic resonance imaging (MRI). Functional neuroimaging provides information on functional characteristics of the brain such as regional blood flow/neuronal activity, cellular metabolism, and neurotransmitter receptor activity.

CT is the oldest of our currently utilized scanning techniques. CT relies on the different densities of brain tissues to attenuate (diminish) multiple X rays at different rates, yielding images that visualize a "slice" of the brain at a certain anatomical level. (This principle is identical to that used in producing conventional X rays with CT utilizing multiple X ray beam generators and detectors.) CT images may be enhanced by contrast media, typically iodine-based, that are injected intravenously. These contrast media are infrequently associated with allergic reactions to the dye. CT is relatively inexpensive, the time needed for its administration is brief (ten minutes), and anxiety responses during the scan are relatively minimal since the scanner is not too confining. Its disadvantages are that it cannot distinguish easily between types of tissues with similar density, and it uses radiation.

MR scans provide representations of brain structures by comparing the responses of various types of brain tissue to a magnetic force generated by a powerful magnet. Based on the water density of each tissue, a different amount of radio frequency energy will be absorbed and then re-emitted. This is measured by an antenna, providing images of brain structures. As with CT scans, contrast may be used with MR to enhance the image. The advantages of MR are its lack of radiation (thereby allowing it to be repeated safely), its excellent visualization of many brain tissues, and the relative lack of allergic reaction to its contrast dye. Its disadvantages are the confining space needed for the scan (which is associated with panic attacks or claustrophobia), greater expense, and—because of the magnetic nature of the stimulus—the inability of patients with cardiac pacemakers or metal in their body to be scanned.

Of the functional imaging techniques, PET (positron emission tomography) has provided the most important research advances. In PET, a radioactive tracer is injected which then emits a positron (a positively charged particle). When the positron collides with an electron, energy is released and detected by the PET scanner. The exact locations where the positrons are released provide a series of scan images. Different chemicals can be radioactively labeled and then injected (or inhaled). Radioactive oxygen will provide scans measuring blood flow (and therefore neuronal activity), since the oxygen will be delivered to brain regions proportional to their blood flow. Radioactive glucose (generally given in a form called fluoro-deoxy-glucose, or FDG) is taken up into cells along with nonradioactive glucose and serves as a marker of metabolic activity since neurons use glucose as their source of energy. PET scans are associated with superbly detailed images. The brief time in which most of the radioactive tracers are active means that each scan is relatively brief and multiple scans can be obtained in a short period of time. PET scans, however, require very specialized equipment, are therefore available only in a few sites, and are very expensive. Therefore, in contrast to MR and CT scans which are commonly used for clinical reasons, PET remains almost exclusively a research technique.

In a more recently developed PET technique, radioactive ligands which bind to specific neurotransmitter receptors can be used to quantify receptor binding capacity and receptor occupancy. This technique has been used most successfully so far with dopamine receptors (most relevant to schizophrenia studies) but has begun to be extended to serotonin research. Over time, it is likely that increasing numbers of receptor systems will be able to be visualized and will revolutionize research into neurotransmitter systems and their functions.

A variation of PET is SPECT—single photon emission computed tomography. SPECT measures the emission of a photon rather than a positron. This difference is associated with poorer spatial resolution (the images are less clear) but is far less expensive and is more available because of the reduced need for specialized equipment.

Finally, two recent technical variations of MRI that are just beginning to be developed are magnetic resonance spectroscopy (MRS) and functional MRI. MRS measures the amounts of certain chemicals, such as phosphorus, in various brain regions by evaluating the response of the chemicals to a standard magnetic force. Functional MRI uses the MR technique to measure neuronal activity by changes in blood flow. As such, if perfected, it would rival PET.

BIOLOGICAL HYPOTHESES OF THE MAJOR
PSYCHIATRIC DISORDERS

Despite over twenty years of energetic effort, no biological hypothesis has yet marshalled enough supporting evidence to definitively explain any psychiatric disorder. (Of course, the same could be said about any model of psychopathology, be it psychoanalytic, behavioral, or cognitive.) Three major factors have precluded better biological hypotheses and more definitive answers. First, our diagnostic categories are generally crude, imprecise, and are likely to subsume more than one entity within any category. If a group of patients with major depression, for example, actually have a variety of disorders, finding consistent biological dysfunctions within the group becomes far less likely. Second, just as no one neurotransmitter can be considered to regulate any specific brain function, it is equally unimaginable that any of the major psychiatric disorders could be caused by one biological abnormality, given the complexity of their presentations. Third, progress in developing the necessary tools for biological investigation such as biochemical tests (e.g., measurements of various neurotransmitters and receptor function) and neuroimaging techniques, including the various types of brain scans, takes time. Since the entire field of biological psychiatry is very young, sophisticated research in the area has not had sufficient time to provide the types of data needed for mature hypotheses.

On the other hand, there is little doubt that disturbed biology plays a part in the vulnerability towards the major psychiatric disorders and that biological abnormalities are evident in the major disorders. Overall, the most consistent and persuasive evidence for the biological hypotheses rests on the twin pillars of genetic studies and the efficacy of medications in treating those disorders. Numerous investigations have confirmed not only that schizophrenia, bipolar and unipolar mood disorders, and panic disorder run in families, but also that genetic transmission specifically is involved to some degree. Regardless of the method by which the genetic contribution is investigated, the evidence is consistent.

Similarly, the documented efficacy of medications in experiments that have controlled for the effects of expectation—double-blind, placebo-controlled trials—also adds to the weight of biological evidence. This is especially true for those disorders such as schizophrenia or acute mania for which no other modalities of treatment are consistently effective. It is not unreasonable to assume that the effectiveness of a biological treatment such as medication reflects the presence of a biological abnormality (although not necessarily a biological etiology— see below). This line of thinking is further strengthened when there is consistent evidence from a number of directions, all of which agree with each other. For instance, since drugs that increase dopamine cause psychosis and dopamine blockers diminish psychosis, a theory that explains psychotic processes by abnormalities in the dopamine system is supported.

However, examining the arguments just set forth with a critical eye reveals the shaky ground upon which the biological hypotheses rest. Genetic contributions are important, even central, in understanding the vulnerability to certain psychiatric disorders. Yet no disorder can be explained solely by a 100 percent genetic vulnerability. Similarly, no laboratory test has ever been shown to be so strongly associated with any psychiatric disorder as to define its presence. Examining the evidence for efficacy of medications, one must confront the fact that placebo response rates for many disorders, although less than that for active medications, are virtually never zero. As an example, 20 to 40 percent of depressed patients will respond to placebo (Klein, Gittelman, Quitkin, and Rifkin, 1980). Furthermore, the rate of response of depressed patients to some short-term psychotherapies, such as interpersonal therapy or cognitive therapy, is significant, in some studies comparable to that for antidepressants (Elkin et al., 1989). Does this imply that those patients who are placebo responders or who respond to nonbiological treatment have a different disorder? Herein lies the weakness in extrapolating from a treatment response to a theory of causation. The observation that a biological treatment is effective implies very little about the "cause" of the disorder, nor does it preclude other modalities from being equally or more effective. Theoretically, there may be many pathways, biological or psychological, towards the same result—that of clinical improvement.

With the caveats just noted, it is worth reviewing the major biological hypotheses of schizophrenia, mood disorders, panic disorder, and obsessive compulsive disorder. However, no hypothesis consistently explains all the research data available for any disorder and none should be considered as more than a working proposal to be refined as more information becomes available. Much evidence both supporting and contradicting these theories is integrally linked to clinical and biological effects of the medications used to treat these disorders. Further details on the medications are presented in subsequent chapters.

Mood Disorders

From the time of the ancient Greeks, who believed that melancholia resulted from the biochemical effects of toxic humors such as black bile, and the tendency of mania and depression to run in families, thereby implicating possible genetic factors, it has long been suspected that mood disorders have a biological basis. The most important of the modern biological explanations, which dominated research from the mid-1960s for the next twenty years, was the monoamine hypothesis. Simply put, it stated that depression is characterized by a deficiency of monoamines, the class of neurotransmitters that includes norepinephrine and serotonin, while mania is associated with overactivity. As so often happens, the initial evidence supporting the hypothesis derived from two observations related to medication effects. First, the two antidepressant classes discovered in the 1950s both functionally increase the amount of norepinephrine or serotonin, albeit by different mechanisms. Tricyclic antidepressants block the reuptake of the neurotransmitters, thereby increasing their availability to the postsynaptic receptor (see Figure 2-4) while the MAO inhibitors prevent their metabolism. Second, reserpine, used to treat hypertension (high blood pressure), was found to cause severe depression in some patients. Reserpine releases neurotransmitters from the intraneuronal vesicles where they are stored, thereby making them easier to metabolize. Thus, two medication classes that increase monoamines alleviate depression while another which decreases them causes depression. Although the initial hypothesis focused on the role of norepinephrine, it was also postulated that either neurotransmitter or the interaction between the two could be abnormal in mood disorders (Bunney and Davis, 1965).

From the late 1960s through the early 1980s, biological research in depression focused on evaluating the monoamine hypothesis. An early hope was that it would be possible to characterize depressions as norepinephrine deficient or serotonin deficient. Hypothetically, the former would then respond to norepinephrine-enhancing antidepressants while the latter would improve when treated with serotonergic antidepressants. Preliminary evidence supported this idea.

As is so common in research, the satisfying nature of the monoamine hypothesis and the early experimental research in support of its clinical applicability unfortunately represented a triumph more of hope and excitement than of replicable clinical science. Multiple methodological problems cast doubt on the original hypothesis and on the early supporting data. Additionally, the findings of the early studies have not been consistently replicated. In the largest study to date, measuring a variety of neurotransmitters and their metabolites, no consistent differences between depressed patients and controls were found at all (Koslow et al., 1983). In that same study, no evidence was found for the existence of subgroups of norepinephrine deficient or serotonin deficient patients (Davis et al., 1988).

More recently, using more sophisticated measures, biological research has focused on other aspects of noradrenergic and serotonergic function (Schatzberg and Schildkraut, 1995; Maes and Meltzer, 1995). These have included examining a number of different neurotransmitter metabolites together, and studying the number and function of a variety of receptors in depressed vs. nondepressed individuals. Another approach to exploring serotonergic influences on depression has been to induce decreases in brain serotonin by acute dietary depletion of tryptophan (the precursor of serotonin) and examining the effect of this decrease in a variety of depressed and nondepressed populations (Miller et al., 1992). Although abnormalities are commonly found in a number of these variables in depressed patients, none is consistent enough to be integrated into a coherent understanding of the role of either norepinephrine or serotonin in mood abnormalities.

Experimental findings aside, a larger objection to the original monoamine hypothesis focused on the time course of response to antidepressants. It may be remembered that antidepressants have the effect of functionally increasing the amount of norepinephrine, serotonin, or both, thereby implying a possible correction of a deficiency of these neurotransmitters. The functional increase in the neurotransmitters occurs within the first day of treatment with the antidepressant. Unfortunately for the hypothesis, patients don't improve with antidepressants for many weeks (see chapter 3). If simple increases in important neurotransmitters were sufficient to correct the presumed deficiency, why do the medications take weeks to work? Additionally, how do we explain the efficacy of certain antidepressants, such as bupropion and others available only in Europe, which have little or no effect on these neurotransmitters? In exploring these questions, it was discovered that antidepressants have different biological effects when taken chronically (e.g., over a number of weeks) than acutely. These chronic effects therefore correlate with the time course of antidepressant response. Chronic changes secondary to antidepressant treatment have been demonstrated for a number of different biological functions, including the rate of synthesis of neurotransmitters, the number of some receptors, the responsivity of the receptors, and intracellular changes such as those in G proteins or second messenger function (Hyman and Nestler, 1993). Because no universal effects common to all antidepressants have yet been demonstrated, it is still unclear which of these changes (if any) are central to the clinical efficacy of the medications.

Although it has been an integral part of the hypothesis, the biology of mania has been relatively ignored. In part, this has been due to the difficulty in recruiting manic patients for research (they are not very cooperative for activities such as blood drawing and urine collections) but also because the effects of the medications used to treat mania, such as lithium, do not fit easily into the model. Additionally, whatever studies in mania have been done are not consistently in favor of the biogenic amine hypothesis.

So far, neuroimaging studies have not helped elucidate the core biological dysfunction in mood disorders. Structural studies have indicated nonspecific decreases in brain tissue and increased ventricles, similar to those found in schizophrenia (Ketter et al., 1994). MRI studies of depressed patients have consistently noted the presence of what are called "UBOs" (unidentified bright objects) that are of uncertain significance and do not seem to be associated with specific clinical findings. Some, but not all, studies using functional measures have found decreased metabolic activity in the frontal areas in the brain, especially on the left side. With greater technical sophistication and the use of neurotransmitter-based PET studies, more relevant findings are likely to emerge.

Where, then, does that leave the monoamine hypothesis of mood disorders? With the benefit of twenty years of research and powerful hindsight, the hypothesis as originally formulated has more evidence against it than for it. No consistent evidence yet exists to support the notion of either a decrease of norepinephrine or serotonin in depression or an increase in mania. Even the likely mechanism of action of antidepressants, the cornerstone of the hypothesis, is different than initially thought. Despite the contradictory results across studies, however, a number of diverse findings still consistently point to a pattern of dysregulation in noradrenergic and serotonergic functions in depression. These abnormalities are not found uniformly enough to aid in diagnosis or to indicate a core dysfunction, but do suggest that when more is known, noradrenergic and serotonergic abnormalities will still be considered central to the pathophysiology of mood disorders.

Schizophrenia

The dopamine hypothesis has been the predominant biological theme of schizophrenia over the last thirty years. In its simplest form, this hypothesis postulates that the disorder results from a functional excess of dopamine in the central nervous system. The term "functional excess" implies that the enhanced activity could result from a variety of means, such as hypersensitive receptors, decreased inhibitory influences, as well as a sheer increase in the amount of dopamine released at synapses. As initially proposed, the hypothesis rested on two lines of evidence (Wyatt, Kirch, and Egan, 1995): First, amphetamines when ingested in large amounts ultimately lead to a paranoid psychosis, resembling paranoid schizophrenia. Also, some schizophrenic patients show a marked worsening of their psychosis if given amphetamines. As one of their major effects, amphetamines cause an increase in the release of dopamine at the synapse, thus potentially linking the symptom change with a biological effect. Second, although their clinical effects were discovered serendipitously, antipsychotics, which are the mainstay of treatment in schizophrenia, seemed to work by blocking postsynaptic dopamine receptors (see chapter 12). Furthermore, there is a strong inverse correlation between the capacity of conventional antipsychotics to block dopamine and the dose of the antipsychotic needed for a clinical effect. In other words, a medication that is a powerful dopamine blocker is usually prescribed in low doses (e.g., 5 mg) to be effective whereas a weaker dopamine blocker must be given in larger doses (e.g., 100 mg) for the same clinical effect.

These lines of evidence supporting the dopamine hypothesis, linking response to treatment with documented effects of the medications and understanding the biology of abused drugs, are powerful indeed. In attempting to corroborate these older findings, the role of dopamine in the etiology of schizophrenia has been more directly evaluated using newer research techniques. The types of measurements examined have included the amount of dopamine metabolites in schizophrenic patients, the number of dopamine receptors in post-mortem specimens of schizophrenic patients, and the number of dopamine receptors in patients determined by PET scans. Overall, the results of these studies are inconsistent (Kahn and Davis, 1995). Unfortunately, much of the research investigating direct evidence for dopamine hyperactivity in schizophrenia has been hampered by the biological effects of the medications. As an example, if increased dopamine metabolites or dopamine receptors are found in schizophrenic patients recently treated with dopamine blockers, does it reflect the disorder or the lingering effects of medication?

Other problems, both theoretical and clinical, cast further doubt on the dopamine hypothesis. First, antipsychotics are effective in a number of clinical states (see chapter 12), not just schizophrenia. Second, amphetamines do not worsen clinical symptoms in all schizophrenic patients. In fact, some seem to improve (Van Kammen et al., 1982). Third, since antipsychotics block dopamine quickly, why does it take many weeks to see maximal improvement with the medication?

Partly in response to these objections, and partly due to the emergence of the atypical neuroleptics (see chapter 12) that consistently alter serotonergic as well as dopaminergic activity, revisions of the classic dopamine hypothesis have been presented (Davis, Kahn, Ko, and Davidson, 1991; Wyatt, Kirch, and Egan, 1995). The first part of the revised hypothesis postulates that schizophrenia is characterized by excessive and insufficient dopamine simultaneously in different parts of the brain. In this hypothesis, excessive dopamine in the mesolimbic system would result in psychotic symptoms. Negative symptoms of schizophrenia such as social withdrawal, blunted affect, and poor motivation (see chapter 5 for details) would represent dopamine deficiency symptoms in the mesocortical dopamine tract, which connects the midbrain to the prefrontal cortex. This would help explain findings such as the improvement of some schizophrenic patients with dopamine agonists, the lack of improvement of some patients with dopamine blockers, and the relative lack of response of negative symptoms to antipsychotics. It has been further postulated that the mesocortical dopamine deficiency could secondarily result in overactivity in the mesolimbic tract through overcompensation or disinhibition, thereby explaining dopamine excess and deficit simultaneously (Weinberger, 1987).

The second revision of the dopamine hypothesis adds the influence of serotonin to both the etiology and pharmacotherapy of schizophrenia. Decades ago, it was discovered that hallucinogens such as lysergic acid diethylamide (LSD) were structurally related to serotonin. More recently, the efficacy of clozapine, an atypical neuroleptic with strong serotonin blocking effects and weak dopamine-2 blocking effects (in contrast to the conventional antipsychotics) rekindled interest in serotonin's contribution to schizophrenia (Roth and Meltzer, 1995). Even more than for dopamine, there is insufficient direct evidence to define a role for serotonin in the biology of schizophrenia. Investigations in the near future will help clarify the issue.

Neuroimaging studies have generally demonstrated structural brain abnormalities in schizophrenic patients. The most consistent of these findings has been enlargement of the ventricles (the areas containing cerebrospinal fluid as opposed to brain tissue) (Lieberman, Brown, and Gorman, 1994). These findings are also seen in first-episode schizophrenic patients, implying that the abnormality is not likely to be due to medication or chronicity of the disorder. However, enlarged ventricles are seen in only some schizophrenic patients and may be found in other disorders too, casting doubt on the specificity of the finding. Although a number of studies have pointed to specific brain regions that may be smaller in schizophrenic patients (especially the hippocampus), these findings are inconsistent.

Using functional brain imaging, the most consistent finding in schizophrenia has been decreased activity in the frontal lobes. As with enlarged ventricles, however, this finding is far from universal. Some studies have suggested hypofrontality especially in those patients with prominent negative symptoms (see chapter 5). Measuring dopamine receptors in the brain of schizophrenic patients prior to neuroleptic treatment by PET is a field still in its infancy.

Anxiety Disorders

Among the anxiety disorders, panic disorder and obsessive compulsive disorder have been the subjects of most of the intensive biological research over the last decade. (See chapter 4 for a discussion of the different anxiety disorders.) Unfortunately, compared to the investigations into the biology of schizophrenia and depression, anxiety research is in its infancy. Therefore, even the most current hypotheses must still be considered very tentative. Since most of the biological research into generalized anxiety has focused on the mechanism of action of the benzodiazepine tranquilizers, which include medications such as diazepam (Valium) and alprazolam (Xanax), it will be discussed in chapter 11 which focuses on these medications.

From the early investigations in the beginning of this century, it has long been suspected that adrenergic chemicals such as epinephrine and norepinephrine play a role in the generation of acute arousal and panic. The symptoms of panic resemble those feelings triggered by acute fear or sudden excitement colloquially known as "the adrenaline rush." More recent research has, in part, continued this approach with the more modern element of focusing on a possible dysregulation of the noradrenergic system in panic causing a functional hyperactivity of the system and consequent symptoms of anxiety. The two other major directions of panic disorder research have been: (1) to identify chemicals that provoke panic attacks and to understand how these effects are mediated; and (2) since hyperventilation or rapid breathing is so common in panic, to understand the relationship between respiratory control and panic disorder.

Most of the attention has focused on the workings of the locus ceruleus, noted above as the part of the brain with the highest concentration of cells utilizing norepinephrine as a neurotransmitter. Animal experiments have demonstrated that when this area of the brain is stimulated, fear responses are provoked; destruction of the locus ceruleus abolishes these responses (Charney et al., 1990). Consistent with these observations, most medications that block panic, such as the cyclic antidepressants (see chapter 4), decrease locus ceruleus activity.

Direct evidence of abnormalities of the adrenergic system in panic disorder, however, is lacking. As examples, panic attacks are usually but not always accompanied by increases in heart rate, blood pressure, and skin temperature. Patients with panic disorder tend not to show heightened cardiac activity (such as high pulse or blood pressure) throughout the day although they may have more intermittent rises in pulse during the course of the day (Shear, 1986). Similarly, although adrenergic agents can cause increased anxiety in panic disorder patients, the results are inconsistent enough to preclude a definitive link between noradrenergic dysfunction and panic (Price, Goddard, Barr, and Goodman, 1995).

A variety of pharmacological agents will reliably provoke panic attacks in panic disorder patients but not in control subjects. Surprisingly, epinephrine seems not to provoke panic. The most well documented panic-producing technique is the infusion of intravenous lactate, which provokes clear panic in 70 percent of panic patients but only rarely in normal controls (Cowley and Arana, 1990). When patients are successfully treated for panic with medications, lactate no longer provokes attacks. Two other agents that seem to provoke significant anxiety or panic are yohimbine (a medication used in the treatment of impotence), and inhaling high concentrations of carbon dioxide. Unfortunately, the mechanisms by which these agents provoke panic are still obscure.

Because panic is often associated with hyperventilation and since carbon dioxide inhalation often provokes panic in susceptible individuals, abnormal respiratory control mechanisms have been proposed as a possible biological vulnerability to panic disorder (Papp, Klein, and Gorman, 1993). Since the locus ceruleus has important connections with the brainstem center regulating respiration, these observations link noradrenergic influences to the breathing abnormalities (Gorman, Liebowitz, Fyer, and Stein, 1989). A recent hypothesis—the suffocation false-alarm theory—has further suggested that panic patients have a hypersensitive suffocation detector that is triggered by small rises in carbon dioxide leading to panic attacks (Klein, 1993a).

As must be obvious from the above, there is no coherent explanation of the biology of panic. It does seem likely that a heightened biological sensitivity and response to internal and/or external cues exists in panic patients, although consistent proof of this does not exist. Thus, symptoms such as spontaneous panic attacks or phobic fear may reflect exaggerated psychological and biological responses to normal stimuli. Aside from our lack of understanding of the mechanisms of provoked panic, it is also not clear that these induced attacks, which provide much of the research data, are valid models for spontaneous episodes. Certain somatic cues during a lactate infusion, for instance, may trigger a learned anxiety response because of prior naturally occurring panic, and not because of the specific provoking agent, thereby making the exploration of the "cause" of the provoked panic attack spurious. As the research progresses, hypotheses encompassing the role of learning, using both biological and psychological constructs, will undoubtedly enhance the richness and validity of the models.

Because obsessive compulsive disorder (OCD) is a disorder for which serious biological investigation began in the 1980s, virtually all research in this area is very recent. Although biochemical abnormalities in OCD have been explored by measuring neurotransmitter function and metabolites, the more important and influential investigations have utilized neuroimaging studies.

The most common biochemical hypothesis of OCD implicates serotonergic dysfunction as a central factor, since all effective medications for the disorder powerfully increase serotonin in the central nervous system (see chapter 4). Yet, as discussed elsewhere, the mechanism of action for any treatment does not inherently suggest an etiology for the disorder being treated. Even theoretically, it is not clear whether OCD is most likely to be associated with excessive or diminished serotonergic function. Experimental studies in this area using a variety of techniques have yielded inconsistent results (Price, Goddard, Barr, and Goodman, 1995). For now, it must be concluded that there is no consistent evidence of baseline serotonergic dysfunction in OCD patients.

The more intriguing biological research and more consistent findings for biological abnormalities in OCD have emerged from neuroimaging research (Baxter, 1994). Overall, the evidence points to abnormalities in an area in the frontal lobes called the orbital prefrontal cortex and in the caudate, a part of the basal ganglia, the area that helps control movement. It is as yet unclear how dysfunction in these areas leads to the symptoms of OCD. The most influential hypothesis suggests the presence of a "circuit" composed of the caudate, orbital cortex, and the thalamus that focuses and drives behavioral routines that are difficult to interrupt. Decreased inhibitory input to this system from the caudate may result in dysfunction, causing the routines to become inappropriately repetitive and noninterruptible, as with obsessions and compulsions. Successful treatment of OCD would increase caudate function (as it seems to do), and diminish the self-sustaining loop quality of the circuit. This would result in increased flexibility of performance, which clinically would be expressed as fewer rituals. Of note, the biological abnormalities such as diminished caudate activity improve with any successful treatment, such as medication or behavior therapy (Baxter et al., 1992). The exact role of serotonin in this hypothesized system is still unclear. However, since serotonergic influences to these regions are present, serotonergic medications might be helpful by indirectly altering the inputs to this dysfunctional system.

SECTION
THREE

3

Mood Disorders

DIAGNOSIS

Major Depression

The evaluation of abnormal moods, especially depression, is the most common reason for psychopharmacological consultation. This stems from a number of different factors. First, mood disorders are relatively common, having twelve-month and lifetime prevalences of 8.5 and 14.7 percent respectively in this country (Kessler et al., 1994). Second, mood disorders are among the most pharmacologically treatable disorders in psychiatry, with extensive documentation of success for over thirty years. But the frequency of consultations stems just as much from two other sources: one is the semantic confusion surrounding the word *depression,* and the other is the increasingly accepted notion of depression as a spectrum of disorders, ranging from severe incapacitating major depressive episodes with melancholia to mild depressive personality features.

Semantically, using one word—depression—in a number of separate ways guarantees both muddled conceptualization and fuzzy communication. The first and colloquial use of the term *depression* treats it as equivalent to or synonymous with the terms *sad, blue, down in the dumps, unhappy, miserable,* and so on. This use of the term, therefore, defines a symptom or feeling state. The second use refers to a specific depressive syndrome—major depressive episode or disorder (MDD) in DSM-IV—which is manifested not only by a mood disturbance but also by a cluster of clearly defined signs and symptoms noted below. Still another use of the term depression refers to a group of depressive syndromes, such as dysthymic disorder, that are less severe than major depressive episode but are characterized by more than just a depressed mood.

Depression as a symptom (also called dysphoric mood) is ubiquitous in virtually all psychiatric disorders. Almost everyone who walks into a therapist's office is unhappy to some degree or they wouldn't

49

seek treatment. The only possible exception to this are patients with
mania and certain forms of schizophrenia and dementia, all of which
are disorders in which insight is lost as part of the psychopathology and
the severe disturbance may be unrecognized by the patient. Traditionally, antisocial patients (or psychopaths as they were called in the past)
were thought to be guilt free as part of their core pathology, but some
recent studies indicate that these patients frequently experience depressed mood, whether they view their problems as consequences of
their own behavior and feelings or because of the unfairness of the
world (Perry, 1985). All other forms of Axis I and II psychopathology
(see chapter 1 for definitions) involve clear measures of distress or depressed mood.

If depressed mood, then, were synonymous with a depressive disorder, virtually all patients seeking psychological treatment would be
seriously considered for antidepressant treatment. Clearly, this is a foolish notion. In the vast majority of cases, antidepressants are useful for
treating depressive syndromes and not depressed moods. In this chapter, therefore, the focus will be on evaluating and treating the spectrum
of depressive disorders (other than depressive personality, which will
be discussed in chapter 7).

Table 3–1 shows the DSM-IV criteria for major depressive episode
or disorder (MDD). Although patients with more than one major
depression are described as having major depression, recurrent, in
DSM-IV, they are also commonly referred to as unipolar depressives
(as distinguished from bipolar patients who suffer from both manias
and depressions—see below). Implicit in the five-of-nine-symptom
criterion is the lack of a pathognomonic symptom for MDD (i.e., a
symptom or sign that is specific for the disorder in question, seen only
in that disorder and in no others). The clearest way of using these criteria is to think of major depression as a syndrome characterized by (1)
an alteration in mood and (2) a cluster of signs and symptoms reflecting alterations in basic biological functioning (sleep, appetite, psychomotor changes) and subjective/psychological functioning (change
in cognition, suicidal ideation, guilt, apathy, and fatigue) lasting two
weeks or more. It is unusual for a patient to exhibit all the signs and
symptoms listed in Table 3-1. DSM-IV requires the presence of only
five of the nine symptoms to meet the criteria. But there is nothing magical about the threshold of five symptoms. Many patients
whose clinical presentations are entirely consistent with a diagnosis of
depression (by natural history, family history, response to treatment,
etc.) may have a mild episode in which only four symptoms are pres-

Table 3–1
Diagnostic Criteria for Major Depressive Episode

A. Five (or more) of the following symptoms have been present during the same two-week period and represent a change from previous functioning; at least one of the symptoms is either (1) depressed mood or (2) loss of interest or pleasure.

Note: Do not include symptoms that are clearly due to a general medical condition or mood-incongruent delusions or hallucinations.

(1) depressed mood most of the day, nearly every day, as indicated by either subjective report (e.g., feels sad or empty) or observation made by others (e.g., appears tearful). **Note:** In children and adolescents, can be irritable mood.

(2) markedly diminished interest or pleasure in all, or almost all, activities most of the day, nearly every day (as indicated by either subjective account or observation made by others)

(3) significant weight loss when not dieting or weight gain (e.g., a change of more than 5% of body weight in a month), or decrease or increase in appetite nearly every day. **Note:** In children, consider failure to make expected weight gains.

(4) insomnia or hypersomnia nearly every day

(5) psychomotor agitation or retardation nearly every day (observable by others, not merely subjective feelings of restlessness or being slowed down)

(6) fatigue or loss of energy nearly every day

(7) feelings of worthlessness or excessive or inappropriate guilt (which may be delusional) nearly every day (not merely self-reproach or guilt about being sick)

(8) diminished ability to think or concentrate, or indecisiveness, nearly every day (either by subjective account or as observed by others)

(9) recurrent thoughts of death (not just fear of dying), recurrent suicidal ideation without a specific plan. or a suicide attempt or a specific plan for committing suicide

B. The symptoms do not meet criteria for a Mixed Episode.

C. The symptoms cause clinically significant distress or impairment in social, occupational, or other important areas of functioning.

D. The symptoms are not due to the direct physiological effects of a substance (e.g., a drug of abuse, a medication) or a general medical condition (e.g., hypothyroidism).

E. The symptoms are not better accounted for by Bereavement, i.e., after the loss of a loved one. The symptoms persist for longer than two months or are characterized by marked functional impairment, morbid preoccupation with worthlessness, suicidal ideation, psychotic symptoms, or psychomotor retardation.

Reprinted with permission from the *Diagnostic and Statistical Manual of Mental Disorders, Fourth Edition.* Copyright 1994 American Psychiatric Association.

ent. For clinical work, the diagnostic criteria are guidelines, not rigid rules.

DSM-IV criteria for major depression are very similar to those listed in DSM-III-R. The only two changes of any note are: (1) the addition of Criterion C requiring significant distress or impairment beyond the simple presence of the symptoms noted in Criterion A; and (2) the distinction from bereavement in Criterion E by utilizing a two-month cutoff following the loss of a loved one after which the presence of depressive symptoms may be considered for a depressive disorder.

The criteria for major depression are mostly self-explanatory. However, a few key points are worth highlighting. The most important is the DSM-IV equivalence of sadness (depressed mood) and lack of interest (apathy) as the mood disturbance. If a patient is very sad, the notion of a depressive disorder suggests itself quickly. It is less obvious when the patient complains of feeling flat, distant, removed, or disinterested. Yet this is the most prominent symptom for many depressed patients. With further probing, these apathetic patients will describe the same depressive symptoms (sleep, appetite disturbance, etc.) as those who are sad.

The second important diagnostic point is the cognitive deficit of depression. Although characterized as a mood disorder, depression is also a cognitive disorder. From indecisiveness to poor concentration to feeling that one's brain is going at half speed, virtually all depressed patients have some change in cognition. Occasionally, this will be the presenting complaint. Therefore, if an indecisive apathetic person comes to therapy, the possibility of a depressive disorder must be considered seriously.

For those therapists who are not experienced in interviews that focus on symptoms (as opposed to the more open-ended psychodynamic approach), the following questions are examples of how to elicit information needed to diagnose major depression.

Have you been feeling down, blue, or depressed lately? Does this feeling wax and wane a great deal within the course of the day or is this feeling present pretty much all of the time? How long has this feeling been going on?

Do you feel as interested as you usually are in activities that are enjoyable to you? (If you know what the patient likes to do, asking about that activity may be very helpful; e.g., Do you feel less like bicycling lately? How long has that been going on?)

Has your appetite or weight changed during this time? In what way? (If the patient lost weight, make sure it was not from conscious dieting.) Over what period of time did you gain (lose) the weight?

Has your sleep pattern changed? (If decreased sleep, is the problem getting to sleep or waking during the night? If the patient wakes up during the night, can he get back to sleep? What time does he wake up? If increased sleep, how many hours of sleep does the patient get? It is important to distinguish this from lying in bed awake.)

Do you feel physically slowed down such that you are really moving more slowly? Do other people notice it? (DSM-IV requires observable changes, not just the self-perception of being slowed down.) Do you feel agitated or restless so that others might notice it?

What's your energy like? Are you tired most or all of the time?

Have you been feeling bad or guilty about yourself lately? Do you feel like a failure? What kinds of things do you feel guilty about? (Guilt about being depressed should not be considered. The content of the guilt is also a probe as to whether the patient has psychotic guilt, a consideration with treatment implications.)

Have you had difficulty concentrating? (Probe to clarify the patient's concentrating capacity—can he do his work, can he read, can he follow television programs?) Is it hard for you to make decisions? Does it feel as if you are thinking more slowly?

Have you been thinking about dying or focusing on morbid thoughts? Do you find yourself wondering if life is worth living? Have you had thoughts of killing yourself? (If yes, ask how specific those thoughts are. Does the patient have a plan? When? How?)

If you do something you usually enjoy, can you still enjoy it? (As with questions about interest, use an example from the patient's own experience.)

If something good happens to you, can you snap out of your mood, even if only for a while?

Is there a particular time of day in which you feel worst? When is that? (Make sure that the diurnal variation, if it occurs, exists on weekends *and* weekdays. Not looking forward to weekday mornings because you hate your job but feeling fine on weekends is *not* melancholia.)

Subtypes of Major Depressive Disorder

DSM-IV specifies subtypes of major depression according to certain clinical features. Some of these subtypes have characteristic responses to somatic treatment while others have a long tradition of being viewed as somewhat separate clinical entities.

Melancholic Depression

Melancholia is a more severe form of major depression, with the term often used synonymously with endogenous depression. (Since endogenous refers to arising from within as opposed to reactive, and our knowledge about the true etiology of depression is shaky at best, the framers of the DSMs wisely avoid this term.) The two central features of melancholic depressions are anhedonia and autonomy of mood. Anhedonia is the loss of interest or pleasure in all activities. Autonomy of mood refers a person's inability to feel better, even temporarily, when something pleasurable happens. The rest of the DSM-IV criteria for melancholia essentially describe a more severe major depression. The presence of melancholic features should always suggest a psychopharmacological consultation since they predict a good response to somatic treatment (American Psychiatric Association, 1993b).

Major Depression with Psychotic Features

Patients with psychotic depression are usually profoundly dysfunctional and severely depressed. In its most typical form, the psychotic features are mood congruent; that is, the psychotic themes are depressive in content. The importance of making this diagnosis is that the presence of psychotic features predicts a relatively poor response to antidepressants alone and a better response to a combination of antidepressants plus antipsychotics or electroconvulsive treatment (ECT) (Schatzberg and Rothschild, 1992).

Atypical Depression

After years of variable definitions, the term atypical depression was officially placed in DSM-IV to describe a characteristic symptom pattern seen in a subset of depressed patients. This term replaces the previous term hysteroid dysphoria which, although colorful and descriptive, was also sexually stereotyped and pejorative. An atypical depression is characterized by mood reactivity (the ability to be cheered up, albeit temporarily, in response to positive events) and two of the following four symptoms: significant weight gain (or increased appetite), hypersomnia, leaden paralysis (heavy leaden feelings in arms or legs), and a pervasive pattern of interpersonal rejection sensitivity. By definition, therefore, these patients tend to have depressions of mild to moderate severity since they cannot have autonomy of mood, a core feature of melancholic depression. Because patients with atypical depression are overly dependent on relationships for adequate self-esteem while simultaneously being overly reactive to rejection, narcissistic and borderline personality features are prominent in their clinical presentations.

The importance of recognizing atypical depression is twofold. First, since these patients frequently are in psychotherapy for their fragile self-esteem and typically poor interpersonal relationships, and because their symptoms are clearly and inextricably intertwined with their personality disorders and traits, it is easy to miss their psychopathology as a type of depression. Second, these patients often respond very well to antidepressants—both monoamine oxidase (MAO) inhibitor antidepressants and probably the serotonergic antidepressants (see below)—with a marked diminution of their depressive response to narcissistic slights (Liebowitz, Quitkin, et al., 1988).

Charlene had always seemed to feel her feelings more intensely than did others. She was bright, friendly, good in school and active in organizations. She considered herself (accurately) to be unusually sensitive, both in the positive sense of understanding the feelings of others and being a good friend, but also in being easily hurt. When others were angry at her—parents, friends, or boyfriends—she would cry and be unable to continue a conversation. This type of sensitivity was ego-dystonic for Charlene. She wished she were more thick skinned and more able to defend herself with a cool head, and not a trembling voice.

As an adult, Charlene functioned well, working in production in the entertainment industry. She was a valued employee, industrious and eager to please her demanding bosses. In relationships, Charlene struggled, becoming overly attached to men who were relatively insensitive to her. Even when it became clear that a relationship would not work for her, Charlene had enormous difficulty breaking up. When the relationships did end, Charlene was typically devastated.

She was still able to work but was teary during the day, hid in bed when she wasn't working, and gained ten pounds. She responded to the support of her many friends with a temporary lifting of her mood.

After hearing about the efficacy of the newer antidepressants from a friend, Charlene sought a medication evaluation with the encouragement of her therapist. Despite her reluctance to take medication, perceiving it a sign of weakness, she agreed to try sertraline. Within three weeks, she noticed a general decrease in a kind of internal anxiety that she had not previously recognized. She felt less concerned about what everybody thought of her. She brooded less about a negative interaction with her irritable boss and stood up for herself without crying with her distant boyfriend. Eventually, Charlene broke up with him, realizing that he was not the right man for her. Although she was deeply sad about the breakup and became tearful talking about it, she stayed active, utilizing the support of her friends. In evaluating the effect of the antidepressant, Charlene missed some of the exquisite sensitivity of her feelings. Overall, however, her enhanced ability to deal with the emotional stresses in her life and relationships with more confidence and less fear far outweighed the negative effects.

Seasonal Depression

This depressive subtype is officially described in DSM-IV as depression with seasonal pattern. The best estimate is that approximately 10 percent of mood disorder patients have a seasonal pattern of recurrence in which the depressive episodes begin at the same time of year in a predictable pattern (Faedda et al., 1993). Those episodes that characteristically begin in late fall or winter and typically remit in springtime are colloquially called seasonal affective disorder (or SAD). Some, but not all of these patients become hypomanic in the springtime. These winter depressions are usually characterized by atypical features (see below) such as increased sleep, increased appetite, and feeling slowed down, not agitated. Eliciting a history of seasonal winter depressions is important since SAD responds to both antidepressants as well as to a unique form of treatment—light therapy (Terman et al., 1989; Dilsaver, Del Medico, Quadri, and Jaeckle, 1990).

Postpartum Depression

DSM-IV describes a postpartum depression as a depressive episode occurring within four weeks of childbirth, characterized by the same symptoms seen in other depressions. However, just as the term *depres-*

sion has been blurred by multiple definitions, so too has the term *postpartum* depression. It is important to distinguish among the three common uses of the term, since the need for medical intervention differs among them.

1. Postpartum blues is a common (50 to 80 percent of all women giving birth) mild depressive syndrome occurring within the first ten days postpartum and characterized by rapid mood swings, crying spells, and a sense of confusion (but without disorientation or serious cognitive changes). The blues are self-limited. The appropriate treatment is support and reassurance that the feelings experienced are normal.
2. Severe postpartum psychosis/depression occurs in 2 per 1,000 births usually starting within the first month postpartum and frequently within the first two weeks. A full depressive syndrome may be present (although it is difficult to evaluate sleep and energy symptoms in a woman who has just given birth) and psychotic features are common. It is vital to diagnose postpartum psychosis because suicidal and infanticidal ideation and acts can occur. Therapists should look for an inability to function, unusual feelings of worthlessness and hopelessness, suicidal or homicidal statements, or any psychotic symptom. This type of psychosis constitutes a potential psychiatric emergency; hospitalization is commonly indicated.
3. Mild postpartum depression is seen in 10 to 15 percent of women within six months after giving birth. These depressions look like mild to moderate major depressive episodes. Some of these women will do well with psychotherapy, education (about being a mother), and support while others need antidepressants in addition (Gitlin and Pasnau, 1989). There is some question as to whether the rate of mild to moderate postpartum depression over many months to one year after childbirth is any higher than that for women of the same age range who are not postpartum (Cooper, Campbell, Day, Kennerly, and Bond 1988).

The use of pharmacological agents during pregnancy and in the postpartum period is a complex issue and is discussed in Chapter 8.

Bipolar Disorder

The other major mood disorder is bipolar disorder (or manic-depressive illness as it was previously called). By definition, patients with bipolar disorder have episodes of mania and depression. The diagnostic criteria for bipolar depression and major depression are the same. When depressed, however, bipolar patients, especially younger ones, are more likely to exhibit hypersomnia (increased sleep), hyperphagia (increased appetite), and psychomotor retardation, in contrast to the more common insomnia, decreased appetite, and agitated depressions seen in unipolar depressions (Caspar et al., 1985).

The DSM-IV criteria for a manic episode are shown in Table 3–2. As can be seen, the diagnostic principles used are the same as for MDD; that is, mania is defined as a period of time in which there is an abnormal mood and a cluster of signs and symptoms.

A severe manic syndrome is called mania, the hallmark of which is increased energy/activity. This energy may be reflected in a euphoric, expansive mood, by irritability, or by a combination of the two. It is helpful to think of someone taking amphetamines who can feel focused, intense, and good, or irritable, paranoid, and uncomfortable. As with major depression, the criteria for mania include physical, observable symptoms (decreased sleep, increased activity and talking), subjective/psychological symptoms (increased self-esteem, racing thoughts), and mixed symptoms (distractibility and poor judgment).

When a florid manic syndrome exists, it is impossible to miss; the person's energy is alternately infectious to those around him and exhausting, irresistible, and obnoxious. By definition, a manic episode always causes significant impairment in the patient's ability to function. Manic individuals act bizarrely enough at work to be fired, obnoxious, impulsive, and frightening enough to destroy relationships, spend a lifetime of savings, or uncharacteristically get into legal trouble.

Manic patients also tend to increase (or start) their consumption of alcohol and street drugs which, of course, exacerbates the impulsive poor judgment characteristic of the mania. Bipolar individuals consistently drink and use drugs more when they are manic than when depressed (Goodwin and Jamison 1990). Although one might reasonably imagine that manic patients drink more alcohol for its sedative effects, to calm down the manic excitement, this is unlikely to be the entire explanation since they also use more cocaine and other stimulants.

Hypomania (i.e., "under" mania) is a mild version of mania. The diagnostic criteria and symptoms of hypomania as listed in DSM-IV are identical to those for mania with the exception of the time criterion—four days in contrast to mania's seven days—and the requirement that the symptoms not be so severe as to cause marked impairment in social or occupational functioning. For clinical pur-

Table 3-2
Diagnostic Criteria for Manic Episode

A. A distinct period of abnormally and persistently elevated, expansive, or irritable mood, lasting at least one week (or any duration if hospitalization is necessary).

B. During the period of mood disturbance, three (or more) of the following symptoms have persisted (four if the mood is only irritable) and have been present to a significant degree:
   (1) inflated self-esteem or grandiosity
   (2) decreased need for sleep (e.g., feels rested after only three hours of sleep)
   (3) more talkative than usual or pressure to keep talking
   (4) flight of ideas or subjective experience that thoughts are racing
   (5) distractibility (i.e., attention too easily drawn to unimportant or irrelevant external stimuli)
   (6) increase in goal-directed activity (either socially, at work or school, or sexually) or psychomotor agitation
   (7) excessive involvement in pleasurable activities that have a high potential for painful consequences (e.g., engaging in unrestrained buying sprees, sexual indiscretions, or foolish business investments)

C. The symptoms do not meet criteria for a Mixed Episode

D. The mood disturbance is sufficiently severe to cause marked impairment in occupational functioning or in usual social activities or relationships with others, or to necessitate hospitalization to prevent harm to self or others, or there are psychotic features.

E. The symptoms are not due to the direct physiological effects of a substance (e.g., a drug of abuse, a medication, or other treatment) or a general medical condition (e.g., hyperthyroidism).

Note: Manic-like episodes that are clearly caused by somatic antidepressant treatment (e.g., medication, electroconvulsive therapy, light therapy) should not count toward a diagnosis of Bipolar I Disorder.

Reprinted with permission from the *Diagnostic and Statistical Manual of Mental Disorders, Fourth Edition,* Copyright 1994 American Psychiatric Association.

poses, then, the distinction between hypomania and mania is in the amount of personal damage caused by the episode. Manias are destructive, hypomanias less so. In part due to a concern about the overdiagnosis of hypomania to many patients with mildly excited states, the framers of DSM-IV also require that hypomanic patients show an unequivocal change in functioning that is uncharacteristic of the person when not symptomatic and that the mood disturbance and functional changes be observable by others. Many experts in the field would argue that these criteria are too stringent, that many patients have mild hypomanic episodes that are more subtle than the criteria require. The concern of these experts is that if the DSM-IV criteria are taken too literally, many patients with mild hypomania will go unrecognized and thus be deprived of effective treatment. As always, in clinical work, diagnostic criteria should be utilized as guidelines and not the revealed truth.

Another clue to the presence of a subtle hypomanic state is the frequent emergence of a depressive episode following the hypomania. In a subtle hypomania, the patient may simply seem to be functioning exceedingly well. If a switch into hypomania occurs while the patient is in therapy, it is easy to assume that the therapy has "clicked." Since virtually all hypomanic episodes are time-limited, however, the period of high energy and functioning will end, and a depression will frequently follow. This pattern—cycles of expanding activities, new plans, and a spurt of self-confidence followed by a collapse of these changes—should make the therapist consider the diagnosis of Bipolar II disorder (see below).

The major subtypes of bipolar disorder are called Bipolar I disorder in which patients suffer full blown manias and depressions, and Bipolar II disorder, characterized by recurrent hypomanias and depressions but without manic episodes. In comparison with Bipolar I disorder, Bipolar II disorder has depressions equal in severity, but manic episodes of lesser intensity.

Patients will sometimes present with features of both mania and depression simultaneously, called a mixed state or mixed mania. Intense dysphoria will be present along with racing thoughts, suicidal ideation with increased energy, depressive delusions with grandiose delusions. DSM-IV requires the presence of full manic and depressive syndromes simultaneously for the diagnosis of a mixed episode. Many observers, including myself, feel these criteria are too rigid (McElroy et al., 1992b). A more reasonable clinical rule would be to look for an admixture of at least a few depressive symptoms along with a manic syndrome. Mixed states can be explosive and destructive—the combination of suicidal despair and manic irritable energy is a dangerous combination for suicide risk. In general, these patients are treated the same as for manic episodes; the first goal of the pharmacological treatment is to decrease the irritable energy and possibility of impulsive behavior.

Rapid cycling describes a subtype of bipolar disorder in which the patient suffers from four or more manic, hypomanic, or depressive episodes in a twelve-month period. Although DSM-IV requires the full time criterion (e.g., two weeks for a depressive episode) for each episode, others have noted that patients with multiple episodes of short duration are indistinguishable from those with full-length episodes (Bauer et al., 1994). Risk factors for rapid cycling include being female, Bipolar II (vs. Bipolar I), and hypothyroid. Most studies indicate that rapid cycling patients are more difficult to treat, with lesser responses to lithium and a generally poorer prognosis, although in some patients, rapid cycling may disappear after a number of years (Coryell, Endicott, and Keller, 1992).

Often, it is vital to obtain information from significant others in the patient's life to evaluate a possible manic episode. Because denial and lack of insight are very common in mania and hypomania, others may observe clear dysfunctional symptoms that the patient denies. It is impossible to overemphasize the seductive qualities of mania or hypomania. Manic patients can be wonderfully coherent for short periods of time and fool even experienced therapists. The use of outside observers (e.g., friends, family members) can be crucial for making an accurate diagnosis.

The questions that follow may help the therapist identify manic symptoms:

Have you been feeling much better than usual? Would you describe your mood as euphoric? Have others commented on how happy you seem? Is this the best you've ever felt? or, Have you been irritable in a speedy way lately, such that you've gotten into more fights than usual?

During this time, have you been feeling terrific about yourself? Did you feel as if you had special powers? (Ask about new-onset "creativity," or telepathy or a new ability to make people do things.)

Have you been sleeping less than usual? How much less? Are you tired?

Have you been talking more than usual?

Do you have the sensation of thoughts racing in your head? Does it feel like you are going at 78 rpm while the rest of the world is at 45 rpm?

Have you had trouble following through on tasks because you were easily diverted to other tasks or because you felt that there were so many interesting things to do you wanted to do them all at once?

Have you been more active than usual—doing more things for longer hours? Like what?

Have you gotten into trouble lately? For example, have you been speeding in your car, having more sexual affairs than usual, or spending more money than usual? (It is always important to compare these activities to the person's *usual* behavior.)

Have these symptoms or activities had a major impact on you, on your job, your relationships?

Have you been making long distance phone calls? Have you been buying lots of things you don't need or have you been buying more items than you need, like six pairs of shoes when you need only one?

NATURAL HISTORY, EPIDEMIOLOGY, AND GENETICS

It is likely that the disorder we call major depression is heterogeneous in nature; that is, it is composed of a number of different subtypes, all of which share the same cluster of signs and symptoms. Because of the presence of multiple subtypes, it is difficult to describe accurately the natural history of major depression. However, depressions are increasingly seen in younger people, with the median age of onset in the late twenties (American Psychiatric Association, 1993b). The mean length of a depressive episode is six months. Increasing evidence, though, suggests that a substantial proportion of patients have episodes lasting one year or more (Keller, Shapiro, Lavori, and Wolfe, 1982). Additionally, 20 percent of depressions last two years or more (Keller, Lavori, Rice, Coryell, and Hirschfield, 1986). Over half the patients with depression will have more than one episode in a lifetime (American Psychiatric Association, 1993b). Those with recurrent depressions average approximately five to six episodes in a lifetime without preventive treatment (Angst, 1973; Grof, Angst, and Haines, 1973).

The mean age of onset in bipolar disorder is in the late teens to early twenties with at least half the patients showing symptoms of the disorder in the teenage years (American Psychiatric Association,

1994b). An average manic episode lasts approximately three months. All the possible sequential patterns of episodes—depression followed by mania followed by euthymia, mania leading into depression, mania alone, and depression alone—can be seen. Bipolar disorder is almost always recurrent, with more than 95 percent of patients having more than one episode in a lifetime (Goodwin and Jamison, 1984). Within the almost uniform pattern of recurrence, the course of bipolar disorder is exceedingly variable, with some patients suffering only a few episodes and others having multiple episodes.

Both unipolar and bipolar mood disorders unquestionably run in families. That is, in the families of both bipolar and unipolar patients, more relatives have mood disorders than are seen in the general population. The risk to the relatives differs, depending on the subtype of the disorder of the patient. The families of bipolar patients show a marked increase in both bipolar (Bipolar I and Bipolar II) and unipolar disorder. In the families of unipolar patients, the increased risk is strongest for unipolar disorder, less so for Bipolar II, and minimal for Bipolar I disorder (Rice et al., 1987). A possible explanation for these findings is that bipolar disorder is the most severe form of mood disorder (resulting from greater genetic vulnerability), conferring a higher risk for all forms of the disorder, whereas the milder unipolar type confers higher risks for only the milder subtypes. Earlier onset of the disorder is usually associated with increased risks in family members (Weissman et al., 1984). Unipolar patients with recurrent episodes are more likely to have relatives with mood disorders than are those with only one episode (Bland, Newman, and Orr, 1986).

PRESENTATIONS OF MILD MOOD DISORDERS

There are a number of mild mood syndromes that should cause a therapist to consider psychopharmacological consultation and treatment. In addition to dysthymia, cyclothymia, and the minor and brief depressive disorders to be discussed in this section, even milder mood syndromes—those inextricably intertwined with personality features—are increasingly treated with pharmacotherapy. These syndromes include depressive personality and rejection sensitivity syndromes (even in the absence of formal atypical depressive features). Because these milder disorders are inherently chronic and viewed by patients and mental health professionals alike as personality based, they will be discussed in chapter 7 with the other personality disorders.

Dysthymia

The core concept underlying the definition of dysthymic disorder is that of a low-grade chronic depressive disorder. The DSM-IV definition requires at least two years of depressed mood most of the time with at least two of the following: (1) poor appetite or overeating, (9) insomnia or hypersomnia; (3) low energy or fatigue; (4) low self-esteem; (5) poor concentration or difficulty making decisions; (6) feelings of hopelessness.

Conceptually, although dysthymia has its roots in the depressive personality described in the past, as it is currently defined in DSM-IV it is appropriately classified as a mood disorder. Four of the six symptom criteria for dysthymia are so-called vegetative symptoms, virtually identical to those defining major depressive episode (although the required time frames differ). Only hopelessness and low self-esteem distinguish dysthymic symptoms from major depression. DSM-IV dysthymia differs significantly from depressive personality disorder (see chapter 7) because the former is predominantly defined by the language of symptoms, not personality attributes. Nonetheless, because its diagnostic criteria include both vegetative features as well as more affective/cognitive symptoms (hopelessness and low self-esteem), dysthymia is a heterogeneous disorder.

Some dysthymic patients have the onset of their disorder during their adult years, while others cannot remember a time when they weren't depressed. Although some dysthymic individuals are successful as measured by occupational status or role performance, dysthymia is, in general, characterized by significant role dysfunction, days in bed, restrictions in social activities, and so on (Wells, Burnham, Rogers, Hays, and Camp, 1992).

Many dysthymic patients suffer from a variety of other psychiatric disorders, including major depression, eating disorders, social phobia, generalized anxiety disorder, and personality disorders (Gwirtsman, 1994). The pattern of dysthymia and major depression within the same individual, with the boundaries between the two disorders often blurred, is called double depression (Keller, Shapiro, Lavori, and Wolfe, 1982). Although this may represent true coexistence of two disorders, it may also stem in part from the overlap in diagnostic criteria.

Although relatively few studies have examined the topic, it is clear that dysthymic patients respond to antidepressants, but probably at lower rates than do patients with major depression (Howland, 1991). (This may reflect the more heterogenous nature of dysthymia). Thus far, controlled treatment studies indicate that dysthymic disorders respond equally to all the major classes of antidepressants; tricyclic anti-depressants, MAO inhibitors, and SSRIs have all been shown to be effective (Gitlin 1995a). Clinical experience, however, including my own, indicates that SSRIs seem to be the most effective class of agents (Hellerstein et al., 1993).

Since no valid predictors of medication response exist for treating dysthymia, an empirical trial of antidepressants is the only way to ascertain which dysthymic patients will respond. A specific indication for antidepressants with these patients may be a lack of progress in psychotherapy, especially for those who are working well in the treatment, attaining insights and shifting cognitions, yet feeling no better in their mood or energy.

Patients with double depression have a waxing and waning course to their disorder with major depressions that are comparatively shorter than those of classic depressives (Keller et al., 1982). These patients may also be more likely to respond to antidepressants than those with pure dysthymia (Akiskal et al., 1980). When treated with antidepressants, some double depressives will show improvement only in the superimposed major depression (leaving the underlying dysthymia unchanged), while others will show amelioration of both disorders.

For his entire life, Sam felt he was missing something that others seemed to possess. During childhood, he was relatively shy, had a few friends, but was never boisterous or mischievous. Because he did well in school and socialized a bit, neither his parents nor his teachers had any significant concerns about his psychological well-being. In high school and early college, he had very few romantic interests because of his self-consciousness and inability to approach women for dates. During this time, he noticed that he seemed to have less physical stamina and energy than others, describing himself as always tired. He claimed to need nine to ten hours of sleep every night and if he had a night in which he slept only seven hours, he would become more irritable. Sam was preoccupied with his sense of inferiority and would rarely take risks because of his absolute conviction that he would fail. Nonetheless, he seemed capable of enjoying himself with good friends although he complained that he never quite felt the intensity of happiness that he perceived others as experiencing.

As an adult, Sam married and became a middle-level manager in a department store. His relationship with his wife was somewhat strained but stable. She continuously complained about how emotionally distant he was with her, his resistance to social encounters, and his pattern of lying in bed on weekends. He had a few friends at work but, as in college, he was convinced that they all had more fun and zest in life than he did.

In his thirties, he sought psychotherapy on his wife's insistence. He acknowledged the general restrictiveness of his psychological and emotional life. Explorations of his early life with his distant rigid parents helped explain his own emotional style but did not change his overall sense of self. Similarly, cognitive/behavioral techniques gave him more mastery over his negative thoughts and feelings but did not change his perceived poor quality of life.

Eventually, he sought a psychopharmacological consultation on the advice of his therapist who identified a family history of major depression—a paternal aunt who had been hospitalized for depression and a paternal great uncle who received ECT in the 1950s. Sam was placed on fluoxetine, with the dose quickly increased to 20 mg daily. For the first three weeks on the medication, Sam felt incredibly energized, talking more, being more active and less resistant to social encounters. Although some of the initial energy faded, he continued to show positive benefit from the antidepressant in his increased activities, decreased sleep (averaging seven hours nightly instead of his previous nine hours), and far greater interest in social encounters.

Like Sam, Ernie, now 60, had always felt a spark missing from his life. He was a successful businessman, having worked his way to a high management position in a large firm. His marriage of thirty years had always been conflictual, in part because his wife correctly felt he was resistant to any spontaneity in their lives. She was also resentful of the recurrent depressive episodes that Ernie suffered. Multiple times during his life, often but not always in response to an external stressor, Ernie would become seriously depressed with anhedonia, sleep and appetite difficulties, and fatigue. Twice in the past, he had needed to be hospitalized because of a serious risk of suicide. Ernie had been in psychotherapy for twenty years and had developed a significant dependency on his therapist. Yet neither his baseline dysthymic disorder nor his recurrent major depressions were altered with treatment. Eight years ago, during a hospitalization for another depression, a consultant strongly recommended antidepressants. Desipramine was started and increased to 150 mg daily. The effect on Ernie's depression was unequivocal—his suicidal ideation dissipated, he began to eat and sleep normally, his mood brightened. Because of the frequency and seriousness of his depressions, Ernie and his therapist agreed with the psychopharmacologist that maintenance, preventive treatment with the antidepressant was appropriate. Over the last eight years, Ernie has continued to brood and be restricted in his affect, but has had no major depressions.

Cyclothymia

Patients described as cyclothymic have a disorder characterized by rapid and frequent bipolar mood swings—that is, they have frequent hypomanic and depressive periods. What distinguishes them from patients with Bipolar II disorder is that the depressions are neither long enough nor severe enough to meet criteria for major depression. As such, cyclothymia can be thought of as a clear bipolar disorder, but that does not fit our other diagnostic "boxes."

Cyclothymic patients, like Bipolar II patients, tend to lead chaotic lives. It may be easy to miss the cyclothymic mood swings and ascribe the cycles of mood and energy to narcissistic disturbances, or flights into health. The key point in distinguishing cyclothymics from patients with personality-based mood swings is the presence of clear behavioral signs of mania (Akiskal, Djenderedjan, Rosenthal, and Khani, 1977). Cyclothymic patients tend to have cycles with shortened sleep, increased spending, increased rapidity of talking, and the grandiose plans of mania which are then followed by a collapse—the hypersomnia, fatigue, apathy, and suicidal ideation of depression. Thus, the patient who spends excessively and compulsively constantly is less likely to have cyclothymia than the patient who spends in spurts and in conjunction with other typical hypomanic symptoms.

Cyclothymic individuals frequently show excellent responses to pharmacological treatment. Treatment strategies are akin to treating bipolar patients (see below). Because cyclothymic episodes tend to be short-lived, the focus of treatment must be prophylactic, to prevent these rapid frequent cycles of highs and lows.

When first seen at age 28 for psychopharmacological consultation, Judy complained of being tired of the chaos in her life. She had been in and out of psychotherapy for years, never staying in treatment for more than a few months. Family members, friends, and lovers had always characterized her as moody and unpredictable, descriptions she felt were accurate. Her usual self was energetic, active, and talkative. However, she described frequent episodes of what she called her "demons," a term she used with both affection and fear. During these episodes, she would become much more energetic than usual, having new ideas and often staying up nights organizing her thoughts for a career change. She would become absolutely focused on these plans and became enraged at anyone (typically her boyfriend or family) who wasn't completely supportive. She would spend hours on the telephone, calling old acquaintances, telling them of her ideas. After a few days of this, Judy seemed to collapse. She would be unable to sustain interest in the very ideas that had so recently possessed her. Although she was able to work, she simply dragged herself around, feeling depressed, guilty, and sleeping ten hours or more nightly. The depressive phases lasted no more than a week, following which she would return to her normal self and try to undo the damage in her relationships. It was at these times that she entered therapy, typically quitting during the next hypomanic phase.

Following a recent episode, Judy saw a new therapist who elicited a family history of bipolar disorder and referred her for a consultation. Two weeks after starting lithium, Judy had another cyclothymic episode during which she stopped treatment. Four months and two episodes later, she restarted lithium. Although she had a number of cyclothymic episodes during the next few months, they were markedly attenuated in severity. Gradually, the episodes became less frequent. Judy then restarted therapy and worked productively and consistently on issues of relationships and self-esteem.

Recurrent Brief Depressions and Minor Depressions

Listed in DSM-IV under the wastebasket term of depressive disorder NOS (not otherwise specified) are two recently identified variants of depression called recurrent brief depression and minor depression. These are depressive disorders that differ from classic major depression by either the brevity of the episodes or the number of symptoms during the episodes.

Recurrent brief depressions are frequently occurring episodes—at least monthly, but not in association with the menstrual cycle. They are identical to major depression in symptoms and in impairment but last two to thirteen days (fourteen days is the minimum time criterion for major depression). Seemingly common in epidemiological studies, the responsivity of these depressions to antidepressants has not been evaluated in controlled studies (Angst and Hochstrasser, 1994). However, given the rather classic depressive symptoms and the disabling nature of the disorder, patients with brief depressions should be strongly considered for psychopharmacological evaluation.

Minor depressive disorder is defined by depressive episodes of similar duration to major depression but with two to four depressive symptoms (as opposed to the requisite five symptoms in the classic disorder). As with brief depressions, patients with minor depressions are common in epidemiological studies and show significant functional impairment. (Judd, Rapaport, Paulus, and Brown, 1994; Broadhead, Blazer, George, and Tse, 1990).

MEDICAL DIFFERENTIAL DIAGNOSIS AND EVALUATION

The list of medical disorders that can mimic depression is very long (see Table 3–3). Therapists do not need to make specific medical diagnoses or recognize subtle medical problems that might be contributing to patients' psychiatric problems. It is important, however, to recognize when an evaluation is necessary. When a patient has a mood disorder, the following signs and symptoms should suggest a medical evaluation by an internist or family practitioner: (1) prominent vegetative symptoms, such as weight and sleep disturbances; (2) no prior history of depression, that is, a first episode; (3) older age; (4) ongoing treatment for a current medical disorder.

Of the medical disorders listed in Table 3–3, the most commonly confused with depression are hypothyroidism, Parkinson's disease, certain cancers, chronic fatigue syndrome, acquired immune deficiency syndrome (AIDS), and disorders related to drug and alcohol ingestion and withdrawal.

Hypothyroidism is a low thyroid condition in which patients may look as if they have a psychomotor retarded depression with hypersomnia, weight gain, and fatigue. They may also have dry skin and hair and a lower voice. The diagnosis is confirmed by blood tests for circulating thyroid hormone (called T4, T4 index, or free T4 index) and the pituitary hormone that regulates the production of thyroid hormone (called thyroid stimulating hormone or TSH).

Table 3–3
Medical Disorders That May Cause Depressive Syndromes

Central Nervous System: Alzheimer's disease, brain tumors, brain abscesses, aneurysms, encephalitis, intracranial hemorrhages, general paresis (syphilis), subdural and epidural hematomas, epilepsy, brain contusion (from head injury), normal pressure hydrocephalus, multiple sclerosis, Parkinson's disease, Huntington's disease, stroke, AIDS

Endocrine: Hyperthyroidism, hypothyroidism, hyperparathyroidism, hypopituitarism, Cushing's disease, Addison's disease

Vitamin Deficiency: B$_{12}$ (pernicious anemia), niacin (pellagra), thiamine

Toxins: Heavy metals (lead, manganese, mercury), toxic wastes

Intoxications: Alcohol, sedatives, hypnotics, tranquilizers, opiates, marijuana, withdrawal syndromes (especially from stimulant drugs)

Metabolic and Others: Remote effects of carcinomas, Wilson's disease, uremia (renal failure)

Chronic fatigue and other postviral syndromes

Parkinson's disease is diagnosed primarily by history and a neurological examination. Parkinsonian patients are most likely to be over 50. The most prominent symptoms are a tremor of the hands that is most noticeable when the patient is at rest but which increases with anxiety and disappears during sleep, and stiffness/rigidity affecting the whole body. These patients have marked psychomotor retardation. When they move, they do so slowly. Parkinson's disease can be confused with depression, and the two disorders are often present simultaneously. Depression occurs in 40 percent of patients with Parkinson's disease (Cummings, 1992). The common coexistence of these two disorders may be related to the changes in brain neurotransmitters, especially dopamine, inherent in Parkinson's disease.

Certain cancers such as pancreatic and some lung cancers cause depression far more often than other equally severe illnesses. Presumably, this is due to biological changes caused by the cancer. These cancers tend to appear in older patients who also show significant weight loss, breathing difficulties, or other medical symptoms.

Chronic fatigue syndrome has been increasingly implicated over the last five years as a possible cause of depressive syndromes. Presumptively viral in origin, the syndrome is characterized by profound fatigue, muscle aches, and depression, and frequently begins with a typical viral syndrome (fever, sore throat, swollen glands, etc.) (Krupp, Mendelson, and Friedman, 1991). There is still much controversy regarding the classification of chronic fatigue syndrome as a depressive variant, a viral syndrome, or a separate psychological disorder (Abbey and Garfinkel, 1991). Antidepressants, typically prescribed at lower doses than used for major depression, seem to be helpful in relieving both the mood and fatigue symptoms in chronic fatigue syndrome (Goodnick and Sandoval, 1993).

Because the HIV virus infects the brain well before overt symptoms of AIDS occur, there are concerns about the nature of depression in HIV-positive individuals: Is it an understandable reaction to a fatal illness, or is it secondary to the presence of the virus in the central nervous system? In contrast to initial concerns, recent studies suggest the risk of depressive disorders in infected HIV-positive gay men is no higher than that seen in a noninfected control group (Perkins et al., 1994). For those HIV-positive men with or without AIDS, antidepressants are effective in treating depression, although many patients are more sensitive to side effects (Rabkin, Rabkin, Harrison, and Wagner 1994). Stimulants—methylphenidate or dextroamphetamine—seem to be helpful specifically for those AIDS patients with mixed apathy/depression syndromes (Fernandez and Levy 1994).

Excessive alcohol and/or drug use, especially barbiturates and high-dose tranquilizers have long been known to mimic depression. A more recently described cause of depression (as well as mania or psychosis) is the use of anabolic steroids, used by body builders to increase muscle mass (Pope and Katz, 1994). Taking an accurate history is, of course, mandatory; often a urine test for drugs can be helpful. It is *impossible* to evaluate an underlying depression while the patient is using street drugs and/or alcohol chronically. The alcohol and drugs need to be stopped for a number of weeks before any evaluation of an underlying depression can be made. (See chapter 6 for further discussion.)

Withdrawal syndromes that occur after stopping stimulating drugs can result in a transient depressive syndrome. Of these stimulating drugs, the most notorious are cocaine and amphetamines. A good history is, as always, vital. As with acute drug-induced mood disturbances, the need for antidepressants cannot be assessed until the patient has been drug-free for at least a few weeks. (See chapter 6 for medications to help reduce drug craving.)

For mania, the most common medical mimics are hyperthyroidism and drug use. Hyperthyroidism is the opposite of hypothyroidism and is characterized by an increased metabolic rate. Hyperthyroid patients have difficulty sleeping, are irritable, restless, and may show poor concentration; they sweat profusely and hate hot weather; their hands tremble and they may lose weight despite eating more than usual. In a specific form of hyperthyroidism called Graves' disease, patients may have bulging eyes. The diagnosis is made by testing for the amount of thyroid hormone in the blood (T4) and sometimes by a thyroid scan.

Street drugs such as cocaine and amphetamine can easily mimic mania. The diagnosis is made by history and urine tests, if needed.

MEDICATIONS CAUSING DEPRESSION

The list of medications that have been reported to cause depression in an occasional patient is endless. But some medications are more likely to cause depression than others. It is most important that the therapist ask all depressed patients whether they are taking any medications. If the answer is yes, a consultation regarding that particular medication's capacity to cause depression is in order.

Historically, the medications purported to be most associated with depression have been the antihypertensives (blood pressure medications). In part, this link reflected the likely depressogenic effects of reserpine, one of the first antihypertensives that is now rarely in use. Additionally, many of the older antihypertensives work by decreasing the amount or effect of epinephrine or norepinephrine in the brain. Since, as explained in chapter 2, norepinephrine and serotonin are neurotransmitters that are important in the regulation of mood, it was theoretically consistent that predisposed individuals might become sluggish or depressed when given some of the older antihypertensives.

Over the last decade, a group of new and qualitatively different classes of antihypertensives have been developed and now dominate the treatment of hypertension in this country. These new antihypertensives—particularly the calcium channel blockers and the angiotension converting enzyme (ACE) inhibitors—both theoretically and clinically seem far less likely to cause depression. Furthermore, recent evidence has suggested that the risk of depression with the older antidepressants, such as the beta-blockers or diuretics, is much less than previously thought (Metzger and Friedman, 1994). At this point, then, antihypertensives should be considered a possible but uncommon cause of depression.

The other medications most likely to cause mood symptoms, either depression, mania, or nonspecific psychotic thinking, are steroids, such as cortisone or prednisone. Oral contraceptives have long been linked with depression in some women. As with the antihypertensives, however, recent evidence casts doubt on this link (Patten and Love, 1993). Whether this reflects simply more accurate research or the different effects of the lower doses of estrogens and progestins (the two hormones found in birth control pills) in more recent preparations is unclear. However, since many women do describe depressed mood (as opposed to a full depressive syndrome) in association with oral contraceptives, it would be reasonable to consider the two linked if a mood change occurs just after a course of birth control pills is begun.

LABORATORY EVALUATION

No agreement exists among psychopharmacologists regarding the minimum mandatory blood tests to be obtained before antidepressants can be safely prescribed. As described previously, certain aspects of the patient's history may suggest a more extensive medical evaluation. For the medically healthy patient who has no history, signs, or symptoms suggestive of a medical disorder, a general screening blood test (often called a Chem panel, which includes measures of liver and kidney function and of chemicals called electrolytes), a blood test for thyroid function called TSH (thyroid stimulating hormone), and an electrocardiogram if the patient is over 40, will suffice. The purpose of these simple and inexpensive screening tests is to ensure that there are no unrecognized medical problems that will either cause depression or mania or interfere with the treatment of either disorder. With the domination of the newer antidepressants in treating depression, many medical practitioners are reducing the requirement for even these few medical tests, reflecting the greater medical safety of the newer agents. Nonetheless, some medical screening or a review of lab tests drawn within the last year is still appropriate either just before or in the beginning of treatment.

A number of lab tests are currently promoted as being able to diagnose depression. At present, none of these tests has been validated as clinically useful in diagnosis. The dexamethasone suppression test (DST), which was used extensively in the early 1980s, adds little of value to a careful history. Certain abnormalities in sleep EEG studies may suggest depression, but the cumbersomeness and expense of the test rarely justifies its use in everyday clinical work. Over the last five years, neuroimaging tests measuring brain structure, blood flow, or metabolism, such as MRI (magnetic resonance imaging), PET (positron emission tomography), MR-SPECT (magnetic resonance spectroscopy), as well as computerized EEG (electroencephalogram) studies have been evaluated as aids to clinical diagnosis. (Chapter 2 provides further details about these scans.) All of these tests are important windows into understanding the abnormal biology of depression and are appropriately utilized in research studies. However, none of them is reliable, valid, and inexpensive enough to be used in everyday clinical situations.

PSYCHIATRIC DIFFERENTIAL DIAGNOSIS

Depression

Since, as previously noted, depressive mood (as opposed to depressive disorders) is seen in the vast majority of individuals seeking treatment, it is important to distinguish depressive states for which psychopharmacological treatment should be considered from other dysphoric states. Classically, the three most important general diagnostic cues that can help make this distinction are (1) the episodic nature, (2) the tendency towards cyclicity, and (3) the characteristic genetic pattern of depression. Therefore, in trying to evaluate whether a particular patient has a disorder that might be treatable by antidepressants, a psychopharmacologist will focus on the timing of symptoms: When did it begin? Have you ever had this before? How many times? How long did it last? Are there particular times of year that you tend to feel like this? The psychopharmacologist will also ask a somewhat detailed family history that focuses not so much on the relationship between the patient and his relatives but on the individual characteristics of the family members. In obtaining a family history, care must be taken to remember the dual nature of the word depression: when a patient describes his mother as depressed, it is vital to know whether this refers to the miserable life she had with her husband, with a chronic sadness but with normal functioning (suggestive of poor marital relations), or a pattern of discrete episodes of apathy, poor functioning, and suicidality.

With the increasing realization on the part of patients and mental health professionals alike that many milder depressive disorders, previously considered unresponsive to pharmacotherapy do in fact, respond to the newer antidepressants, the classical questions just described are less useful than in the past. Patients with chronic mild depressive disorders without any hint of cyclicity or even a family history of significant depressive disorders are sometimes successfully treated with the newer serotonergic antidepressants or other agents. Given the lack of thoughtful research studies in this area, our ability to predict who among this milder, less typically depressed population might respond to antidepressants is exceedingly poor.

Even with the number of dysphoric states that are truly unresponsive to antidepressants seemingly shrinking, it is still worthwhile to describe those disorders easily confused with depression. They include mourning, demoralization, adjustment disorders with depressed mood, premenstrual syndrome, and dementia syndromes (including Alzheimer's disease).

Mourning

Patients who are mourning frequently complain of the same symptoms as those seen in major depression. Early in the mourning process, therefore, the distinction is difficult. Traditionally, it was thought that in mourning the preoccupation revolves around the person who has died with self-references focusing on the effect of the loss. In depression, the person becomes obsessed with his own feelings to the exclusion of thinking about the person who has died. Normal mourning also decreases in intensity after a number of months whereas depression may not. However, prominent depressive symptoms in those who are recently bereaved may indicate that mourning has emerged into a true depressive disorder. As an example, those patients with a significant number of depressive symptoms only two months after the death of a spouse are likely to have past histories of major depression and are at high risk to show continued depressive symptoms one and two years later (Zisook and Shuchter, 1993). Given these findings, patients in mourning—especially if they have a past history of depression—who do not show at least some resolution of depressive symptoms within a few months after a loss should be further evaluated for a depressive disorder.

Demoralization

The person in a state of demoralization has given up hope of improvement. This is frequently seen in association with a variety of chronic medical and psychiatric disorders. At first glance, it is easily confused with depression. The key difference is that demoralization is not necessarily associated with vegetative symptoms, but more with depressive cognitive distortions and attitudinal symptoms. Patients who become demoralized following a major depression from which they have recovered may present an extremely difficult therapeutic problem. Demoralization does not respond to antidepressants. Because of the similarity between the two disorders, however, an empirical trial of antidepressants is often necessary.

John was a 38-year-old man who came for treatment of his chronic depressive state, which had lasted for five years. He had been a highly successful businessman in his twenties until a cocaine addiction eroded his judgment. During his years of business success, he lived in a grand manner and exhibited many features of a narcissistic character. His first manic episode seems to have been precipitated by his cocaine use. Over the next four years, despite his not using any street drugs, he had two manic and one depressive episodes by which time his fortune and his marriage were gone. After the second manic episode, he was started and continued on maintenance lithium. In the four years before seeing me, he had experienced a constantly depressed mood, despite continuing on his lithium treatment, supplemented by a variety of antidepressants, none of which were effective. He lived in a small apartment, subsisting on money begrudgingly given to him by his parents. His only attempt at working was interrupted by a manic episode during which he was hospitalized. This last episode humiliated him and he lived in constant fear of another episode.

In discussing his current state, John noted that he ate and slept normally and was capable of enjoying things, although not to the degree he experienced previously. He had no diurnal variation and could concentrate well enough to read novels, although he claimed to be unable to read journals relating to business. He could not imagine starting his career again at the bottom and building his way back up. He continually mourned his past—his financial success, his marriage, and his status—feeling that he would never be able to be successful again. He was additionally terrified that any attempt to work would precipitate another manic episode.

It was clear that John did indeed suffer from bipolar disorder (as well as narcissistic personality disorder) but that his current state was more consistent with demoralization, rather than a major depression. For John, the appropriate treatment at this point would be psychotherapy, along with his maintenance lithium. Had he not been previously treated with antidepressants (albeit unsuccessfully), a trial of antidepressants, despite the lack of vegetative signs, would have been appropriate.

Adjustment Disorder with Depressed Mood
This dysphoric state is distinguished from depression by its relative paucity of vegetative symptoms, nonautonomous mood (i.e., the mood is responsive to events in the environment), and temporal proximity to the obvious major stressor. Similar to mourning, a disorder that initially presents as an adjustment disorder may evolve into a major depression.

Premenstrual Syndrome
The most obvious feature of premenstrual syndrome (called premenstrual dysphoric disorder in DSM-IV) is its relationship to the menstrual cycle. Since it is surprisingly difficult for patients to accurately assess their moods retrospectively, a mood chart filled out prospectively over two cycles is often helpful to ascertain whether the depressive syndrome varies according to the menstrual cycle. Chapter 8 reviews premenstrual syndrome and its treatment in detail.

Dementia Syndromes
Dementia generally and Alzheimer's disease specifically have been the object of increased scientific and public interest as part of a growing awareness of psychiatric disorders of the elderly. One of the most important distinctions that must be made is between "true" dementia, such as Alzheimer's disease, and "pseudodementia," the reversible cog-

nitive symptoms seen in depressions in the elderly. Some features that help distinguish between depression and dementia are shown in Table 3–4. No single sign or test reliably distinguishes between the two disorders. Further complicating the clinical distinction between the two disorders, prominent depressive symptoms are seen in a substantial proportion of patients with Alzheimer's disease (Wragg and Jeste, 1989). Additionally, those elderly depressed patients with severe cognitive deficits are at high risk to develop classic irreversible dementia over the three years following the depression, implying that the "pseudodementia" was, for these patients, an early sign of the emerging dementia (Alexopoulus, Meyers, Young, Mattis, and Kakuma, 1993). Despite this diagnostic confusion, if, after a thorough evaluation, a depressive disorder is suspected (with or without a comorbid dementia), it should be treated with antidepressants.

Mania

A personality type recognized earlier in the century but not described in more recent texts is that of hyperthymic (or hypomanic) personality in which the symptoms of mania exist as personality attributes. These people are the proverbial used car salesman types—talkative, bombastic, grandiose, optimistic, and cheerful. They may also exhibit excessive risk taking and reduced need for sleep. Since there is no research on these patients, it is unclear whether this represents a personality type or a subsyndromal mania.

The other personality types that look like bipolar disorder are the chaotic personality disorders—histrionic, narcissistic, borderline, and antisocial types in which "bipolar" (i.e., high and low) mood swings are

Table 3–4
Differentiating Pseudodementia (of Depression) from Dementia

Depression	Dementia
Past personal history of depression	No past personal history of depression
Family history of depression	Family history of dementia
Vegetative signs prominent (sleep and appetite disturbance)	Cognitive deficits out of proportion to vegetative signs
Diurnal variation (symptoms worse in morning)	Sundowning (symptoms worse in the evening)
Gives up easily during cognitive testing	Attempts to cover up deficits during cognitive testing

typical. As with distinguishing misery from depression, the most difficult cases are those in which a chaotic personality *and* a bipolar disorder coexist.

Describing the characteristics of happiness in order to distinguish it
from hypomania may seem peculiar. Yet the question arises frequently,
especially in the ongoing treatment of bipolar patients. Most typically,
the patients' spouse will call the therapist complaining that the patient
is exhibiting signs of hypomania. The patient will then angrily deny it,
blaming the spouse for not wanting him to be happy. Table 3–5 lists
some ways to distinguish between the two states.

> Barbara was a 29-year-old married woman with a clear history of
> bipolar disorder. Prior to a course of maintenance lithium therapy, she
> had a number of very severe depressions, one manic and one hypo-
> manic episode, and many short-lived mood swings. During her manic
> episode, which occurred in September, she left her husband and
> moved to a different city, citing marital discontent. After the episode
> resolved, she returned to the marriage. During the hypomania, which
> also occurred in September two years after the mania, marital rela-
> tions were severely strained but no separation ensued. Barbara started
> lithium treatment in January of the next year and initially did well,
> with a clear diminution of her short mood swings. In September, nine
> months after starting lithium, she became increasingly dissatisfied
> with her marriage, pointing to a number of problems which, she cor-
> rectly pointed out, had existed for many years. She made plans to
> move to a different city, insisting that the relationship was untenable

Table 3–5
Distinguishing Hypomania from Happiness

Hypomania	Happiness
Cheerfulness switches easily to irritability when the person is crossed	Mood is even and not so easily perturbed
Drivenness in energy	Able to settle down
Less sleep than normal	Full night's sleep
Grandiosity leading to poor judgment	Good judgment
Frequently preceded by or followed by depression, usually of psychomotor retarded hypersomnic type	No predictable relationship to depression
Typically cyclical, frequently timed to a specific time of year	Generally not seasonal
Family history of bipolar disorder	No family history of bipolar disorder

and she could never be happy with her husband. At this time, she was compliant with lithium, slept seven hours a night, denied racing thoughts, and showed no obvious signs of mania. Because this marital crisis occurred in September, Barbara's husband was concerned that the problems were due to another hypomanic episode, a conclusion that understandably infuriated her. Because of logistical problems, Barbara did not plan to move until February. By January, however, her anger had substantially dissipated and she abandoned her plans for separation. The quality of the marriage returned to its baseline. By February, she felt strongly that she had experienced a mild hypomania (which had been partially muted by the lithium) during which her dissatisfactions with the marriage were fueled by a manic irritability and anger. She has had no subsequent hypomanias in the last three years and the marriage has continued as before.

PSYCHOPHARMACOLOGICAL TREATMENT

The number of first-line medications for treating mood disorders has expanded to twenty-one antidepressants within at least five different classes, three mood stabilizers, and electroconvulsive treatment (ECT). Unfortunately, our ability to predict a positive response for an individual patient to any one of these treatment options has not kept pace with the growing number of medications. For an occasional clinical problem there may be one, or at most a few, rational treatment options; for example, when a bipolar patient on an antidepressant becomes acutely manic, the only reasonable initial approach would be to stop the antidepressant. But for most other clinical situations, a variety of alternatives may be equally valid. For instance, a first major depressive episode can be treated with any of the cyclic antidepressants with equal likelihood of success. Increasingly, therefore, important pharmacological decisions are correctly made in a practical, rather atheoretical manner: which medications have the least objectionable side effects and are simplest for that particular patient?

A thorny clinical problem in prescribing antidepressants is deciding how aggressive the pharmacotherapy should be—that is, how many medication trials should be given? For patients with relatively severe mood disorders, such as major depression with melancholia or bipolar disorder, it is appropriate to continue pharmacotherapy until an effective reasonably well-tolerated treatment is found. Yet, for the milder disorders, such as dysthymia, depressive personality, or rejection sensitive individuals, it is less clear how aggressively to pursue the treatment. If the first two trials of a serotonergic antidepressant have been cut short because of side effects, should a third be tried? If full trials of two anti-depressants have been ineffective, should a third be given? Should combination treatment be utilized (see below)? The decision is ultimately made by patient, psychopharmacologist, and therapist, typically based on the clinical conviction that "biological factors" are a significant part of the patient's problems.

In the organization of this section, the treatments for major depression and bipolar disorders are separated. Although the symptoms of unipolar and bipolar depression are phenomenologically similar and the therapeutic options are identical, the "drug decision trees" for these two major types of depression differ. This stems from two clinical observations: First, bipolar and unipolar depressives differ somewhat in their response to mood stabilizers (see below). Second, and more important, antidepressants have the potentially adverse effect of causing mania or rapid cycling in bipolar patients, a risk not shared by unipolars.

Pharmacotherapy of Major Depression (Unipolar Depression)

Table 3–6 shows the broad classes of psychopharmacological treatment options for an acute depressive episode. For the majority of depressed

Table 3–6
Psychopharmacological Treatment Options for Depression

Basic Antidepressant Classes

First-line agents:
   Selective serotonin reuptake inhibitors (SSRIs)
   Novel new agents: Bupropion (Wellbutrin), Venlafaxine (Effexor), Nefazodone (Serzone)
   Cyclic antidepressants: Tricyclics (TCAs)
Second-line agents:
   Monoamine oxidase (MAO) inhibitors
   Electroconvulsive therapy (ECT)

Other Options

Mood stabilizers (lithium, valproate, carbamazepine)
Stimulants
Light therapy
Antianxiety agents:
   Alprazolam
   Buspirone

patients, the five basic classes shown are equally likely to be effective. A full trial (enough dosage for a sufficient period of time, see chapter 9 for details) of any of the medication treatments will be effective in 60 to 65 percent of patients (Davis, Wang, and Janicak, 1993). Sometimes, patients tend to equate bothersomeness of side effects with efficacy, so that a very sedating medication will be thought of as more powerful, or an antidepressant well tolerated will be considered mild. The capacity to cause side effects does not correlate with efficacy. If any generalization is appropriate, it is that the more powerful the side effects, the less likely it is that the patient will comply with treatment. Decreased efficacy will then ensue.

Only four clinical features predict a specific response to any antidepressant class or strategy. (See Table 3–7.) For depression with psychotic features, an antidepressant plus a neuroleptic (antipsychotic) or ECT are the appropriate first-line treatments. Depression with atypical features (see above for definition and description) responds better to MAO inhibitors than to the tricyclic antidepressants. Clinically, SSRIs also seem very effective in this population. Winter depression responds both to antidepressants—probably from all classes—as well to light therapy. Finally, there is some evidence, albeit conflicting, that for the most severely melancholic hospitalized depressed patients, tricyclics may be somewhat more effective than the SSRIs (Roose, Glassman, Attia, and Woodring, 1994).

First-Line Agents

For all other patients without these specific features, since all treatments are equally likely to be effective, overall ease of treatment plays an enormous role in the specific pharmacotherapy chosen. Because of this, ECT and MAO inhibitors, each of which has cumbersome aspects to its use, are rarely first-line agents. Therefore, the first antidepressant prescribed is typically either an SSRI, one of the novel new agents listed in Table 3–6, or a tricyclic antidepressant.

Table 3–7
Depressive Subtypes with Specific Pharmacotherapies

Depression with psychotic features
Depression with atypical features
Seasonal (winter) depression
Melancholic hospitalized depression

Table 3–8 shows the major factors that are considered in deciding which specific antidepressants to prescribe initially. As in deciding which antidepressant classes should be considered as first-line agents, side effects and ease of administration are the most important factors to be considered in choosing a specific antidepressant. Noncompliance to medication regimens is startlingly high for both psychiatric and nonpsychiatric treatments (see chapter 14), and side effects and difficult medication regimens are major causes (although not *the* major cause) of noncompliance. The appropriate strategy, then, is to find a medication the patient can take correctly and will tolerate at an appropriate dose for a sufficient amount of time to cause a positive clinical response. Since all antidepressants have some potential side effects, and are theoretically equally effective, the psychopharmacologist's task is to ascertain the side effects that will be most disruptive *for that particular patient,* and then to choose an antidepressant that is least likely to cause them (see chapter 9 for details on side effects of specific antidepressants). Examples of this approach would be:

1. A 42-year-old accountant whose depression is characterized by hypersomnia and psychomotor retardation does not need to be sedated. Therefore, a more stimulating antidepressant such as fluoxetine (Prozac) or desipramine (Norpramin) would be reasonable first choices, while doxepin (Sinequan), a sedating tricyclic, would not be.

Table 3–8
Factors Used in Choosing a Specific Antidepressant

Primary Considerations

Side effect profile
Ease of administration
History of past response
Safety/medical considerations
Specific subtype (if applicable; see Table 3–7)

Secondary Considerations

Neurotransmitter specificity
Family history of response
Blood level considerations
Cost

2. For a 27-year-old dancer, weight gain might be the most distressing of potential side effects. Therefore, any of the newer agents, none of which are consistently associated with weight gain, would be more reasonable choices than any of the tricyclics which are routinely associated with weight gain. If the patient was neither particularly anxious nor slowed down, sertaline (Zoloft) might be chosen as a first antidepressant.

3. A 70-year-old retiree with an agitated depression and postural unsteadiness/poor balance from arthritis and/or other causes is at high risk to fall if he takes a medication that causes postural hypotension (a drop in blood pressure upon standing up). Here too, any of the newer agents cause far fewer blood pressure changes than any of the tricyclics and would be reasonable first choices. Because of the agitation, this patient might be given paroxetine (Paxil), one of the least stimulating SSRIs.

Naturally, this approach, logical though it may be, does not always work. The accountant may find fluoxetine too stimulating, requiring a switch to a somewhat less stimulating SSRI. The retiree may find paroxetine or any of the newer agents too stimulating and may need to take nortriptyline, the tricyclic with the fewest hypotensive effects.

As is apparent in these examples, the newer antidepressants as a group unquestionably have fewer side effects than the tricyclics. Because of the lower side effect burden, doses can be raised more quickly with the newer antidepressants. Additionally, the SSRIs specifically can be given in once-daily dosing with many patients able to start on a full therapeutic dose on the first day, thereby simplifying the treatment regimen and enhancing compliance. Because of these considerations, the first antidepressant prescribed is typically one of the newer agents.

A history of a past response is another important consideration in choosing an antidepressant. However, in evaluating the past response, it is important to evaluate the likelihood of the causal link between the past treatment and the remission of a prior episode. For instance, a patient who "responded" to imipramine after one day is likely to have had a placebo response, while improvement six months after beginning an antidepressant suggests a spontaneous remission (see chapter 1 for further discussion). Another exception might be made if the past successful treatment caused significant side effects. As an example, a patient's depressive episode seven years ago may have responded to amitriptyline (Elavil) but with sedation as a very unpleasant side effect. In that case, the current episode might be best treated with an antidepressant that is chemically similar to amitriptyline (trying to repeat its therapeutic effect) but which is less sedating—such as nortriptyline.

The different capacities of the antidepressants to cause or interact with medical conditions are also important. As an example, patients with certain preexisting cardiac electrical abnormalities are at risk to have that abnormality worsen with tricyclics, an effect generally not seen with the newer agents. In this situation, the prescribing physician would choose one of the newer antidepressants, such as an SSRI or bupropion (Glassman and Preud'homme, 1993).

Lethality in overdose is sometimes a consideration in antidepressant choice. All the newer antidepressants are, in general, safe when taken in overdose. All tricyclics and MAO inhibitors are potentially lethal in overdose. However, if the possibility of overdose is high, hospitalization should be given serious consideration, regardless of the medication's safety.

If the patient has one of the depressive subtypes noted in Table 3–7, then these features would suggest the initial course of treatment.

At one time, it was thought that it might be possible to subtype depressions as norepinephrine-deficient or serotonin-deficient. (See chapter 2 for a review of neurotransmitters and biological theories of depression.) The choice of medication could then be based on the different capacities of each antidepressant to enhance norepinephrine or serotonin to increase the neurotransmitter that was abnormally low. This approach ultimately was demonstrated to be clinically not viable. However, many clinicians have observed that depressed patients with prominent irritability, anger, rejection sensitivity (even if they do not have DSM-IV defined atypical depression), or marked mood reactivity respond better to antidepressants with strong serotonergic effects, such as the SSRIs and venlafaxine.

It is uncommon for a psychopharmacologist to have the luxury of knowing that a close relative of the patient has responded well to a specific medication for the same depressive syndrome, but if this information is available, it should be considered strongly. The research evidence for this approach is somewhat sparse but a great deal of common sense suggests it highly.

The relationship between blood levels of most antidepressants and therapeutic response is inconsistent (see chapter 9 for details). Only four of the cyclic antidepressants—imipramine, nortriptyline, desipramine, and possibly amitriptyline—show any consistent correlation between blood level and efficacy. If a patient does not improve while taking one of these medications, measuring the blood level can tell the psychiatrist whether the patient metabolizes medications very quickly (and thus needs higher doses) or is on too much medication with the possibility that a lower dose would help. One of these antidepressants might therefore be prescribed if the patient is likely to be treatment resistant so that the dose can be adjusted more accurately. Because blood levels of antidepressants are *not* always helpful (since for most antidepressants the range of therapeutic values has not been established), they are not drawn routinely.

Finally, medication cost is a factor in antidepressant choice. The newer antidepressants are much more expensive than most of the tricyclics. In some clinical situations—when a patient has no insurance for medication costs, or is part of a managed care program in which the less expensive medications are required to be prescribed first—this is a relevant consideration. From another vantage point, however, even though the newer antidepressants are more expensive in cost per day, they are not associated with higher costs when other factors, such as numbers of physician visits, laboratory tests, days in hospital, and compliance are considered (McFarland, 1994). As more decisions about health care financing are made by examining total costs, and not just the piecemeal costs in isolation, concerns about the per pill price of the newer antidepressants may diminish.

Second-Line Agents

Monoamine Oxidase (MAO) Inhibitors

Although used far less commonly than either the newer antidepressants or cyclic antidepressants, MAO inhibitors are still occasionally prescribed. Both patients and mental health professionals who are unfamiliar with MAO inhibitors tend to view them as strange and dangerous drugs, to be prescribed only in emergent and desperate situations in which the risks of these medications are warranted. The risks of hypertensive reactions with MAO inhibitors are real and worthy of detailed explanation and concern (see chapter 9 for details). Yet with proper patient preparation, these medications are no more dangerous than the cyclic antidepressants. The lore of the MAO inhibitors' danger stems from the 1960s, before the cause of the hypertensive reactions (ingestion of tyramine-containing foods) was known. Without the basic dietary restrictions necessary with these medications, a number of patients during that time had strokes and died. At that time, both psychiatrists and patients appropriately viewed MAO inhibitors as dangerous. Today, it is simply not true. A psychiatrist knowledgeable about these medications treating a reasonably cooperative patient is a safe combination that confers few special risks beyond those associated with tricyclic antidepressants.

Table 3–9 lists the reasons a psychopharmacologist might consider prescribing an MAO inhibitor.

As with the cyclic antidepressants, a history of past response and possibly a family history of response should be given consideration in favor of MAO inhibitors. Many patients who previously responded to MAO inhibitors, however, also seem to respond to serotonergic antidepressants (SSRIs and venlafaxine) and frequently want to try the latter medications first in order to avoid the difficulties of the MAO inhibitors. MAO inhibitors are also commonly prescribed for patients who have not responded to a number of the first-line antidepressants. Anecdotally, and in many uncontrolled trials (since so few controlled treatment studies on this topic exist), a significant proportion of cyclic antidepressant nonresponders will show a clear response to MAO inhibitors (McGrath et al., 1993).

Depression with atypical features (discussed earlier in the chapter) or depression associated with marked interpersonal sensitivity constitute two of the strongest indications for choosing an MAO inhibitor (Liebowitz et al., 1988; Davidson, Giller, Zisook, and Overall, 1988). Similar to those with a past history of response to MAO inhibitors, many of these patients will try serotonergic drugs first. Patients with mixed panic disorder and depression also show good responses to MAO inhibitors, but are typically prescribed other antidepressants first (Kayser et al., 1988).

When choosing between the three MAO inhibitors for treating depression (see Table 9–8), the choice of medication rests on clinical lore and side effect considerations. Chapter 9 details the differences among these three medications.

Table 3–9
Factors Used in Deciding to Prescribe a Monoamine Oxidase Inhibitor

History of past response
Depression with atypical features (or with marked
interpersonal sensitivity)
Nonresponse to first-line antidepressants
Family history of response
Mixed panic disorder and depression

Electroconvulsive Treatment (ECT)

Without question, the controversy surrounding ECT continues to be the most sensitive in psychiatry's attempt to present somatic treatments of psychiatric disorders to other mental health professionals and the general public. (I am ignoring the debate about psychosurgery for intractable depression and obsessive compulsive disorder since these surgeries are not performed frequently enough in this country to engender much debate.) As with the MAO inhibitors, the residue of past problems with ECT has obscured the vast body of data collected over the last twenty years documenting ECT's efficacy and safety. Chapter 13 discusses ECT in detail.

For patients with acute major depression, there are a few specific indications for ECT. The most well-documented of these are psychotic depression (DSM-IV major depressive episode with mood-congruent psychotic features) and depression with catatonic stupor for which ECT is highly effective (American Psychiatric Association, 1993b). Another indication for ECT in major depression is in treating patients with severe depressions, typically with melancholic features, who have failed to respond to adequate trials of one or more antidepressants. Finally, patients with certain medical problems may be treated more safely with ECT than with antidepressants. An example of this would be a patient with unstable cardiac disease for whom the potential risk of blood pressure changes or alterations in cardiac rhythms seen with antidepressants is unacceptable. Since ECT is administered under controlled conditions (see chapter 13), including the presence of an anesthesiologist and anesthesia lasting only minutes, it is likely to be safer.

For most of her 69 years, Ethel had been energetic, optimistic, capable. Three times during her life, however, she had become profoundly depressed—once after giving birth to her first baby (but not after the second), once in her early forties, and six months ago. During each of these episodes, she became completely dysfunctional. She would lose 10 to 15 pounds, have classic early morning awakening, be unable to see friends, and would spend most of her time agitated and complaining of intolerable anxiety that was not significantly relieved by tranquilizers. Although insisting she wanted to die, Ethel made no suicide attempts. Her first episode had not been treated; a nanny took care of her newborn while family members watched over Ethel for ten months until she spontaneously improved. When she became depressed a second time, the family sought psychiatric help. Inpatient treatment in a hospital was unhelpful until she was given ten ECT treatments to which she responded completely. However, the ECT experience was disturbing to both Ethel and her family; they resented the lack of communication with the doctor, the lack of careful supervision they had expected, and the memory loss she experienced. (See chapter 13 for a discussion of ECT and memory loss.) Now, with a third depression, they reluctantly sought out a psychiatrist specializing in psychopharmacology.

At the initial consultation, the psychiatrist felt ECT was one of many options. Because of their past experience, both Ethel and her family wanted to try antidepressants. Over the next four months, nortriptyline, a cyclic antidepressant, and then phenelzine, an MAO inhibitor, were prescribed at adequate dose for six weeks each. (Two other antidepressant trials had been cut short by side effects.) By this time, Ethel had lost more weight and was talking increasingly of dying. It was explained to Ethel and her family that, although other medications, either individually or in combination, could be tried, the likelihood of a good response was now far less than with ECT. After a great deal of discussion with the psychiatrist and education about the techniques and possible side effects, Ethel ambivalently agreed to ECT. A series of eight ECT treatments again resulted in a complete remission. With the use of unilateral ECT (see chapter 13), the memory loss was significantly less than during her previous ECT treatments. Nortriptyline was restarted as a continuation treatment (see below) for the next six months and then tapered without incident.

Other Options

Mood Stabilizers

The most common clinical situation in which mood stabilizers, especially lithium, are considered to treat an acute unipolar depression is when the patient has a strong family history of bipolar disorder and describes hypersomnic, hyperphagic depressions that are characteristic of bipolar depression. Here one may hypothesize that the patient is at risk to have an unexpressed bipolar disorder, that is, the patient is genetically bipolar but has not yet had an initial manic episode. In this situation, however, many psychopharmacologists would prescribe an antidepressant with lithium, or lithium alone, as an initial treatment. Overall, lithium is not the equal of antidepressants in treating depression (Jefferson, Greist, Ackerman, and Carroll, 1987).

The other mood stabilizers used in treating bipolar disorder, especially valproate and carbamazepine, are also occasionally prescribed in treating acute unipolar depression. The same general guidelines utilized in choosing lithium for depression would be used. Typically, though, these medications are tried after an unsuccessful lithium trial.

Stimulants

Stimulants, such as methylphenidate (Ritalin) or d-amphetamine (Dexedrine) are sometimes prescribed alone to treat depression. Although they are less effective than standard antidepressants, they are often prescribed for those patients who have either not responded to or could not tolerate more conventional antidepressant treatment (Chiarello and Cole, 1987). Stimulants are also prescribed for apathetic, elderly patients or those with significant medical problems (Satel and Nelson, 1989). When used with these patients, low dose stimulants cause a rapid antidepressant response, increase energy, and foster a reconnection between the patient and his environment (Masand, Pickett, and Murray, 1991).

Light Therapy

When light therapy is described, it may sound like the fringiest of fringe treatments, but it is well documented as an effective treatment for winter depression (Terman et al., 1989). Patients sit one and a half to three feet from high-intensity lights (similar to the lights used to grow indoor plants or, of course, sunlight) for 30 minutes to four hours daily, depending on the light intensity. During this time, they may read, watch TV, pay bills, or anything else as long as they keep their eyes open. Typically, a marked reduction of the depressive symptoms is seen within days, far shorter than the usual two- to three week lag time for antidepressants to work. There is controversy as to whether the lights need to be administered during a specific time of day, with inconsistent evidence that light therapy administered in the morning may be more effective than that given in the evening (Blehar and Rosenthal, 1989). If the morning use of lights does not help (or is not practical because of the patient's work schedule), it is reasonable to switch to evening light before abandoning light as a viable treatment. Common side effects from light therapy are headache, eyestrain, and feeling wired (Levitt et al., 1993). There is no evidence thus far that light therapy causes any long-term damage to the eyes.

Antianxiety Agents

Despite a number of large-scale studies in the 1980s indicating the efficacy of alprazolam (Xanax) for treating depression, it is currently considered a weak second-line option when prescribed alone (Rickels et al., 1987). When it is effective, it is likely to be with those individuals with prominent anxiety or panic coupled with a mild depressive disorder. Similarly, buspirone occasionally effectively treats depression with anxious features (Rickels, Amsterdam, Clary, Puzzoli, and Schweizer, 1991).

Strategies Used in Treatment-Resistant Depressions

If a patient does not respond to one antidepressant, how does a psychopharmacologist then proceed? Before this question can be addressed, however, nonresponse to an adequate trial of a cyclic AD must be distinguished from a trial that is cut short by side effects. For instance, a patient who cannot tolerate any dose of fluoxetine because of agitation should be switched to a less activating SSRI. At this point, the patient is not an antidepressant nonresponder; he should be correctly conceptualized (and treated) as receiving an inadequate trial because of side effects. In this kind of situation, trying a number of medications within the same class or different classes would be appropriate to find one medication that the patient can tolerate. The patient may still not respond to that medication, but it is important to distinguish between a nonresponder and someone whose medication trials have been cut short because of side effects.

Although a thorough review of the many possible strategies for treating patients who do not respond to an antidepressant is beyond the scope of this book, it is worth describing the most common options. Table 3–10 shows the available general strategies, as well as specific augmentation and combination possibilities (Price, 1990).

Optimization refers to continuing the same antidepressant but for a longer period of time or at higher dose. As explained in chapter 1, some patients can be safely—and effectively—treated with higher doses than those recommended in the PDR. Switching to a different antidepressant (substitution) is also a commonly used option. If a patient takes a reasonable dose of the initial antidepressant for a long enough period of time (referred to as an adequate trial), it makes sense for the second antidepressant to be in a different class than the first. Although research studies in this area are virtually nonexistent, it is more reasonable to follow an unsuccessful SSRI trial with a tricyclic, or one of the other new antidepressants rather than another SSRI.

Combination strategies are those in which each of the two medications prescribed is, by itself, a potentially effective antidepressant. Combining an SSRI with a tricyclic antidepressant is a common strategy of this kind. Augmentation treatment occurs when the second treatment added to an antidepressant is, by itself, not an effective antidepressant but has been demonstrated to boost the effectiveness of the antidepressant. T_3 is the most well known augmenting agent. (See below for details.) For clinical purposes, combination and augmentation strategies are considered together.

Table 3–10
Treatment Options for Treatment-Resistant Depression

General Strategies

Optimization
Substitution
Combination
Augmentation

First-Line Augmentation/Combination Strategies

Lithium
T_3
SSRI/tricyclic
Stimulant (not with MAO inhibitors)
Tricyclic/MAO inhibitor

Second-Line Augmentation/Combination Strategies

Buspirone
Antidepressant/antipsychotic
MAO inhibitor/stimulant (to be used with extreme caution only)

Adding lithium to an antidepressant from any class is the most well validated augmentation strategy. Prescribing lithium in this adjunctive way can cause a marked clinical improvement in unipolar depressed patients within days to a few weeks (Joffe, Singer, Levitt, and Mac-Donald, 1993). The adjunctive effect of lithium seems unrelated to the lithium blood levels, in contrast to its use in bipolar disorder. Despite the success of lithium as an adjunctive treatment in research studies, many clinicians (myself included) as well as open studies do not find it as effective as expected (Thase, Kupfer, Frank, and Jarrett, 1989).

T_3, a thyroid hormone, has been used with variable success to effect a response when added to a previously ineffective antidepressant. Although it is always mentioned prominently as an effective adjunctive treatment, the evidence for its efficacy is somewhat contradictory (Gitlin, Weiner, Fairbanks, Hershman, and Friedfeld, 1987). Still, it does seem to work in some treatment resistant patients within three weeks (Joffe et al., 1993). There are no established predictors of response to adjunctive T_3. Side effects are virtually nonexistent, thereby making it a low-risk strategy.

Combining antidepressants across classes, most commonly an SSRI with a tricyclic or bupropion, is among the most common strategies for patients who fail to respond to a single agent. Although few good research studies have evaluated this strategy, many clinicians find this approach to be among the most effective (Nelson, Mazure, Bowers, and Jatlow, 1991). However, because the SSRIs as a group (especially fluoxetine and paroxetine) increase the blood levels of other antidepressants when prescribed together, doses must be adjusted and tricyclic blood levels measured when this combination is employed (Preskorn et al., 1994).

Stimulants, such as methylphenidate (Ritalin) or d-amphetamine (Dexedrine), are commonly added as an adjunctive treatment to antidepressants from any class except the MAO inhibitors (Satel and Nelson, 1989). When used as an adjunctive treatment, stimulants may cause either a simple increase in energy or a more global boost in antidepressant efficacy.

Less used now than ten years ago, combining a cyclic antidepressant with an MAO inhibitor is still a useful strategy for those not responding to a single agent. Although the PDR warns against this combination, it has been used for many years by many practitioners and examined in a few careful studies. When combined properly, there are no more side effects than when the individual medications are prescribed and there is no increased danger of a hypertensive episode (Razani et al., 1983). Among the MAO inhibitors, tranylcypromine should be used with increased caution when combined with a tricyclic. The two antidepressants may be started together or the MAO inhibitor may be added to the cyclic antidepressant. Adding the cyclic antidepressant to the MAO inhibitor should not be done, since this confers a risk of provoking a hypertensive or hyperthermic (high temperature) toxic reaction (see chapter 9). Double-blind studies have not shown increased efficacy for combination treatment over single-agent treatment, suggesting that it may be significantly effective for only a minority of patients.

Combining an SSRI and an MAO inhibitor is absolutely contraindicated, causing life-threatening serotonin syndrome with high fever and low blood pressure and should never be attempted (Sternbach, 1991).

Among the second-line strategies, buspirone has been shown anecdotally to augment antidepressant efficacy in a few open case series (Joffe and Schuller, 1993). Combining an antidepressant with an antipsychotic is appropriate in treating psychotic depression and for depressed patients with profound agitation or anxiety. This particular combination treatment, however, is sometimes overused by primary care physicians who sometimes treat mildly anxious or agitated patients with one of the combination preparations, Triavil and Etrafon, both of which contain perphenazine, an antipsychotic, and amitriptyline, an antidepressant. Since antipsychotics confer the risk of tardive dyskinesia (see chapter 12), it is rarely justified to treat patients in this way until more benign treatments have been tried. Furthermore, if both an antipsychotic and an antidepressant are needed simultaneously, it is far better to prescribe two separate medications so the dose ratio can be varied and one can be discontinued while the other maintained if needed.

Finally, in cases of severely depressed, extremely treatment-resistant patients, MAO inhibitors and stimulants may be cautiously prescribed with the possibility of both effectiveness and safety (Feighner, Herbstein, and Damlouji, 1985; Fawcett, Kravitz, Zajecka, and Schaff, 1991). Because of the risks inherent in this treatment combination (hypertensive reactions), it should only be attempted by a very knowledgeable psychopharmacologist and with selected patients.

Continuation Treatment of Unipolar Depression

Once a depressed patient treated with somatic therapy improves, how long should the treatment continue to prevent a relapse? Compared to acute treatment, appropriate techniques of continuation treatment have been virtually ignored in clinical research. Of the handful of studies published, all agree that patients switched to a placebo after remission of clinical symptoms relapse at a far higher rate than patients continued on antidepressants (Prien, 1987). Although most continuation studies have used cyclic antidepressants as the active treatment, it is reasonable to assume similar results for SSRIs and MAO inhibitors. Unfortunately, the majority of these studies do not help answer the question of the appropriate length of continuation therapy. Clinical wisdom has long suggested that the medication be maintained until the episode would have ended without treatment. Since the mean length of a depressive episode is six to eight months, a tradition of treatment extending for that length of time has been established, again with virtually no studies validating this practice. One study, however, demonstrated that patients who were symptom free for at least sixteen weeks (four months) did not relapse significantly when switched to placebo, thus indicating that four months of euthymia was sufficient for most patients (Prien and Kupfer, 1986). Generally, doses used in continuation treatment should be the same as for acute treatment.

Similarly, successful treatment of acute depression with ECT should be followed by continuation therapy with either antidepressants or lithium since ECT alone is followed by an unacceptably high rate of relapse.

If maintenance treatment is deemed not appropriate at the time continuation treatment is ending, the medication should be tapered and discontinued, not stopped suddenly. Sudden discontinuation of antidepressant treatment may precipitate an unpleasant (but not dangerous) withdrawal syndrome, characterized by nausea, insomnia, increased dreaming, sweating, nervousness, diarrhea, and flu-like symptoms lasting two to six days. Tapering the medication over at least one week and preferably two to three weeks will minimize or eliminate the possibility of this syndrome occurring. More importantly, though, a tapering of the antidepressant (compared to sudden discontinuation) will afford the opportunity of observing whether a relapse will occur *before* the medication is completely withdrawn. When an antidepressant is tapered over six weeks, a depressive relapse will generally be manifested as a mild, gradual return of symptoms, following which the medication dose can be raised. If the medication is stopped suddenly, a full depressive syndrome may result.

Maintenance Treatment of Unipolar Disorder

Table 3–11 lists the most important factors to be considered in deciding whether maintenance treatment is appropriate for patients with unipolar depression. Unlike bipolar disorder, in which the likelihood of a patient experiencing just one episode in a lifetime is minimal, a substantial number of unipolar patients may have just one lifetime episode. Therefore, there is virtually no justification for maintenance treatment after a first unipolar depressive episode. However, once the pattern of recurrence is established, it is likely to persist. Patients at higher risk for recurrence include those with dysthymia, other nonaffective psychiatric disorders, chronic medical problems, as well as a history of prior episodes (Consensus Development Panel, 1985). In utilizing the factors in Table 3–11, certain clinical situations are clear: Ernie, for instance, who was presented earlier in this chapter, had multiple major depressions over thirty years, three of which required hospitalizations, and during two of which suicide was a major risk. He was thus a likely

Table 3–11
Factors Used in Considering a Maintenance Treatment in Unipolar and Bipolar Mood Disorders

Frequency of recurrences

Severity of episodes, in functioning, suicidality, effects on relationships and/or job

Responsivity of the episodes to treatment

Speed of onset or episode: Does it gradually get worse over weeks or explode into profound depression or mania within days?

Capacity of patient to retain insight (ability to self-monitor) as episode begins

candidate for maintenance treatment. Just as clear would be the 52-year-old man who has had two depressions separated by fourteen years, both of which were precipitated by major life events (one divorce, one death of a parent); both depressions responded well to a combination of psychotherapy and antidepressants without hospitalization or loss of ability to function. Most practitioners would not recommend preventive treatment in this situation.

Other clinical situations, of course, are more complicated. Patients with infrequent episodes may have depressions that are life-threatening in their suicidal severity, or may respond to no treatment except ECT. What if the patient has had only three episodes in fifteen years but developed psychotic thinking early in each episode, with profound loss of insight and then resistance to treatment until it was involuntary and much psychological, interpersonal, and vocational destruction has ensued? The factors in Table 3–11 are guidelines to be discussed by the patient, the psychotherapist, and the psychopharmacologist. Exploring the possibility of maintenance treatment should provoke the discussion of the early warning signs of depressive (or manic) episodes. Using patients' experiences and teaching them to be better self-monitors promotes mastery and diminishes the helplessness that is frequently experienced when they consider taking a medication to prevent psychiatric problems that are not controlled by psychological means.

It is increasingly necessary to consider the appropriate length of maintenance treatment for a chronic disorder like dysthymic disorder. The factors noted in Table 3–11 are unhelpful with a nonepisodic disorder. Since no studies have yet examined this issue, a reasonable guideline is for the patient to continue on the antidepressant for a year after improvement before considering medication withdrawal. Unfortunately, clinical experience indicates that most dysthymic patients relapse after antidepressant withdrawal and need to resume the previously effective agent.

All cyclic antidepressants and lithium are effective preventive treatments in recurrent major depression (American Psychiatric Association, 1993b). Because the medication that was effective as an acute antidepressant will usually be prescribed as the maintenance treatment, lithium is less commonly prescribed and may be underappreciated as an effective preventive therapy. In the longest study examining maintenance treatment, antidepressant preventive efficacy continued up to five years, with patients switched from active medication to placebo in the fourth or fifth year relapsing at a high rate despite having been well while taking imipramine for the prior three years (Kupfer et al., 1992). Although less well studied, a full dose of the antidepressant—that is, the dose that was required for acute clinical effect—is likely to be the most effective preventive dose (Frank et al., 1993).

Occasionally, a patient who responds well to ECT acutely and then relapses regularly when treated with a prophylactic antidepressant is given maintenance ECT typically administered as one treatment per month (Thienhaus, Margletta, and Bennett, 1990).

PHARMACOTHERAPY OF BIPOLAR DISORDER

Treatment of Acute Manic Episodes

There are a number of appropriate, effective strategies for the treatment of a manic or hypomanic episode. It is important to remember, though, that a substantial number of manic (not hypomanic) episodes will need to be treated in hospital because of the destructive aspects of mania—its damaging effect on jobs, relationships, and savings, and the high likelihood of profound social embarrassment and potentially dangerous actions based on impulsiveness, irritability, and poor judgment.

Table 3–12 lists the somatic treatments for acute mania. While lithium and the antipsychotics are the most well documented by sheer longevity, first-line antimanic treatments include two anticonvulsant mood stabilizers, valproate and carbamazepine, as well as neuroleptics and the benzodiazepine tranquilizers. The greatest advantage of the mood stabilizers over other medications in the treatment of mania is their quality of "normalizing" the patient's mood. In comparison to neuroleptics or tranquilizers, patients do not generally complain of feeling "drugged" from mood stabilizers when they are prescribed in appropriate doses. The major disadvantages of the mood stabilizers

Table 3–12
Treatments for Mania and Bipolar Disorder

Treatment	Acute	Maintenance
Mood stabilizers	★	★
Lithium	★	★
Valproate	★	★
Carbamazepine	★	★
Neuroleptics	★	0
Benzodiazepine tranquilizers	★	0
Clonazepam	★	0
Lorazepam	★	0
Electroconvulsive therapy (ECT)	★	0
Verapamil	?	?
Clozapine	?	?

★ = Evidence of efficacy
? = Possible efficacy
0 = No evidence of efficacy

compared to the other first-line agents is their relatively slower onset of action. Full therapeutic effects are rarely seen within the first week and it may take up to three weeks or more for a full therapeutic effect to be manifested. This is especially true in outpatient settings where dose adjustments cannot realistically be obtained on a daily basis, as they can in hospital.

The choice of a specific mood stabilizer in treating acute mania is currently based on comparative risks and benefits for each, including prior response (if available), side effect profiles, and need for blood tests. (See chapter 10 for details.) Although lithium is still the most commonly used mood stabilizer prescribed for acute mania, the two anticonvulsants—valproate (Depakote) and carbamazepine (Tegretol)—are used with increasing frequency. Of the two mood stabilizers, the evidence is most persuasive for valproate which was recently shown to be equivalent to lithium in treating acute mania (Bowden et al., 1994).

Antipsychotics have been used for decades to treat acute mania. Their major advantage is speed of efficacy, with therapeutic effects seen within hours to days. However, they cause many more side effects than do mood stabilizers (see chapter 12)—sedation, neurological symptoms, dizziness, neuroleptic malignant syndrome, and so on. Additionally, patients have a more negative subjective response to antipsychotics than to mood stabilizers, often describing the feeling as having a "blanket on their brain." One frequently sees a manic patient on, for instance, chlorpromazine (Thorazine) who is sedated, stiff, and motorically slowed while still trying to talk at excessive speed and in a scattered speech. This contrasts pointedly with mood stabilizers' greater "normalization of mood," and patients' satisfaction with them.

Sedating antipsychotics, such as chlorpromazine, and nonsedating antipsychotics, such as haloperidol (Haldol), are equally effective in treating mania. Higher doses of the nonsedating medications can be used since the dose is not as limited by the sedation. However, there is no good evidence that very high doses of antipsychotics are more effective than moderate doses in treating mania.

Benzodiazepines, the dominant class of antianxiety agents (see chapter 11), are frequently prescribed either alone or with mood stabilizers to treat acute mania. Documentation of efficacy is best for lorazepam (Ativan) and clonazepam (Klonopin) (American Psychiatric Association, 1994b; Chou, 1991). Patient acceptance of these tranquilizers is generally high since, other than sedation, they do not cause the same side effects as neuroleptics. It is not known whether the antimanic properties of lorazepam and clonazepam are shared by all the other benzodiazepines.

Frequently, an acutely manic patient will be started on a mood stabilizer and a more quickly acting antimanic agent—a neuroleptic or a benzodiazepine—simultaneously. (Often, a patient will be started on a mood stabilizer, a benzodiazepine and a neuroleptic together in order to minimize the doses of the latter). In these situations, an attempt is made to lower the dose of the benzodiazepine and antipsychotic or to stop them completely during the second through fourth week of treatment as the mood stabilizer takes effect.

Occasionally, patients failing to respond adequately to one mood stabilizer have a second one added. Rarely, a patient may be placed on all three mood stabilizers simultaneously.

A number of other medications are occasionally used to treat mania including verapamil (Calan), clonidine (Catapres), and propranolol (Inderal) (Chou, 1991). For the most treatment-resistant patients, clozapine, the atypical neuroleptic (see chapter 12), has been shown to be effective (Kimmel, Calabrese, Woyshville, and Meltzer, 1994).

Electroconvulsive treatment is an extremely effective treatment for acute severe mania (Mukherjee, Sackeim, and Schnur, 1994). However, relatively few manic patients will give the required informed consent for its use; thus, it is not as commonly utilized as its efficacy would suggest.

Continuation Treatment of Manic or Hypomanic Episodes

Following the guideline of continuing treatment for the same length of time as the natural history of the episode, manic episodes should be treated for approximately six months. After that time, if maintenance treatment is not appropriate, the medication should be tapered and discontinued. During continuation treatment, however, it is often possible to decrease the amount of medication. If not done previously, antipsychotics or benzodiazemines may be tapered and withdrawn while the mood stabilizer is continued.

Bipolar Depression—Acute and Continuation Treatment

Although bipolar and unipolar depression shows great clinical similarity, treatment decisions between the two groups differ, because of the risks of treating bipolar patients with antidepressants. When bipolar patients are given antidepressants, a significant proportion will become hypomanic or manic (Wehr and Goodwin, 1987). (The risk is difficult to quantify since some bipolar patients would shift from depression to mania as the natural course of their disorder regardless of whether antidepressants were prescribed.) In addition to the potentially destructive effects of the manic episode, the patient is also put at risk for a postmanic depression. A further risk for some bipolar patients is that the use of antidepressants may cause rapid cycling, which, as noted above, may be associated with a poorer prognosis.

Most experienced clinicians would initially treat Bipolar I patients with mild to moderate depression with a mood stabilizer, either lithium, valproate, or carbamazepine. It is reasonably well demonstrated that some bipolar patients will respond to lithium with an acute antidepressant response (Zornberg and Pope, 1993). This response, however, may take up to 6 weeks to be evident. Carbamazepine and valproate are also likely to effectively treat bipolar depression although the evidence for their efficacy is far less than for lithium (American Psychiatric Association, 1994b). Even if the patient does not improve on the mood stabilizer, an antidepressant can then be added. The mood stabilizer is likely to decrease the risk of an antidepressant-induced mania, although not completely. Similarly, those patients already on a mood stabilizer whose depressions are moderate to severe are typically prescribed antidepressants.

For those bipolar patients who are severely depressed, a mood stabilizer and an antidepressant can be started simultaneously. This strategy increases the risk of precipitating mania (since the lithium is not given the same chance to work before antidepressants are administered) but may accelerate the antidepressant response. All antidepressants effective in treating major depression are also likely to treat bipolar depression successfully. The paucity of studies comparing one antidepressant to another in treating bipolar depression precludes any reasonable generalizations about comparative efficacy. In one of the few systematic examinations of this issue, patients with anergic features (being slowed down and hypersomnic) showed a better response to MAO inhibitors compared to tricyclics (Himmelhoch, Thase, Mallinger, and Houck, 1991).

Although all antidepressants share the capacity to trigger a post-depressive manic episode, the comparative risks of pharmacologically inducing a manic episode across antidepressant classes is still unknown. There is soft evidence that, compared to a tricyclic antidepressant, bupropion may be less likely to induce mania (Sachs et al., 1994a). Some observers even posit a role for bupropion as a mood stabilizer (Haykal and Akiskal, 1990). No systematic studies have compared the SSRIs to other antidepressant classes.

Finally, as with unipolar depression, ECT is an important viable alternative for severe bipolar depression. Lithium must be stopped during the time of ECT treatment to avoid a neurotoxic reaction (confusion, disorientation, marked memory loss) seen when these two treatments are used simultaneously.

The only difference in strategies for treating depressions in Bipolar II versus Bipolar I patients is that many clinicians are less likely to treat Bipolar II patients with a mood stabilizer alone, preferring a mood stabilizer plus an antidepressant as a first option. Some clinicians prescribe antidepressants alone to treat Bipolar II depression. Unfortunately, even though hypomania is by definition less destructive than mania, Bipolar IIs are probably at equal risk to experience pharmacological (hypo)-mania compared to Bipolar I patients. Compared to Bipolar I patients, those with Bipolar II disorder are at higher risk for rapid cycling (Coryell, Endicott, and Keller, 1992).

Continuation treatment is as important for bipolar depression as it is for unipolar depression. If a bipolar patient is on a mood stabilizer plus an antidepressant, it is reasonable to attempt to decrease or discontinue the antidepressant before six months (the usual continuation period for unipolar depression) since the mood stabilizer may have its own continuation effect. This strategy would minimize the amount of time a bipolar patient takes antidepressants with the attendant risks.

Maintenance Treatment of Bipolar Disorder

Compared to unipolar patients, bipolar patients are far more likely to be treated with maintenance pharmacotherapy. The reasons for this are rooted in the known natural history of the disorder, reviewed earlier in this chapter: (1) the increased cycle frequency in bipolar versus unipolar disorder, (2) the rarity of bipolar patients who suffer just one episode in a lifetime, (3) the more destructive effects of manic or hypomanic episodes on relationships, jobs, bank accounts, self-esteem. Because of these factors, virtually all Bipolar I patients and most Bipolar II patients should properly be on maintenance pharmacotherapy at some point in their disorder. But when?

The same factors used to evaluate maintenance treatment in unipolar disorder (see Table 3–11) are used for bipolar disorder. However, since bipolar disorder is more recurrent and destructive, the same evaluative process will generally suggest a preventive treatment. The most difficult clinical decision in treating these patients occurs early in the course of the disorder after the first episode. A recent panel of experts concluded that after a single manic episode, maintenance treatment should be made available to patients, although different patients would be expected to make different decisions regarding preventive treatment (American Psychiatric Association, 1994b). The rationale for preventive treatment after a first episode is clearly based on the assumption of a second potentially highly destructive episode in the life of a young person (the mean age of onset of bipolar disorder is the early twenties) whose self-esteem and social reputation are not established and are subject to major disruption. As an example, a second-year medical student who has had a hospitalized manic episode that was embarrassingly obvious to the faculty, nurses, and staff at the hospital in which he was training may be able to avoid having that episode affect his dean's letter (written to potential residency programs). But if he suffers a second episode before the end of medical school, it may well have an irreversible effect on his career path.

For most patients, however, it is generally after the second episode that the discussion of preventive treatment arises. At that time, the patient can no longer be so sure that the first episode was an extraordinary fluke that could never happen again (as many patients want to believe). Also, the cycling frequency—the length of time between the onset of the first and second episodes—may be crudely calculated. While the decision about maintenance treatment rests on a best judgment using the factors outlined in Table 3–11, for most patients who experience two major episodes, the benefits of preventive treatment generally outweigh the burdens of treatment. In setting appropriate expectations for maintenance treatment whenever it is started, patients need to be aware that even with optimal pharmacotherapy, some mood swings are likely. It is often at the point of starting a maintenance therapy that psychotherapy may be particularly valuable in helping the patient deal with the inherent uncertainty in having a lifelong recurrent mood disorder.

Without question, lithium is still the most commonly prescribed and most well documented maintenance treatment for bipolar disorder. Although many patients continue to experience either persistent mood swings or manic or depressive episodes while taking lithium, it is effective in the majority of cases in diminishing manifestations of the disorder. Lithium's efficacy can be shown by its effect in (1) decreasing the number and frequency of episodes, (2) diminishing the intensity of the episodes, (3) shortening the length of episodes, and (4) decreasing the more subtle and transient mood swings seen between episodes (Goodwin and Jamison, 1990). In controlled studies, lithium seems equally effective in preventing manic and depressive episodes, although many patients complain about minor depressive symptoms. Predictors of a poor response to prophylactic lithium are rapid cycling, mixed states, drug abuse, multiple prior episodes, and a pattern of having depressive episodes precede rather than follow manic episodes (Prien and Potter, 1990).

Since lithium treatment is monitored by lithium levels (the concentration of lithium in the blood), it is imperative that the maintenance level be established and followed consistently (see chapter 10 for details). Optimal lithium levels vary between individuals: levels between 0.6 and 0.8 are recommended for most patients (American Psychiatric Association, 1994b). Some patients require higher levels (e.g., 1.0 to 1.2) for effective prophylaxis and tolerate these higher levels, while other patients, especially the elderly, may show a good response at levels of 0.4.

For those patients who show an inadequate response to lithium or for whom lithium side effects are intolerable, either of the two other mood stabilizers—valproate and carbamazepine—may be prescribed. Although neither drug can approach lithium in its sheer documentation of efficacy, a few studies and much clinical experience attests to their effectiveness as preventive treatments (Calabrese, Bowden, and Woyshville, 1995). No well-controlled studies comparing any two of the three major mood stabilizers exist and their comparative efficacy is unknown.

Another strategy occasionally used in the maintenance treatment of bipolar disorder is combining two or more partially effective treatments. Any combination of the three mood stabilizers may sometimes be prescribed together (as opposed to substituting one for the other) when a patient has a partial response to one agent.

Patients with frequent breakthrough manic or psychotic symptoms are often treated with adjunctive maintenance antipsychotics with some success. Yet this approach must be used with caution because of the risk of developing tardive dyskinesia (see chapter 12) when a mood-disordered patient takes antipsychotics for a significant length of time (Sernyak and Woods, 1993).

Less commonly, bipolar patients with frequent breakthrough depressions are, by necessity, treated with maintenance antidepressants, typically added to a mood stabilizer such as lithium. Although this approach is sometimes effective, it confers the risks of increasing the number of manic episodes and potentially inducing rapid cycling. Both the psychopharmacologist and the psychotherapist *must* be alert to these possibilities and intervene quickly if a manic episode or rapid cycling emerges.

Patients with truly treatment-resistant bipolar disorder are sometimes effectively treated with clozapine, the atypical neuroleptic (Banov et al., 1994). Rapid cycling patients may respond to high-dose thyroid treatment (Bauer and Whybrow, 1990). Finally, any patient not responding to conventional treatment should be further evaluated for unrecognized substance abuse or noncompliance.

4

Anxiety Disorders and Insomnia

L IKE THE WORD *depression, anxiety* refers to a number of different entities. Anxiety may be considered a normal, transient feeling that has adaptive properties when it signals danger; it is a symptom seen in a wide variety of disorders; and it refers to a group of disorders in which the symptom of anxiety forms a dominant element. Concepts regarding pathological anxiety have shifted continuously over the last hundred years depending on both the types of patients studied and the causal models of the investigators. As concepts of anxiety have changed, so, of course, have our notions of how best to classify these disorders. Freud, for instance, shifted the focus from physical to psychological symptoms and distinguished anxiety neurosis from the more global disorder, neurasthenia. In Freud's use of the term, anxiety neurosis consisted of what we would now call both panic disorder and generalized anxiety. In modern times, the most important distinction was made during the 1960s when anxiety neurosis was split into panic disorder/agoraphobia and generalized anxiety because of the evidence of differential response to both behavioral and pharmacological treatments.

More recently, toward the goal of increasing diagnostic specificity, anxiety syndromes have been further divided into related but officially separate disorders. Panic disorder, previously split from generalized anxiety, was then split again into panic with and without agoraphobia. Yet substantial overlap between anxiety disorders continues in DSM-IV. As an example, panic attacks, the core symptom of panic disorder, are also seen as core features of social phobia, specific (a.k.a. simple) phobia, and post-traumatic stress disorder (PTSD), with the diagnostic distinction based on a host of other features such as situational cues that may be associated with the attack, or prior history (a required part of the diagnosis of PTSD). Moreover, the borders between anxiety disorders continue to be somewhat blurred. For instance, how should we diagnose the individual who was comfortable with air travel until age 26 when he had two panic attacks on an airplane, has never had another panic attack, but now avoids flying. Is this a specific airplane phobia or panic disorder with limited agoraphobia? (Liebowitz, 1992).

Conversely, it would be premature to assume that the diverse disorders currently classified as anxiety disorders form a single related group of entities. In many ways, there are marked differences: obsessive compulsive disorder bears little resemblance to post-traumatic stress disorder, and both stand in marked contrast to the phobias and panic disorder. As with so many other aspects of diagnostic nosology, the DSM-IV anxiety classification scheme simply represents our best current guess. Classification is clearly a process in evolution.

In this chapter, the disorders to be considered are panic disorder with or without agoraphobia, generalized anxiety disorder, specific and social phobias, obsessive compulsive disorder, and post-traumatic stress disorder. More detail will be provided for those disorders for which medications play a more prominent role in treatment. Since the same medications are used to treat insomnia and anxiety disorders (especially generalized anxiety), this chapter will also briefly cover the common causes of and pharmacological approaches to insomnia.

DIAGNOSIS

Panic attacks, hallmark features of a number of different anxiety disorders, are characterized by discrete episodes of intense fear/anxiety, peaking quickly and associated with a variety of physical, dissociative, and cognitive symptoms. Table 4–1 shows the DSM-IV diagnostic criteria for a panic attack. Panic attacks share similar qualities whether they are triggered by an environmental stimulus or not, and regardless of the disorder with which they are associated. Attacks with intense anxiety and the same time course as listed in Table 4–1 but with fewer than four symptoms are referred to as limited-symptom attacks.

DSM-IV panic disorder is characterized by recurrent unexpected panic attacks (i.e., the attacks are not associated with a situational trigger), and one month or more of at least one of the following: (a) persistent concern about having additional attacks; (b) worry about the implications of the attack (e.g., going crazy or having a heart attack); (c) a significant change in behavior related to the attacks, such as changing jobs, even if the patient denies concerns about having another attack. Despite the requirement that attacks be unexpected, most patients with panic disorder can identify situations in which panic attacks are likely. In contrast to DSM-III-R, in DSM-IV no specific number of

Table 4–1
Diagnostic Criteria for Panic Attack

A discrete period of intense fear or discomfort, in which four (or more) of the following symptoms developed abruptly and reached a peak within 10 minutes:

(1) palpitations, pounding heart, or accelerated heart rate
(2) sweating
(3) trembling or shaking
(4) sensations of shortness of breath or smothering
(5) feeling of choking
(6) chest pain or discomfort
(7) nausea or abdominal distress
(8) feeling dizzy, unsteady, lightheaded, or faint
(9) derealization (feelings of unreality) or depersonalization (being detached from oneself)
(10) fear of losing control or going crazy
(11) fear of dying
(12) paresthesias (numbness or tingling sensations)
(13) chills or hot flushes

Reprinted with permission from the *Diagnostic and Statistical Manual of Mental Disorders, Fourth Edition*. Copyright 1994 American Psychiatric Association.

panic attacks is required for the diagnosis of panic disorder, only a pattern of recurrence (therefore at least two) and the presence of associated symptoms. Panic disorder defines the more symptomatic point on the continuum of the larger group of individuals who experience unexpected anxiety attacks less frequently or with limited symptoms (Eaton, Kessler, Wittchen, and Magee, 1994).

Those panic patients who constrict their activity, usually to avoid situations from which they fear they cannot escape or get help or in which they feel another panic attack might occur, are diagnosed as having panic disorder with agoraphobia. Examples of commonly avoided situations include being outside the home alone or being in a car or in crowded areas such as movie theaters or supermarkets. It is presumed that in these patients, who comprise half of all panic patients, agoraphobic symptoms develop after the panic attacks (Eaton, Kessler, Wittchen, and Magee, 1994). Among those with agoraphobia who present for treatment, 95 percent have a current or past history of panic disorder (American Psychiatric Association, 1994a). Yet epidemiological studies, which evaluate patients without regard to whether or not they have sought treatment, document a relatively large number of people with agoraphobia without panic symptoms (Robins et al., 1984). The cause of this discrepancy between clinical and epidemiological studies is unknown, but may reflect the difficulty that clinically inexperienced interviewers, used in the latter studies, have in distinguishing among related clinical disorders. Consistent with this, individuals in one epidemiological study who were diagnosed as agoraphobic without panic were reinterviewed by more experienced clinicians. The majority of these individuals were rediagnosed as having simple (specific) phobias or fears with constricted activities on that basis as opposed to agoraphobia (Horwath, Lish, Johnson, Hornig, and Weissman, 1993).

Specific phobia (known in DSM-III-R as simple phobia) is a fear of a specific object or situation. When confronted with the stimulus, the patient becomes markedly anxious in a manner identical to a panic attack. Blood-injury phobia (fear of witnessing blood or injuries), claustrophobia, or fears of airplane travel are typical examples.

Social phobia (also known as social anxiety disorder) is distinguished from other phobias in DSM-IV, as it was in DSM-III-R. Patients with social phobias specifically fear situations involving observation or scrutiny by others to a degree that interferes with social or occupational functioning. Common fears are those of public speaking, urinating in a public lavatory, or of hand trembling while writing a check. Similar to panic disorder, social phobia exists on a continuum, with many patients who do not meet the full DSM-IV criteria nonetheless showing significant impairment from their symptoms (Davidson, Hughes, George, and Blazer, 1994). Two types of social phobia should be distinguished. In the limited form, usually described as performance anxiety, patients fear public speaking or performing. As an example, a professor's career would be limited by a phobia of speaking at conferences or of lecturing. The second type of social phobia is a generalized social anxiety which interferes with a broader range of social activities such as meeting new people, talking to salespeople, or discussing a work-related issue with the boss. In both types of social phobia, exposure to the feared situation brings on anxiety similar to that seen in specific phobias or panic. Anticipatory anxiety and avoidant behavior are common. Thus, a patient with a social phobia manifested by fear of urinating in a public place may completely restrict any sort of significant travel, thus seeming agoraphobic when the primary fear is that of urinating in a public lavatory, not of being away from home.

In obsessive compulsive disorder (OCD), the vast majority of patients present with a combination of both obsessions and compulsions.

Obsessions are persistent ideas, thoughts, or impulses that are intrusive and inappropriate, and that cause anxiety. Compulsions are repetitive, ritualized behaviors the goals of which are to decrease anxiety. Although many individuals have mild compulsions or rituals (superstitious rituals such as not walking under a ladder are examples), obsessive compulsive disorder is characterized by significant functional impairment, marked distress, and/or spending more than one hour daily (and often far more) on the rituals. Even with the increasing public awareness of OCD as a treatable disorder, many OCD patients are embarrassed by their symptoms. Because of this, unless specifically asked, patients often come into treatment complaining of other symptoms, only to reveal their secret obsessions and compulsions many months later. Remarkably, in some studies, the time from beginning of symptoms to first treatment is frequently more than ten years (Rasmussen and Tsuang, 1986).

According to the DSM-IV definition, both the obsessions and compulsions are recognized as the product of the person's own thinking (in contrast with psychotic thoughts which are experienced as alien). Attempts are made to neutralize or undo the thoughts, typically by a compulsion that is grossly excessive compared to the fear. Patients who are obsessed by the thought that they have run someone over with their car may return to the spot fifty or more times, consuming incredible amounts of time to reassure themselves that no body is lying in the street. Unfortunately, the compulsions that attempt to relieve the obsessional anxiety are never more than trivially and transiently successful.

Classically, patients with OCD have insight into the irrationality of their obsessions and compulsions. However, recent studies indicate that this level of insight is both incomplete and varies over time (Foa and Kozak, 1995). Therefore, in the DSM-IV definition of OCD, individuals are only required to recognize the excessiveness or unreasonableness of the symptoms at some time during the course of the disorder.

The other major change in DSM-IV OCD is the definition of mental rituals as compulsions. These are rituals that are performed internally, the goals of which are identical to behavioral rituals—to ward off the distress associated with the obsessions. Examples of mental rituals are reciting special words or prayers, repeating numbers, mental counting, and so on.

Among the obsessions, fear of contamination, fear of harming oneself or others, and symmetry are the most common (Foa and Kozak, 1995). An example of an obsession of having harmed another is a mother who is afraid she might hurt her baby (without any desire to do so, having loving feelings towards the child, and having no history of violent behavior at all) or a man who fears he has left the gas on while using the stove. The most common compulsions are those of checking, cleaning, and mental rituals. Not surprisingly, patients with contamination obsessions typically have cleaning rituals. An example of a typical symmetry ritual might be a patient who is unable to get dressed unless all his clothes are lined up perfectly and grouped in clusters of seven (which he feels has some magical ability to ward off bad events).

Post-traumatic stress disorder (PTSD) is defined in DSM-IV by a cluster of symptoms following exposure to an extreme traumatic stressor. The person may have experienced, witnessed, or been confronted with an event that involved actual or threatened death, serious injury, or threat to physical integrity of self or others. The person's response is characterized by intense fear, helplessness, or horror. An additional group of symptoms that last at least one month are characterized by: (1) reexperiencing of the traumatic event, such as flashbacks, intrusive thoughts, recurrent dreams; (2) persistent avoidance of stimuli associated with the trauma and numbing of general responsiveness, such as avoiding thoughts or conversations about the event, feelings of detachment from others, and restricted affect; and (3) symptoms of increased arousal, such as irritability, hypervigilance, and exaggerated startle response.

Generalized anxiety disorder (GAD) is the least specific of the anxiety disorders. The DSM-IV criteria for GAD require at least six months of excessive anxiety and worry that the person finds difficult to control. The anxiety occurs most days, is focused on a number of events or activities, and is characterized by at least three of the following: restlessness or being keyed up, being easily fatigued, difficulty concentrating, irritability, muscle tension, and sleep disturbance. GAD cannot be diagnosed if the focus of the anxiety consists of symptoms of another Axis I disorder. Thus, the anticipatory anxiety that typically develops during ongoing panic disorder would not be classified as GAD. DSM-IV generalized anxiety differs from DSM-III-R in the requirement that the worries be uncontrollable, and because many of the uncommon physical symptoms have been eliminated from the diagnostic criteria.

Because it is often seen coincident with other Axis I disorders, some experts feel that GAD is simply a nonspecific complication of other disorders and therefore should not be delineated as a separate category. Other observers object to the diagnostic separation between panic and

GAD, noting that the differences between the two may be more quantitative than qualitative (Basoglu, Marks, and Sengun, 1992).

Yet substantial evidence suggests the presence of and the clinical need for an anxiety disorder that is predominantly characterized by excessive worry and nonspecific anxiety symptoms (Brown, Barlow, and Liebowitz, 1994). For instance, approximately one quarter of GAD patients presenting for treatment have no other psychiatric diagnosis (Brawman-Mintzer et al., 1993). Consistent with this, most clinicians, myself included, regularly see patients without panic, depression, or other disorders who are chronic worriers with many somatic anxiety symptoms. Even among the large group of GAD patients who have other mood or anxiety disorders, the GAD often has an earlier age of onset. Often, when the other disorders are successfully treated in these patients, the more pervasive generalized anxiety persists, implying the existence of a distinct chronic anxiety disorder.

Eliciting symptoms of anxiety disorders is often easy, as with specific phobias or generalized anxiety. Sometimes, though, patients will present for treatment and focus on other problems, leaving disabling syndromes a hidden, embarrassing part of their lives. As previously mentioned, obsessive compulsive disorder frequently stays hidden. Panic disorder is always recognized by patients as a problem, but not always as a psychiatric one (see below). To help elicit information relevant to diagnosing the anxiety disorders, the following questions may be helpful.

Panic Disorder: Have you ever had sudden attacks of anxiety or fear that were extremely uncomfortable? Describe what it felt like. (At that point, one can ask about specific panic symptoms, such as shortness of breath, trembling, and the like.) How long did it take until the symptoms peaked? How long did the entire episode last? How often has this occurred? Is there one specific situation in which these episodes occur or do they occur seemingly out of the blue? Do you worry a lot about having another of these attacks? Have you changed the routine of your life because of your concern?

Agoraphobia: Do you avoid certain situations now because you fear having a panic attack? Which situations?

Social Phobia: Do you get very nervous when you have to do things in front of other people, such as writing or eating or speaking in public? Is it bad enough to make you avoid the situations? If you cannot avoid the situation, how nervous do you get? Do you get very anxious when you have to interact with new people? Is the anxiety so bad that you avoid these interactions?

Obsessive Compulsive Disorder: Do you ever have thoughts that you can't seem to get rid of, thoughts that occur over and over in your mind like a tape that is stuck? What thoughts are these? Are there certain behaviors that you feel compelled to do over and over? Do you have to do them a certain number of times? Are there certain sayings, prayers, or numbers that you are compelled to repeat in your mind? What would happen or what are you afraid would happen if you resisted doing these rituals? How much time do you spend on a daily basis with these activities?

Generalized Anxiety Disorder: Do you think of yourself as a nervous person? How long has this been so? Do you worry a lot? About what kinds of things? Can you stop or control the worrying? Is the anxiety bad enough to interfere with sleep or concentration? Do you see yourself as irritable or tense most of the time?

NATURAL HISTORY, EPIDEMIOLOGY, AND GENETICS

Because our diagnostic categories for anxiety disorders have changed dramatically over the last three decades, many important clinical questions relating to the natural course, prevalence, and amount of genetic loading of these disorders are difficult to answer. Therefore, this section relies primarily on the more recent studies which, unfortunately, are limited in the information they yield on topics such as long-term outcome. Additionally, it is not yet clear whether each anxiety disorder has its own genetic pattern (with some showing little heritability) or whether there are more broad-based inherited vulnerabilities such as "phobia proneness," with other variables determining which anxiety disorder is expressed.

Panic disorder, occurring in 2 to 3 percent of the population, tends to arise in the late teens to mid-twenties and is twice as common in women as in men (Kessler et al., 1994; Wittchen and Essau, 1993). It is unusual for it to arise after age 40. The natural course of panic disorder is variable. Most commonly, it waxes and wanes, with total remission uncommon. Often, patients describe months to a few years in which panic attacks are frequent, followed by a period of time with few attacks, although mild panic or agoraphobic symptoms may persist (Pollack et al., 1990). Later, often after years, the attacks recur in full force. Another group of patients seem to have chronic unremitting symptoms of panic with or without agoraphobia.

The consistent finding that there is an increased rate of panic in the families of panic patients indicates the familial nature of the disorder (Weissman, 1993). Furthermore, the increased concordance seen in monozygotic (genetically identical) as opposed to dizygotic (genetically related but not identical) twins indicates that at least part of the risk is genetically determined (Skre, Onstad, Torgersen, Lygren, and Kringlen, 1993).

Panic patients frequently have other psychiatric disorders, the most common of which is generalized anxiety disorder. Major depressive episodes, which may occur before, coincident with, or following the panic disorder, are also common, seen in 50 to 70 percent of panic patients (Breier et al., 1984). The likelihood of a depression which occurs after the onset of the panic disorder is related to the length of time the patient has had panic disorder (Lesser et al., 1988). Additionally, both childhood separation anxiety disorder and alcoholism may also be seen more frequently in panic patients, although this is less certain.

Specific phobias, which occur more in women by a 2 : 1 ratio, are common, although many of these patients never seek treatment. They have a relatively early age of onset, frequently in childhood. Compared to other anxiety disorders, specific phobias tend to have a more benign course. Genetic influences probably play a role in the development of only some specific phobias, such as blood-injury phobias (Marks, 1986).

Social phobia typically arises in childhood or in the teenage years and seems to be a chronic unremitting condition when not treated (Schneier, Johnson, Hornig, Liebowitz, and Weissman, 1992). In contrast to the findings of earlier studies, social phobia is rather common, affecting over 10 percent of the population, with rates somewhat higher in women (Kessler et al., 1994). Social phobia is certainly familial, although genetic contributions are moderate at best (Fyer, 1993). However, there seems to be some heritable component to aspects of social anxiety such as discomfort when eating with strangers or when being watched working (Torgersen, 1979). Patients with social phobias are at higher risk for other anxiety disorders, depression, and alcohol abuse.

Obsessive compulsive disorder (OCD) begins in the late teens or early twenties, although childhood OCD is far from rare (Rasmussen and Eisen, 1992). Additionally, many patients with OCD recall having minor obsessions or compulsions as children which were not severe enough to significantly interfere with functioning. Recent studies indicate that it is far more common than had been previously thought, with a lifetime prevalence of 2.5 percent and an approximately equal sex ratio (Robins et al., 1984). A common pattern of the disorder is chronic mild symptoms interspersed with acute exacerbations. However, a minority of patients have a progressive downhill course in which the symptoms gradually take over more and more of their lives. OCD is certainly familial, with family members of patients showing higher rates of obsessions and compulsions (including both mild symptoms and the full disorder, indicating the continuum nature of OCD) and possibly other anxiety disorders (Black, Noyes, Goldstein, and Blum, 1992). There seem to be no familial or genetic contributions to the expression of the disorder; for example, the child of a parent with contamination obsessions and cleaning rituals may be obsessed with symmetry and exhibit mental compulsions.

Patients with OCD are at high risk to have other psychiatric disorders, the most common of which are major depression (seen in 50 percent of patients) and other anxiety disorders, especially panic disorder, social phobia, and specific phobia (Piggott, L'Heureux, Dubbert, Bernstein, and Murphy, 1994). In contrast to the results of earlier studies, fewer than 10 percent of patients with OCD have obsessive compulsive personality disorder, indicating a clear distinction between the two disorders (Baer et al., 1990). In a subtype of OCD, usually estimated as 5 to 10 percent of the total OCD population, patients exhibit either chronic tics or Tourette's syndrome, a disorder arising in childhood and characterized by multiple tics (see chapter 8). In these cases, it is likely that the tics, obsessions, and compulsions are manifestations of a unitary disorder, as evidenced by higher rates of Tourette's syndrome among relatives of patients with OCD and tics (Pauls, Alsobrook, Goodman, Rasmussen, and Leckman, 1995).

Estimates of the prevalence of PTSD range between 1 and 8 percent (Helzer, Robins, and McEvoy, 1987; Kessler, Sonnega, Bromet, Hughes, and Nelson, 1995). Much remains to be learned about the long-term outcome of these patients, although studies of World War II veterans indicate that the symptoms may persist for decades after the stressor (Sutker, Allain, and Winstead, 1993). These patients may be at risk to have higher rates of alcoholism, depression, and anxiety while their families show high rates of alcohol abuse (Davidson, Swartz, Storck, Krishnan, and Hammett, 1985; Southwick, Yehuda, and Giller, 1993).

For generalized anxiety disorder (GAD), the overall estimates are that between 4 and 6 percent of the population have the disorder. GAD is twice as common among women as among men (Wittchen, Zhao, Kessler, and Eaton, 1994). As noted above, most patients with generalized anxiety disorder have at least one other psychiatric disorder. GAD is somewhat heritable, although probably less so than some other anxiety disorders (Kendler, Neale, Kessler, Heath, and Eaves, 1992). The age of onset of GAD seems to be in the late teens or early twenties. Its course is variable, with many patients showing a chronic pattern of symptoms, albeit with a waxing/waning quality over many years (Rickels and Schweizer, 1990).

MEDICAL DIFFERENTIAL DIAGNOSIS

Because so many anxiety symptoms, especially those of panic, are physical, patients with anxiety disorders often see a variety of medical specialists before seeking mental health consultation. In one early study, 70 percent of a group of panic patients had seen more than ten physicians (Sheehan, Ballenger, and Jacobsen, 1980). Even after extensive medical evaluation has uncovered no medical disorder, and after many months of psychiatric education and treatment, some panic patients still need reassurance that they are not having heart attacks, impending strokes, or other catastrophes.

As with depression, a host of medical disorders can cause anxiety symptoms simulating generalized anxiety, panic, or both (see Table 4–2). The most commonly considered disorders, which are discussed below, are acute myocardial infarction (heart attack), hyperthyroidism, hypoglycemia, mitral valve prolapse, pheochromocytoma, and drug-related syndromes.

A look at the classic symptoms of a panic attack makes the common fear among panic patients of having a heart attack understandable. It would be difficult for anyone to experience a sudden episode characterized by shortness of breath, dizziness, palpitations, chest pain, and fear of dying without at least considering that a heart attack is in progress. The patient's age, a normal electrocardiogram, and a lack of signs of cardiac dysfunction help clarify the diagnosis.

Hyperthyroidism, characterized by anxiety, weight loss, sweatiness, tremor, heat intolerance, and tachycardia (fast heartbeat) can be confused with generalized anxiety. The prominence of the physical symptoms compared to the anxiety and easily obtained blood tests of thyroid function will distinguish between the two disorders.

Table 4–2
Medical Disorders and Drugs that May Cause Anxiety Disorders

Cardiovascular:	Drug withdrawal:
Mitral valve prolapse	Alcohol
Cardiac arrhythmia	Opiates/narcotics
Congestive heart failure	Sedatives/hypnotics
Hypertension (high blood pressure)	
Myocardial infarction (heart attack)	Endocrine:
Pulmonary embolus (blood clot)	Carcinoid syndrome
	Cushing's syndrome
Respiratory:	Hypoglycemia
Asthma	Hypoparathyroidism (low calcium)
Emphysema	Hyperthyroidism
Hyperventilation	Pheochromocytoma (adrenal
Hypoxia (low oxygen)	tumor—see text)
	Premenstrual syndrome
Drugs:	
Anticholinergic medications	Neurological:
Aspirin	Epilepsy
Caffeine	Huntington's disease
Cocaine	Migraine headaches
Decongestants	Multiple sclerosis
Hallucinogens	Pain
Steroids	Vertigo
Stimulants (including diet pills)	Wilson's disease

Patients often ask about hypoglycemia as a cause of panic disorder. Although the symptoms of the two conditions are indeed similar, panic attacks rarely occur in a characteristic relation to meals—three to five hours after eating—as would be true with hypoglycemia. When panic patients are tested for hypoglycemia by glucose tolerance tests, they are virtually never found to have low blood sugar. Additionally, when hypoglycemia is induced in panic patients, the symptoms are experienced as different from panic attacks (Uhde, Vittone, and Post, 1984).

Mitral valve prolapse (MVP) may be associated with panic disorder. The mitral valve connects the left atrium of the heart with the left ventricle. In MVP, when the heart contracts, the valve is abnormally pushed back into the atrium. This may be heard with a stethoscope as a click or seen in an echocardiogram (a test that uses sound waves to "visualize" the heart). MVP is found in 3 to 5 percent of the population, often undiagnosed and typically asymptomatic. In some patients, however, it is associated with palpitations or fatigue. Although the evidence is far from definitive, patients with MVP may be at slightly higher risk for panic disorder while patients with panic disorder may be at slightly higher risk for mitral valve prolapse (Margraf, Ehlers, and Roth, 1988). At present, no hypothesis adequately explains the link between these two conditions. Does mitral valve prolapse cause panic symptoms? Do panic attacks somehow predispose patients to mitral valve prolapse? Are the two linked genetically? Regardless of the association, the presence of the prolapse does not change either the treatment or prognosis of panic disorder.

Pheochromocytomas are rare tumors of the adrenal glands that can cause discrete episodes of hypertension and anxiety symptoms by releasing excessive amounts of catecholamines such as adrenaline. Physical anxiety symptoms in these episodes are similar to those seen in panic disorder. The psychological symptoms, however, are less common in pheochromocytomas. For instance, feelings of terror, fears of losing control, anticipatory anxiety, and agoraphobia are unusual with adrenal tumors (Starkman, Zelnick, Tesse, and Cameron, 1985). Also, pheochromocytomas are rare compared to panic disorder. If a pheochromocytoma is clinically suspected, blood and urine tests can help make the diagnosis.

Drug use or withdrawal may be a sole cause of the symptoms or can exacerbate an ongoing anxiety disorder. Caffeine, which may cause symptoms of generalized anxiety or panic, is the most commonly used anxiety-producing drug, in part because it is often not regarded as strong enough to cause problems by the same people who consciously use it as a stimulant! Those who consume large amounts of caffeine to stay awake, such as students at exam times or shift workers who have a disruption of normal sleep-wake cycles, may complain of anxiety unaware that they are drinking five to ten cups of caffeinated beverages, including coffee and soft drinks. Patients with panic disorder are also more sensitive to caffeine (Charney, Heninger, and Jatlow, 1985). Many, but not all, have already stopped drinking coffee before seeking care. For those who haven't, however, tapering and ultimately discontinuing caffeine intake is mandatory. Although caffeine only rarely actually causes panic disorder, it may certainly make it worse.

Other stimulants, such as cocaine, amphetamines, diet pills, and nasal decongestants (which typically contain pseudoephedrine or other stimulants), can also cause or exacerbate anxiety. Blood and urine tests and/or asking the patient directly are the only ways to ascertain whether drugs are causing the anxiety symptoms. In cocaine abuse, characteristic signs such as coming late to appointments, missing appointments, and inconsistent money spending patterns will be present.

Drug withdrawal, primarily from sedatives or tranquilizers, can also cause anxiety symptoms. Alcohol is the classic substance that causes withdrawal anxiety, but benzodiazepine withdrawal, especially from the short-acting drugs such as alprazolam (Xanax) and triazolam (Halcion) is increasingly common (see chapter 11 for more details). A good history is the key to the diagnosis.

MEDICAL AND LABORATORY EVALUATION

As noted above, many patients with anxiety disorders and most panic patients will already have had an extensive medical evaluation before seeking mental health care. For those who have not, it is appropriate that they consult an internist to exclude an undiagnosed medical disorder as a cause of the anxiety. Medical evaluations also help reassure those patients who are most frightened by the physical nature of their symptoms.

Basic laboratory tests to rule out obvious medical problems include many of the same tests recommended for evaluating depression. These include the general screening blood tests, thyroid function tests, and an electrocardiogram. If a specific diagnosis is being considered, further tests will be obtained.

PSYCHIATRIC DIFFERENTIAL DIAGNOSIS

Because it is seen in so many psychiatric disorders, anxiety as a symptom can be easily confused with an anxiety disorder. Even more difficult is detecting an anxiety disorder in patients who have more than one source of anxiety. As an example, a patient with a mixed personality disorder characterized by feelings of inadequacy and fearfulness may also develop a panic disorder which may then be complicated by the anticipatory anxiety of another attack. Further confusing the diagnostic problem is the common occurrence of a patient with more than one anxiety disorder—for instance, panic disorder and generalized anxiety. Unfortunately, some of the clues that are helpful in distinguishing depression as a symptom from depressive disorders—family histories, the cyclical or episodic nature of the disorders—are not as useful for anxiety. Although evidence for the familial nature of anxiety disorders is increasing, as noted above, it is still unclear whether there are inherited vulnerabilities to specific disorders as opposed to a general vulnerability to anxiety disorders. Thus, knowing a patient's family history may not always help distinguish between social phobia and agoraphobia. Furthermore, the natural history of many anxiety disorders is simply not as clear as it is for depression. Therefore, until our knowledge about anxiety disorders increases substantially and our diagnostic system has more validity, distinguishing these disorders from others in which anxiety is a symptom will continue to be difficult. At present, the most distinctive symptoms that are helpful in diagnosing anxiety disorders are patterns of avoidance, discrete episodes of anxiety symptoms, and ritualistic behaviors.

In distinguishing panic disorder from other disorders in which anxiety is a major feature, the important clues are the crescendo nature of panic, the discrete nature of the attacks, the occurrence of some attacks that are spontaneous, and the agoraphobia that typically ensues. Panic disorder often coexists with other disorders, especially generalized anxiety and depression. Both social and specific phobias can be distinguished from panic by the specific situations that provoke the anxiety in the former. This distinction, however, may be difficult to draw for patients whose panic attacks are sometimes triggered by certain situations (such as being in a supermarket or driving). Hypochondriacal patients and panic patients share an exquisite body sensitivity and fears of catastrophic physical events. Hypochondriacs, however, do not describe clear panic attacks and do not become agoraphobic; they dwell exclusively on their physical symptoms, not on their anxiety as do panic patients.

Agoraphobia and social phobia differ in that patients with the latter disorder fear doing something humiliating or embarrassing as opposed to fear of having a panic attack itself. In reality, this differentiation is not always easy to make, since in some socially phobic patients a fear of the anxiety symptoms themselves may gradually evolve, thereby blurring the distinction. Avoidant personality (see chapter 7) and social phobia frequently coexist and may be difficult to distinguish because of the overlapping nature of their diagnostic criteria. In many ways, this distinction is irrelevant since treatment approaches are probably similar.

Obsessive compulsive disorder may be confused with major depression since ruminative thinking occurs frequently in the latter. Patients with depressive ruminations, though, do not generally perceive their thoughts as ego-dystonic or senseless as do those with OCD. Depressed patients will also have the other characteristic signs of their disorder such as sleep and appetite disturbances or diurnal variation, symptoms that are not present in uncomplicated obsessive compulsive disorder. The two disorders often coexist. Some schizophrenic patients will present with true compulsions. The presence of the typical features of schizophrenia other than delusional thinking will help distinguish it from obsessive compulsive disorder. However, a subgroup of patients with obsessive compulsive disorder may have psychotic thinking, due either to a loss of insight into the senselessness of their compulsions and their obsessive thoughts, or because of a comorbid schizotypal or delusional disorder (Eisen and Rasmussen, 1993). Loss of insight as the only psychotic symptom should be considered on a continuum, from OCD with poor insight to OCD with delusional disorder for those patients who have a completely delusional belief in the meaning of their symptoms.

Obsessive compulsive spectrum disorders are a group of disorders with features similar to OCD, but characterized by neither classic obsessions nor compulsions. The net cast by this term varies in its scope, ranging from a few disorders to over two dozen. The core aspects defining obsessive compulsive spectrum disorders are the presence of obsessive/compulsive features (anorexia nervosa, bulimia nervosa, body dysmorphic disorder, hypochondriasis, delusional disorder) or impulsive features (paraphilias, kleptomania, pyromania, pathological gambling) (McElroy, Phillips, and Keck, 1994). Among this broad range of disorders, those that seem most related to OCD are trichotillomania (compulsive hair pulling), onchyphagia (compulsive nail biting), and body dysmorphic disorder. Some evidence suggests the efficacy of SSRIs and clomipramine for OCD spectrum disorders, although the medications are less consistently effective than is typically seen with OCD. Although the spectrum concept has some inherent merit (similar to affective spectrum disorders, discussed in chapter 9), lumping as diverse a group of disorders as borderline personality disorder, autism, kleptomania, and OCD in this fashion in the absence of solid data linking them may broaden the concept into a meaningless mass (Rasmussen, 1994).

For clinical reasons, distinguishing between generalized anxiety disorder (GAD) and similar syndromes such as adjustment disorder with anxious mood is not very important since the treatment options are identical. Thus, a disorder characterized by generalized anxiety symptoms but lasting less than six months (which is the time cutoff for GAD) may be called anxiety disorder NOS by DSM-IV, but should be treated the same as GAD.

Many patients present with a mixture of anxiety and depression that is associated with significant distress or impairment, but with neither group of symptoms sufficiently prominent to be diagnosed as either major depression, dysthymia, generalized anxiety disorder, or panic disorder. This disorder, called (not surprisingly) mixed anxiety-depressive disorder, has been placed in the Appendix in DSM-IV as a proposed criteria set requiring further study. Patients with mixed anxiety-depression typically lack the pervasive anhedonia and apathy of depressed patients and do not show the pervasive excessive worry and tension of anxiety patients, yet share some features of each (Zinbarg et al., 1994). It is still unclear whether, with further follow-up, these patients would ultimately show more typical anxiety or depressive disorders. Because of the recency of this proposed diagnostic category, treatment approaches (should it be treated more like a depression with anxious features or an anxiety disorder with some depressive symptoms?) is unknown. For now, then, it would suffice to simply recognize this disorder as cutting across our diagnostic boxes, and to consider a variety of treatment approaches in an empirical fashion.

PSYCHOPHARMACOLOGICAL TREATMENT

Using psychopharmacological agents to treat anxiety is an ancient concept. Since the dawn of history, chemicals such as alcohol and opiates have been used to deaden feelings, diminish arousal, and induce calm. What is new, though, is the range of options available for treatment as well as the beginning of a more targeted approach to anxiety that links a specific medical treatment to the distinct anxiety disorder being treated. Certainly, as noted in the beginning of the chapter, our current diagnostic distinctions are neither as clear-cut nor as useful for predicting specific treatment responses as we would hope. (The exception to this rule is OCD for which only a few specific medications are first-line treatments, with the other agents generally not very useful.) One type of medication may be effective for three or four of the anxiety disorders we have discussed. For instance, the MAO inhibitor class of antidepressants and probably the SSRIs are effective in treating panic disorder, social phobias, and post-traumatic stress disorder. Yet other diagnostic distinctions are important in predicting medication response. Cyclic antidepressants and SSRIs are fine first treatments for panic disorder but not for generalized anxiety. Overall, the broad range of reasonable first- and second-line options for most anxiety disorders is a strength, allowing choice in case of nonresponse or side effects, but demanding skill in knowing how to prescribe a broad range of treatment alternatives.

As in the first half of this chapter, therefore, psychopharmacological strategies will be organized by specific diagnostic categories. Specific phobias will not be discussed further since there is no evidence that medications are useful in their treatment.

Acute Treatment of Panic Disorder

The notion that panic patients differ from those with other anxiety disorders in their treatment responses was first suggested in 1964, when Klein reported that antidepressants were effective for patients with discrete episodes of panic and subsequent constriction of activities (Klein, 1964). Since then, the treatment options have greatly expanded. Two medication classes—cyclic antidepressants and the benzodiazepines, especially alprazolam—are well documented as effective in treating panic, while two other classes—SSRIs and MAO inhibitors—are clinically effective, albeit without as much research documentation. Table 4–3 shows the advantages and disadvantages of these four medication groups. Because of the number of viable first-line options for treating panic disorder, choosing any one medication depends on the specific needs of the individual patient.

Table 4–3
Advantages and Disadvantages of Antipanic Medications

Medication	Advantages	Disadvantages
Cyclic antidepressants	Well established Once-daily dosage	Delayed onset of action Stimulant side effects (with some) Other side effects
Benzodiazepines	Rapid onset of action Effective against anticipatory anxiety Few side effects	Drug dependence, withdrawal problems Sedation, cognitive side effects
Selective serotonin reuptake inhibitors (SSRIs)	Once-daily dosage Relatively few side effects	Delayed onset of action Stimulant side effects
Monoamine oxidase inhibitors	Possible increased antiphobic effects	Delayed onset of action Dietary restriction, risk of hypertensive reaction Other side effects

Among the four major medication groups commonly prescribed for panic disorder, the cyclic antidepressants, especially imipramine, are the most well documented to have significant antipanic properties. Despite convincing proof, most of the cyclic antidepressants are likely to be effective in treating panic disorder. Reports on both trazodone and amoxapine are somewhat inconsistent, although some patients will respond to them.

Advantages of using the cyclic antidepressants for treating panic are their long history of successful use, once-daily dosing, usually at night, and their lack of addiction or withdrawal potential. Unfortunately, since panic patients tend to be exquisitely sensitive to side effects of any medications, they frequently have problems with the cyclic antidepressants, especially in the beginning of treatment prior to a therapeutic response and before accommodation to the side effects has occurred. Panic patients are also far more likely than are depressive patients to have an unwanted and uncomfortable stimulant response to the more noradrenergic cyclic antidepressants, such as desipramine and imipramine (Pohl, Yeragani, Balon, and Lycaki, 1988). This stimulant response, which can occur even at very low dose, is characterized by insomnia, agitation, and restless discomfort which is perceived, understandably, as the medication exacerbating the original problem. Lowering the medication dose temporarily, waiting, switching to a less stimulating antidepressant, or adding a beta-blocker which blocks many of these side effects are all useful strategies for decreasing the stimulant effect. Adding a benzodiazepine tranquilizer early in treatment along with a cyclic antidepressant can also be useful by decreasing the stimulant response and because of its own capacity to decrease panic. However, as with the general use of benzodiazepines for panic, it may be difficult to withdraw the patient from the tranquilizer, even if the cyclic antidepressant is continued (Woods et al., 1992).

Other than the cyclic antidepressants, benzodiazepines are the other very well documented class of anti-panic medications. Alprazolam (Xanax) is the best studied, with consistent efficacy also seen with clonazepam (Klonopin) and lorazepam (Ativan). Other benzodiazepines are also likely to be effective but have not been evaluated as carefully. As a treatment for panic, benzodiazepines have a number of advantages. They are as effective as the antidepressants; their antipanic effects are evident quickly, often within the first week, and faster than the effects usually seen with antidepressants; they effectively diminish the anticipatory anxiety that accompanies panic since they are tranquilizers; they cause none of the typical antidepressant side effects such as dry mouth, stimulant effects, blood pressure changes, and the like; and tolerance to their antipanic effects does not seem to occur.

Over the last few years, however, the drawbacks of the benzodiazepines have become more apparent. The most important of these is their capacity to create both pharmacological and psychological dependence. Also, withdrawal symptoms may be extremely troublesome, especially with the shorter-acting medications such as alprazolam (see chapter 11 for a detailed discussion of this). These withdrawal symptoms can be manifested either by rebound anxiety upon discontinuing the medication or by interdose breakthrough symptoms or "mini-withdrawals" that occur just before the next scheduled dose, typically four hours after the last dose. Withdrawal difficulties are minimized somewhat by the use of the longer-acting agents such as clonazepam. The other major drawback of benzodiazepines is the common side effect of sedation.

Despite a relative lack of good studies evaluating their efficacy, SSRIs are prescribed for panic disorder with increasing frequency (Black, Wesner, Bowers, and Gabel, 1993). Their advantages, similar to when they are used for depression, are their relative lack of side effects. Unlike the benzodiazepines, they are neither sedating nor are they associated with dependence or withdrawal symptoms. Unlike the tricyclics, weight gain, sedation, anticholinergic symptoms, and blood pressure changes are rare with SSRIs. However, the stimulant effects seen with SSRIs can be very troublesome for panic patients. Because of this, despite the lack of comparative studies, the less stimulating SSRIs, such as fluvoxamine or paroxetine, may hold an advantage in treating panic. When the more stimulating SSRIs are prescribed for panic disorder, initial doses are typically much lower than those used for depression. As an example, fluoxetine is often started at 2.5 to 5 mg daily (using the liquid preparation.) All SSRIs are likely to be effective if the patient can tolerate the drug.

Among the other new antidepressants, bupropion is unlikely to be successful in treating panic. Venlafaxine is probably effective, but nefazodone's capacity to treat panic is unknown. Given the similarity of both drugs to other effective agents, however, positive responses with some patients are likely.

Despite evidence of their effectiveness, MAO inhibitors are almost never used as first-line treatments for panic disorder, and are typically the last treatment tried. Assuredly, this is due to the cumbersomeness of the dietary restrictions necessary when they are prescribed (see chapter 9). In my experience, compared to depressed patients, those with panic also become more frightened about the diet and the possible consequences if the wrong food is ingested. Additionally, the common side effects seen with MAO inhibitors, such as postural dizziness or insomnia, seem to be more disturbing to panic patients than to depressed patients. Nevertheless, MAO inhibitors can be exceedingly useful antipanic medications. In the best study comparing a cyclic antidepressant to an MAO inhibitor, the two treatments were equally effective although the MAO inhibitors were slightly better in diminishing phobic symptoms (Sheehan et al., 1980). Unfortunately, there has been no recent interest in further evaluating MAO inhibitors as antipanic agents. Although phenelzine (Nardil) is the most well studied of the MAO inhibitors, the other two medications in this class, tranylcypromine and selegiline, are also likely to be effective.

When patients with panic disorder combined with agoraphobia and anticipatory anxiety are treated by any of these medications, not all the symptoms improve together. By definition, the universal effect of all antipanic medication is to decrease or abolish the panic attacks themselves. Medication effects on the phobic and anticipatory anxiety symptoms are more variable. Once the panic attacks cease, many patients will gradually re-expand their activities by themselves, thereby creating their own "naturalistic" behavioral desensitization program over weeks and months, which then treats both their phobic and anxiety symptoms. Other patients need more structured intervention with at least some formal behavioral therapy following the successful treatment of the panic attacks.

Given these considerations, on what basis does a psychopharmacologist decide whether to prescribe a cyclic antidepressant, a benzodiazepine, or an SSRI as a first treatment for a panic patient? (I am ignoring MAO inhibitors here since they are never prescribed as a first agent for panic.) Because all three are effective in groups of patients, most physicians choose a medication based on their best clinical judgment and the preference of the patient. Despite the relative paucity of studies evaluating their efficacy, SSRIs are probably the most common first-line agents among psychopharmacologists because of their high patient acceptance. If stimulation effects preclude a high enough dose of an SSRI, adjunctive use of a benzodiazepine may be beneficial, especially since all the antidepressants take weeks to decrease panic. If an SSRI is either ineffective or not tolerated, a tricyclic, such as nortriptyline or desipramine, or a benzodiazepine, typically alprazolam or clonazepam, may be used. Although some psychopharmacologists are wary of benzodiazepines as a first treatment because of their potential for dependence, others think the risk is exaggerated and prescribe them regularly as initial treatments for panic.

Although three quarters of panic patients obtain significant relief from one of the above medications, residual symptoms—either occasional panic attacks or phobic avoidance—continue in up to 50 percent of adequately treated patients. When this occurs, a number of comorbid diagnoses or other symptoms frequently associated with panic may be complicating the clinical picture. As an example of the latter, patients who suffer from a combination of anticipatory anxiety, generalized anxiety, and panic may not always (understandably) accurately distinguish between the sources of their discomfort. They may complain about continued symptoms, thinking these are "prepanic" feelings when they are due to anticipatory anxiety—worrying about panic. Since higher doses of antidepressants will not necessarily help this type of anxiety, the distinction is clinically vital. The most appropriate intervention in this situation would probably be cognitive-behavior therapy, although some psychopharmacologists might add a benzodiazepine if the original antipanic drug was an antidepressant. Another condition that may complicate the evaluation and treatment of panic patients is depression. Those patients whose depression does not remit along with the panic may describe social withdrawal and not wanting to leave the house; thus what looks like agoraphobia may actually be a manifestation of untreated depression. The third disorder that may coexist with panic and be associated with treatment failure is social phobia. These patients may show a greater response to MAO inhibitors (see below).

Among alternative medication treatments for panic disorder, the anticonvulsant valproate is infrequently prescribed but occasionally effective (Keck, Taylor, Tugrul, McElroy, and Bennett, 1993). Surprisingly, carbamazepine, the other anticonvulsant commonly used in psychopharmacology, has not been shown to effectively treat panic disorder. Clinically, combination treatment has become increasingly common, especially combining an antidepressant (either an SSRI or a cyclic antidepressant) with a benzodiazepine. Propranolol, a betablocker (see chapter 11), is occasionally prescribed for treating panic, but with limited success (Munjack et al., 1989). It should be reserved for use in treatment-resistant cases, typically prescribed in combination with more effective medications. Although buspirone is ineffective in treating panic when prescribed alone, it is occasionally helpful when used in combination with more standard agents.

Even though she was always a high-energy person, accomplished academically and then vocationally, with many friends and long-term relationships, Carolyn had struggled with anxiety episodes since high school. With her first panic attack at age 19, she was convinced she was having a heart attack, like her grandfather who had died of heart disease two years earlier. To her surprise, all medical tests were normal. For the next six months, she had intermittent episodes, similar to the first one but never as bad. Although she continued with all her usual activities, Carolyn became incapable of doing things alone, a marked contrast to her usual independence. She needed to be with her boyfriend if she drove anywhere, or went anywhere new. Eventually, the attacks subsided and Carolyn went on with her busy life.

Similar bouts occurred three other times in her twenties. When she sought help, the diagnosis of panic disorder was made. The doctor initially prescribed imipramine, but Carolyn hated it and stopped it quickly, complaining of spaciness, weight gain, and dry mouth. Because of this experience and because of her feeling that she should be able to conquer these episodes without drugs, Carolyn resisted taking medications. By her third bout of panic disorder, however, she agreed to take alprazolam, with doses gradually increasing to 1.5 mg daily. Within days of starting the medication, Carolyn felt somewhat better. Ultimately, she had a good response, but disliked the anxiety she felt between doses and the need to take the medication three times daily. Additionally, she continued to have both mild depressive symptoms and daily early morning dread upon arising. Switching from alprazolam to clonazepam (a more long-acting benzodiazepine) eliminated the inter-dose anxiety but did not change the early morning anxiety or the mild depressive symptoms. After initial resistance to the suggestion, she ultimately agreed to a trial of the SSRI paroxetine, which was started at a quarter of a tablet daily. (Luckily, Carolyn was very good at cutting pills.) Within three weeks, Carolyn had increased the dose to one-half pill daily (10 mg) and felt qualitatively better, with a decrease in her morning anxiety and the elimination of her depression. When last seen, she was beginning to taper her clonazepam very slowly while staying on the paroxetine, feeling occasional mild anxiety without cause but no other symptoms.

Continuation and Maintenance Treatment for Panic Disorder

The natural history of panic disorder is exceedingly variable. Some patients have single or widely spaced bouts of the disorder with normal functioning between episodes. Other patients, however, seem to show more chronic symptoms with low grade anxiety and agoraphobic symptoms alternating with acute exacerbations during which panic attacks increase in severity and frequency. Because of this variability, it has been difficult to construct thoughtful recommendations for continuation and maintenance treatment. Compounding the problem is the virtual absence of controlled maintenance treatment studies. Therefore, recommendations for longer-term treatments are based primarily on best clinical guesses. For most patients, a course of antipanic medication should be continued for six months to one year following clinical remission of symptoms before a slow tapering of the medication is attempted. Although the antipanic effects of the medications begin within weeks of starting antipanic treatment, improvement of other symptoms such as phobic avoidance or some anticipatory anxiety may not begin for months (Pollack and Otto, 1994). Of note, effective doses of antidepressants and benzodiazepines for panic disorder stay constant during the many months following symptom remission, suggesting a lack of tolerance to their effect (Schweizer, Rickels, Weiss, and Zavodnik, 1993). If symptoms emerge during the tapering period, the dose is generally increased to the lowest effective dose and continued for another three to six months when a second tapering should be attempted. Discontinuation of alprazolam is particularly difficult for panic patients, even when the medication is tapered over a number of weeks (Rickels, Schweizer, Weiss, and Zavodnick, 1993). (Benzodiazepine discontinuation is discussed further in chapter 11.) Antipanic medications should not be tapered at a time of significant psychological stress such as moving to a new house, starting a new job, separation, or divorce.

Longer-term (one to six years) naturalistic follow-up studies indicate that successfully treated patients show relapse rates of at least 50 percent after medication discontinuation. The most reasonable candidates for maintenance treatment are those patients who have a history of unremitting panic disorder for many years or decades and who have had at least two attempts at tapering their medication that have been unsuccessful because of the reemergence of panic attacks. Tricyclic antidepressants may be particularly problematic in long-term treatment, and many patients may discontinue the medication because of side effects (Noyes, Garvey, Cook, and Samuelson, 1989).

Social Phobia

Distinguishing between the limited and the more generalized types of social phobia is vital since the two subtypes differ in their medication responsiveness. For patients with the limited performance anxiety sub-type of social phobia, beta-blockers are the most well documented treatment (Liebowitz et al., 1985). Either propranolol or atenolol (which causes less sedation and fatigue) is likely to be effective. Typically, the medication is taken on an as-needed basis, usually a half hour or an hour before a public performance. MAO inhibitors may also be effective for performance anxiety, although the evidence is less clear, in part because many studies have not distinguished between performance and generalized types of social phobia. If MAO inhibitors are used for performance anxiety, they must be taken as a maintenance medication. Benzodiazepines are also sometimes prescribed on an as-needed basis with anecdotal success.

The generalized form of social phobia can be effectively treated by a variety of medications shown in Table 4–4. Among these, the most well-documented treatments are MAO inhibitors (Liebowitz et al., 1992). Phenelzine has been used in most studies although tranyl-cypromine is also likely to be effective. When treatment is successful, patients will describe a marked increase in the sheer number of social situations they will allow themselves to enter. One person may now accept dates, another may accept a position of leadership previously avoided because of the necessity of interacting more with others. The level of improvement is independent of any baseline depression. In my experience, even when the MAO inhibitors are helpful, other interventions—social skills training, psychodynamic therapy, confronting associated use of alcohol—are usually necessary for the best clinical response.

Table 4–4
Pharmacotherapies for Social Phobia

Medication Class	Evidence of Efficacy
Monoamine oxidase inhibitors	+++
Benzodiazepines	++
Selective serotonin reuptake inhibitors	++
Buspirone	+
Beta-blockers	+

+++ = Definite efficacy
++ = Probable efficacy
+ = Possible efficacy

Bob, now 22, had always been shy. In school, he was unable to participate in class discussions because of overwhelming anxiety when called upon to speak. This interfered with his grades, which, given his intelligence, were lower than expected. He felt like a failure in comparison with his siblings and was convinced he was a disappointment to his high-achieving parents. Throughout school, he was able to make a few friends with whom he could play sports, but he had no girlfriends. He described how he would be attracted to a girl from afar, yet when he approached her to start a conversation, he would become paralyzed with fear, turn bright red, and say no more than a few words before walking away in anguish. While in high school, he was seen in psychotherapy by a therapist who focused on self-esteem issues and helped Bob improve his social skills. Although Bob liked the therapist and felt better about himself and less criticized by his parents, he was still unable to approach girls or participate in class discussions. By the end of his freshman year of college, Bob was drinking a half bottle of wine a night, insisting that it was the only way he could relax and be less than profoundly self-conscious with others. His growing dependence on alcohol frightened him and he re-entered therapy. His therapist suggested a psychopharmacological consultation, in which social phobia was diagnosed and tranylcypromine (Parnate) was recommended. After reaching a dose of 40 mg daily, which took six weeks to accomplish because of significant postural hypotension, Bob noted a marked increase in his ability to be with others without feeling overwhelmed with anxiety. He was able to talk to girls and feel only moderately nervous. In class, although still hesitant to speak up, he was able to do so at times. Despite his clear improvement, however, he did not diminish his alcohol use for many months because of his fear of being without it. Moreover, Bob found that he still focused on his feelings of failure. Because of this, he continued in psychotherapy, which benefited him greatly. One year after starting the medication, he felt far more confident and stopped psychotherapy, but continued on the tranylcypromine, still feeling unready to try going without it.

Benzodiazepines, especially clonazepam and alprazolam, have also been used successfully to treat social phobia (Davidson, Tupler, and Potts, 1994). As with their use in panic disorder, benzodiazepine withdrawal after successful treatment for social phobia is associated with high relapse rates (Gelernter et al., 1991). My own clinical experience is that, because of their anxiety, patients with social phobia may use excessive doses of benzodiazepines, a problem not found with SSRIs or

MAO inhibitors. Furthermore, patients with social phobia and alcohol abuse (a relatively common combination) should not be treated with benzodiazepines, especially given the other available treatment options.

SSRIs have been demonstrated as effective treatments for social phobia in a number of noncontrolled trials and a few small double-blind studies (Jefferson, 1995). Fluoxetine has been the most well studied but at least three different SSRIs have shown some efficacy, indicating the likelihood that all agents in this class would be beneficial. Similar to the treatment of panic disorder, many clinicians prescribe SSRIs first for social phobia because of their benign side effect profile and high patient acceptance.

Buspirone and beta-blockers are second-line treatments for social phobia. Buspirone may have some efficacy for generalized social phobia but is unlikely to help performance anxiety (Schneier et al., 1993). Beta-blockers are probably not very effective in treating generalized social phobia, although a few patients respond. Cyclic antidepressants have not been investigated in any systematic manner for treating generalized social phobia.

Not enough is known about the natural history of social phobia to make any concrete suggestions regarding continuation and maintenance treatment. My own experience is mixed. When medication is effective, some patients seem to be able to develop social skills and social confidence. They can then stop taking the medication without the return of unmanageable symptoms in social situations. Others experience the return of the same paralyzing symptoms after discontinuing the medication, necessitating its resumption. In the absence of any studies, the same guidelines used with panic disorder are reasonable: six months to one year after a good clinical response, a tapering of the medication is indicated.

Obsessive Compulsive Disorder

From a disorder that, less than ten years ago, was pharmacologically responsive to only one medication, which was unavailable in this country, OCD can now be treated by a variety of available agents. This unquestionably reflects the release of a group of medications that strongly enhance brain serotonin. In fact, all well-documented first-line pharmacotherapies for OCD, listed in Table 4–5, are strongly serotonergic—clomipramine and the four SSRIs. (Despite consistent evidence for the efficacy of all five agents, not all are FDA approved for treating OCD. See chapter 1 for further details.) No other medications can be considered as even remotely effective as these for treating OCD, although theoretically, other strongly serotonergic agents such as venlafaxine (Effexor) might also be effective. At the same time, the limitations of these medications are equally apparent. Although 50 to 70 percent of OCD patients respond to any one of these agents, rarely do the symptoms of the disorder disappear. Rather, in OCD studies, response is often defined as a 35 percent decrease in symptoms, meaning that residual symptoms may be prominent in patients officially designated as treatment responders. For many of these patients, however, a 40 to 50 percent decrease in symptoms qualitatively improves their lives so that they may function despite the residual obsessions and compulsions. The response to these medications is independent of the presence or severity of depressive symptoms. Even though they are all effective, among the first-line agents for OCD listed in Table 4–5, the oldest of the medications, clomipramine, may be the most effective (Greist et al., 1995b). In general, clomipramine is also associated with the greatest number of side effects. OCD patients, though, seem to tolerate medications better than do patients with other disorders treated with the same agents. Consistent with this, despite causing more side effects than the other agents, clomipramine is not associated with high dropout rates when prescribed for OCD.

Thus, for a first choice, any of the first-line agents would be appropriate, with clomipramine slightly more effective and the other agents showing fewer side effects. An appropriate trial of OCD pharmacotherapy for maximum response should be at least ten weeks, longer than generally required to see an antidepressant response with the same agent. A nonresponse to any one of these medications does not predict a poor response to another.

Optimal doses for treating OCD are in some dispute. It has generally been assumed, based on both clinical experience and some early studies, that higher doses of SSRIs than are prescribed for depression were required for treating OCD. Two recent studies, however, indicate that more typical doses of both fluoxetine and sertraline are generally as effective as higher doses (Tollefson et al., 1994b, Greist et al., 1995a).

For those patients who have not responded to one of these first-line agents, a number of adjunctive agents (to be added to the first treatment) or other treatments to be used instead, are available (see Table 4–5). The most important adjunctive treatment, which is not listed in the Table, is unquestionably behavior therapy which is well documented as a powerful treatment for OCD in its own right and probably has additive effects to pharmacotherapy (Greist, 1994).

All the adjunctive treatments, except for neuroleptics, augment serotonergic function. Despite many anecdotal reports and open studies, none of the serotonergic adjunctive treatments have been demonstrated as effective in double-blind studies (Goodman, McDougle, Barr, Aronson, and Price, 1993). Neuroleptics are effective in the subgroup of patients with OCD plus tics, but probably not in OCD patients without tics (McDougle et al., 1994). Neuroleptics are also typically considered for those OCD patients with psychotic or schizotypal features, despite a lack of convincing studies validating the efficacy of this approach.

The second-line treatments listed in Table 4–5 have each been demonstrated as effective in small samples of patients. Other than clomipramine, tricyclic antidepressants should be considered ineffective for treating OCD.

Table 4–5
Pharmacotherapies for Obsessive Compulsive Disorder

First-Line Agents

Clomipramine (Anafranil)
Fluoxetine (Prozac)
Fluvoxamine (Luvox)
Paroxetine (Paxil)
Sertraline (Zoloft)

Adjunctive Agents

A second serotonergic agent
Neuroleptics (for those with tics)
Buspirone (Buspar)
Fenfluramine (Pondimin)
Lithium
Trazodone

Second-Line Agents

Monoamine oxidase inhibitors
Clonazepam (Klonopin)
Buspirone (Buspar)

Third-Line Treatment

Cingulotomy

Long-term treatment studies for OCD are virtually nonexistent. Anecdotally, most patients show an increase in symptoms if not an overt relapse when effective pharmacotherapy is withdrawn.

Joseph had always been anxious and somewhat fastidious. As a child, he had had an unusual number of superstitious rituals, but these were simply assumed to be quirks of childhood. In fact, Joseph had had clear rituals as a child and adolescent which he successfully hid from his parents. These compulsions and their accompanying obsessions would flare up for months at a time but then recede and be present in relatively mild form for years. Recently, his need for order seemed to increase to extraordinary proportions. Instead of just turning the water off after watering his lawn, he tightened the knob and then returned to check it at least five times in the course of the evening. He was concerned, he said, that if the water leaked, the ground would become flooded, which might result in a weakening of his house's foundations. His habit of checking on his children while they were asleep, which had always consisted of glancing into their rooms, had now escalated into taking their pulse, examining their breathing, and rearranging their blankets to make sure they would not suffocate. Not surprisingly, they awakened during these checks. Before leaving the house, Joseph was now compelled to check and recheck the oven, the windows, and the doors so many times that it took him thirty minutes or more to go from his house to his car. He was aware of the irrational nature of his rituals yet felt powerless to resist them.

Initially seen in psychodynamically oriented psychotherapy, Joseph explored his catastrophic fears and his difficulty in being soothed. The rituals, however, continued unabated and even worsened somewhat. A psychopharmacological consultant recommended fluoxetine in doses increasing to 80 mg daily. Four weeks after starting the medication, Joseph felt a decrease in the compulsion to repeat these rituals. Over the next month, the time spent on his rituals decreased by more than half. On the recommendation of the consultant, Joseph sought further help from a behavior therapist who constructed a program of response prevention. Within three months, the compulsions were further diminished. Although occasional obsessions and compulsions remained, they had far less power than before and generally did not interfere with Joseph's ability to function.

One year later, having retained the benefits of treatment, Joseph slowly tapered his fluoxetine. After decreasing his fluoxetine dose to 10 mg daily, his obsessions and compulsions began to return. He quickly increased his dose to 40 mg daily and returned to behavior therapy for six more sessions, with a decrease in his symptoms. He continues on fluoxetine 40 mg daily.

Finally, there is a small but consistent series of reports on the use of psychosurgery (cingulotomy) as a treatment for treatment-resistant paralyzing obsessions and compulsions. The surgery is limited to cutting neuronal tracts between part of the frontal lobe and the cingulate gyrus (in the limbic system). Although I have no personal experience with this treatment, studies suggest a significant improvement in 25 percent of patients, all of whom had failed to respond to multiple aggressive pharmacological and behavioral treatments, with an additional 15 percent showing some improvement (Baer et al., 1995). Clearly, this is a treatment of last resort. Yet intense, severe obsessive compulsive disorder can make life unliveable, as anyone who has treated these patients can attest. Occasionally, extraordinary measures need to be considered.

Post-traumatic Stress Disorder

Of all the anxiety disorders for which medications may be helpful, post-traumatic stress disorder (PTSD) has been the least investigated. In part, this stems from our belated attempts at defining the syndrome. Even more, though, it reflects the conceptualization of PTSD as etiologically related to a profound life event and diagnosed only in relation to that event. It is a counterintuitive notion (although not necessarily correct) to consider using medications to treat a reactive disorder. Increasingly, however, a variety of medications have been demonstrated to be effective in treating PTSD. At the same time, most experts consider pharmacotherapy to be a secondary, adjunctive treatment for PTSD, to be added to the psychotherapy that is indicated in all cases. Moreover, most studies indicate a generally modest effect of pharmacotherapies for PTSD (Davidson, 1992).

In treating acute PTSD, the goal of pharmacotherapy is simply to help diminish the arousal and insomnia that dominate the clinical picture at this time. For chronic PTSD, however, a variety of options are available with no obvious method to choose among them at this time. Appropriate medications include tricyclic antidepressants, MAO inhibitors, benzodiazepines, mood stabilizers such as carbamazepine (Tegretol), clonidine (Catapres), buspirone (Buspar), and the SSRIs (Sutherland and Davidson, 1994). With the possible exception of fluoxetine, the therapeutic effects of all these agents are greater for decreasing the intrusion and hyperarousal symptoms than for the emotional numbing and avoidance. In contrast, fluoxetine (and presumably other SSRIs) may diminish avoidant and numbing symptoms as well as arousal symptoms (van der Kolk et al., 1994). If the avoidance symptoms are seen as secondary protective mechanisms that stem from the primary hyperarousal and intrusive symptoms, most medication effects in PTSD are analogous to those seen in panic disorder in which the panic (hyperarousal) responds to medication but the phobic avoidance (like the numbing and avoidance aspects of PTSD) must often be treated separately. Continuing the analogy, successful pharmacotherapy of PTSD may make psychotherapy more productive as feelings become less overwhelming and reconnecting with the emotional world less threatening.

Several factors should be considered in deciding among the medication choices: (1) the presence of associated depression would suggest the choice of an antidepressant; (2) a history of cocaine or alcohol abuse dictates against prescribing an MAO inhibitor (because of the dietary restrictions); (3) the prominence of explosive outbursts and/or head trauma might suggest prescribing carbamazepine because of its effect on neurological or episodic syndromes; (4) a history of alcohol or sedative/hypnotic abuse would suggest avoiding benzodiazepines. The usefulness of neuroleptics for PTSD is unclear. Many of the psychotic-like symptoms of the disorder should best be considered dissociative phenomena and not true psychosis. Neuroleptics should be considered primarily for those patients with true psychotic symptoms unrelated to traumatic themes or for those with extremely destructive behavior.

Generalized Anxiety Disorder

Because it is a syndrome with its borders rather blurred, treatment for generalized anxiety focuses on decreasing the symptom of anxiety, rather than on manifestations of a truly specific disorder. Therefore, in this section, we will discuss the pharmacological treatment of generalized anxiety, adjustment disorder with anxiety, and situational anxiety together. Currently, two types of medications are rational first choices—the benzodiazepines and buspirone. Seven other medication classes are prescribed, but as second-line treatments. Table 4–6 shows these medication groups.

By far, the benzodiazepines are the most commonly prescribed and most effective antianxiety medications currently available. As with their use in panic disorder, their advantages in treating generalized anxiety are impressive: they are effective when taken on an as-needed basis or when taken regularly; when taken chronically, they generally do not lose

Table 4–6
Medications for Generalized Anxiety

First-Line Agents

Benzodiazepines
Buspirone

Others

Cyclic antidepressants
Monoamine oxidase inhibitors
Selective serotonin reuptake inhibitors
Barbiturates
Nonbarbiturate tranquilizers
Antipsychotics
Antihistamines

their effectiveness; they have no long-term adverse effects on any organ; and, when taken in overdose by themselves, they are extremely safe.

Unfortunately, all these positive points lulled a great many people, physicians included, into considering benzodiazepines as perfect medications rather than excellent ones. Thus, fifteen years ago, when it was the most popular antianxiety drug prescribed, diazepam (Valium) received a great deal of negative publicity for its capacity to cause withdrawal symptoms. More recently, both alprazolam (Xanax) and triazolam (Halcion) have been criticized in the popular press for withdrawal phenomena in the case of the former and cognitive symptoms with the latter. (Since 1990, most of the media criticism has shifted to fluoxetine [Prozac], with which the identical cycle has occurred: hope for an effective new agent, then wildly unrealistic expectations leading to unwarranted excoriation when it became clear that this effective medication was not a savior for all that ails humankind.) All the criticisms have some basis in fact. Nonetheless, overall, benzodiazepines are still the best medications available to treat anxiety—when prescribed for the right people in the right doses for an appropriate length of time.

All benzodiazepines are equally effective as antianxiety agents. They are all somewhat sedating (as opposed to tranquilizing—see chapter 11), with clonazepam slightly more sedating than the others. In picking a specific benzodiazepine, the most important factor is the goal of the medication treatment. (Chapter 11 provides a detailed discussion of this topic.) If the purpose is to decrease anxiety during a period of extreme stress lasting for weeks and months, a long-acting medication, the effects of which will continue throughout the day, is best. Diazepam and clonazepam are examples of this type. If patients who need ongoing relief from anxiety are given a short-acting medication, they will need multiple doses throughout the day and will usually suffer from anxiety between doses as the effects of the medication wear off. On the other hand, patients who need treatment on a more intermittent basis—for example, during a particularly stressful day—will generally do better with a shorter-acting tranquilizer, such as alprazolam or lorazepam. Those who need only intermittent relief and take a long-acting benzodiazepine often complain of feeling drugged for many hours after the anxiety-provoking situation has passed. Frequently, however, patients will tell a psychopharmacologist at their first meeting that they took diazepam in the past for as-needed relief and did well with no hangover or untoward lingering effects. In these circumstances, it makes more sense to yield to patients' own individual experience than to treat them "according to the numbers."

Just as when they are prescribed for panic, the most important drawback to the benzodiazepines as antianxiety agents is their capacity to produce dependency and withdrawal symptoms when they are stopped. Here too, the short-acting medications are more likely to be a problem. Because of their potential for dependency, patients with a history of drug problems, especially with sedating drugs, such as alcoholics, should be treated with benzodiazepines only with extreme caution.

The other disadvantages of the benzodiazepines are their capacity to cause sedation and decrease cognitive capacity (see chapter 11 for details). With patients who operate heavy machinery or drive cars for a living, sedation may be a potential hazard, especially in the beginning of treatment before tolerance to the sedating effects of the benzodiazepines has occurred. Cognitive deficits are manifested primarily by a diminished ability to learn and recall new information. These effects are probably maximal in the initial stages of treatment.

Buspirone (Buspar), the other first-line antianxiety medication, is chemically unrelated to the benzodiazepines. It is completely nonsedating and shows no additive effects when combined with alcohol, thereby making it safe in many circumstances in which the benzodiazepines might pose a hazard. It is nonlethal when taken in overdose, holds no addictive potential whatsoever, and no withdrawal effects are seen at any dose when it is stopped abruptly. As a corollary to its nonsedating nature, however, buspirone is not effective in inducing sleep. Furthermore, it cannot be used on an as-needed basis; it is only effective if it is taken on a regular basis for at least one week. In this way it resembles antidepressants more than the benzodiazepines. The major concern with buspirone is its efficacy. Although the early studies comparing it to a variety of benzodiazepines demonstrated that the two classes of medications were equally effective, recent studies, as well as my experience and those of many colleagues, indicate that patients do not respond nearly as well to buspirone. Additionally, patients who have taken benzodiazepines in the past respond less well to buspirone (Olajide and Lader, 1987). Thus, the decreased recent response to buspirone may, in part, be due to its increasing use in patients with previous exposure to benzodiazepines. Whatever the cause, clinical experience casts some doubt on its efficacy. It may be an excellent choice, however, for sober alcoholics who complain of anxiety.

Although prescribed infrequently, cyclic antidepressants are effective agents for treating generalized anxiety. Imipramine has been used the most and seems as effective as diazepam in a number of research studies (Rickels, Downing, Schweizer, and Hassman, 1993). However, the use of tricyclics in treating generalized anxiety and short-term anxiety has been clinically limited by their side effects and the two-to-six-week delay in clinical improvement. Another approach often used by internists and general practitioners is to prescribe low doses of sedating antidepressants such as doxepin (Sinequan) or trazodone (Desyrel) to anxious patients in order to improve sleep and cause mild daytime sedation. When used in this way, the side effect of the medication (sedation) is being used for a therapeutic purpose. Few psychopharmacologists use sedating antidepressants as a sole treatment for anxiety.

Neither MAO inhibitors nor SSRIs have been systematically studied as treatments for generalized anxiety disorder without depression. This is especially unfortunate given the evidence of efficacy for both antidepressant classes in treating panic disorder. If SSRIs are prescribed for generalized anxiety, it would make more sense to prescribe either fluvoxamine (Luvox) or paroxetine (Paxil) initially since they are the two least stimulating agents in their class. For both MAOIs and SSRIs, my own clinical experience has been positive in a few treatment-refractory cases.

Barbiturates have been used to treat anxiety for over eighty years. Like the benzodiazepines, they are available in both short- and long-acting forms, thereby providing flexibility. Unfortunately, they are extremely addictive medications and can cause a serious withdrawal syndrome which includes grand mal seizures. In contrast to the benzodiazepines, they are also easily lethal when taken in overdose. For all these reasons, barbiturates are rarely prescribed for anxiety. Occasionally, a patient may experience some benefit beyond what might be seen with benzodiazepines when given an occasional dose of one of the shorter-acting barbiturates.

During the 1950s and early 1960s, a group of tranquilizers were released that formed a bridge between the barbiturates and the benzodiazepines. The most commonly prescribed of these was meprobamate (Miltown); the most notorious was methaqualone (Quaalude) which is no longer available in the United States. These medications, initially thought to be much safer and less addicting than the barbiturates, turned out to be neither. As with the barbiturates, there are few reasons to prescribe them at this time except for the occasional benzodiazepine-intolerant patient.

Beta-blockers are also occasionally used for generalized anxiety. They may be most effective with those patients whose anxiety symptoms are predominantly physiological—tremor, sweating, and fast heartbeat—with fewer psychological symptoms. Among the beta-blockers, propranolol (Inderal) has been used the most and is, unfortunately, also associated with the highest rate of side effects. At medium to high dose, propranolol can cause significant fatigue, insomnia, and nightmares. Antianxiety efficacy of the other beta-blockers has been rarely studied.

The other two classes of medications occasionally prescribed for anxiety symptoms are antipsychotics and antihistamines. The antipsychotics may successfully tranquilize and/or sedate some patients. However, the risk of significant side effects, including tardive dyskinesia, should make their use unusual. If they are used for otherwise unmanageable anxiety, the more sedating antipsychotics such as chlorpromazine are generally prescribed. Antihistamines are sedating medications that are occasionally taken by patients whose potential for addiction precludes the use of benzodiazepines.

Continuation and Maintenance Treatment of Generalized Anxiety

When antianxiety medications are prescribed briefly, as with adjustment disorders or for situational anxiety, continuation treatment is not a relevant issue. When the need for the medication no longer exists, it should be discontinued. Except when they have been taken intermittently, medications should virtually always be tapered since rebound symptoms, albeit short-lived, can be seen even after a few weeks of treatment with a short-acting benzodiazepine (Rickels, Fox, Greenblatt, Sandler, and Schless, 1988).

Many patients who suffer from chronic anxiety (typically more than one year) need not take tranquilizers continually. When placebo is substituted for diazepam in a double-blind manner with anxious patients who have been successfully treated, approximately half of them will not become anxious for the first month following drug discontinuation (Rickels, Case, Downing, and Winokur, 1983). Unfortunately, a majority of these patients will have a gradual return of symptoms within one year (Rickels, Case, Downing, and Friedman, 1986). When reexamined three years later, one quarter of patients who had originally successfully tapered their medication had returned to benzodiazepine use because of recurrent symptoms (Rickels, Case, Schweizer, Garcia-Espana, and Fridman, 1991). The implication of these findings is that even chronic anxiety waxes and wanes in intensity over months and years and that many patients can be managed by the intermittent use of benzodiazepines with good chance of benefit.

There is, however, a subgroup of chronically anxious patients who derive consistent relief from a stable dose of benzodiazepines taken over many years and who quickly become more anxious upon medication withdrawal, even if it is correctly tapered to avoid withdrawal effects. If there is no evidence of tolerance (the need for progressively larger doses), it is appropriate to continue these patients on their stable and safe dose of medication.

INSOMNIA

Sleeping problems affect one third of the population, most of whom never seek treatment (Mellinger, Balter, and Uhlenhuth, 1985). Since many psychiatric disorders are associated with insomnia, the proportion of sleeping problems in psychiatric outpatients is certainly higher. Insomnia, however, is a symptom and not a disorder. Therefore, reasonable treatments, pharmacological or otherwise, cannot be discussed before noting the most common causes of insomnia.

Diagnosis

Since there are no agreed-upon definitions of insomnia, it makes the most sense to describe it as a subjective sensation of sleeping poorly.

Most patients will complain that they do not sleep enough hours, although others report sufficient sleep that does not feel restful or refreshing. Another definition of insomnia, sometimes described as clinically relevant insomnia, adds the proviso of a daytime consequence of the sleep problem, such as daytime sleepiness. The great majority of people (but not all—see below) complaining of insomnia have genuine difficulties sleeping as documented by the findings of a sleep electroencephalogram (EEG), which documents with precision how long it takes patients to fall asleep, how many times they awaken, and how long they sleep.

When patients complain of poor sleep, they describe one or a combination of three patterns: difficulty falling asleep; disrupted sleep during the night, which is usually described as awakening multiple times and taking variable amounts of time to go back to sleep; or early morning awakening—getting up one or more hours before it is necessary or usual and being unable to go back to sleep. Although there are some stereotyped links between certain psychiatric disorders and patterns of insomnia, such as depression with early morning awakening or anxiety with difficulty falling asleep, there is enough variability to view this scheme with skepticism.

Table 4–7 lists the common causes of insomnia. Classification of sleep disorders has been in flux over the last decade, with each scheme using somewhat different terms for the same disorder. Whatever the classification system, the first distinction to make is between transient, externally generated causes of insomnia and more persistent types. Persistent insomnia, usually defined as lasting one month or more, should be divided into cases due to a specific cause and those reflecting a true primary sleep disorder. The most common sleep disorders are those related to transient, short-term, or situational stresses. These might be due to interpersonal conflicts, job stresses, moving from one house to another, changing jobs, or anxieties about health. Jet lag is also a common cause of transient insomnia.

Insomnia that persists beyond a few weeks may also be due to stress (interpersonal difficulties are certainly known to extend beyond a few weeks!) but is more likely to reflect some underlying disorder. Underlying psychiatric disorders are the most common etiology (35 percent) of persistent sleep problems in patients presenting to sleep disorder centers (Nofzinger, Buysse, Reynolds and Kupfer, 1993). Therefore, a patient who complains of persistent insomnia should be questioned about other depressive or anxiety symptoms (see chapter 3 and above for appropriate questions). Both unipolar and bipolar depression, mania or

Table 4–7
Common Causes of Insomnia

Transient

Situational stress
Jet lag

Persistent

Secondary to other conditions:
  Many psychiatric disorders—e.g., major depression, generalized anxiety, mania, etc.
  Drug and alcohol use
  Psychiatric medications, e.g., some antidepressants
  Medical disorders
  Medications for medical disorders
  Pain syndromes
Primary sleep disorders
  Sleep apnea
  Nocturnal myoclonus
  Restless legs syndrome
  Primary insomnia
    Psychophysiological insomnia
    Subjective insomnia (sleep state misperception)
    Idiopathic insomnia
    Inadequate sleep hygiene

hypomania, generalized anxiety, panic disorder, obsessive compulsive disorder, and post-traumatic stress as well as other psychiatric disorders can present with insomnia. Psychotic disorders such as schizophrenia virtually always present with insomnia, although these disorders are less common in outpatient practices.

The use of drugs and alcohol is another important cause of insomnia. Alcohol itself has powerful effects on sleep. Everyone is aware of how drinking helps induce sleep onset. Fewer people know that the same alcohol that helps them get to sleep will increase the likelihood of their awakening a few hours later due to alcohol's capacity to fragment and disrupt normal sleep patterns. When patients who have been drinking regularly stop, rebound insomnia will likely ensue, frequently setting up a desire to resume drinking in order to sleep—a strategy that exacerbates the problem. Similarly, if sleeping pills are stopped suddenly, rebound insomnia as well as nightmarish dreams are extremely common (see chapter 11 for details). It may seem that these situations would be easy to ascertain: patients would tell their therapists that they stopped drinking or taking sleeping pills and then had insomnia. More commonly, though, patients either hide the use of alcohol or hypnotics from the therapist or seem to have blocked this knowledge from themselves as well.

Stimulants, both illicit like cocaine and amphetamines and licit like caffeine drinks, can also cause insomnia. As with the use of sedatives, tranquilizers, and alcohol, patients may not be forthcoming about these substances unless asked.

Many medications appropriately prescribed for psychiatric purposes can also cause insomnia. Because they are often prescribed for disorders that are also associated with sleep disruption, the role of the medications can be obscured. Most common among these are antidepressants, especially the SSRIs, bupropion (Wellbutrin), MAO inhibitors, and the more stimulating tricyclics such as desipramine. Nighttime akathisia, caused by antipsychotics, may cause insomnia in some patients. Additionally, both a number of medical disorders (such as pain syndromes, a variety of respiratory ailments, and so on) as well as some of the medications used to treat them can also cause insomnia.

Among primary sleep disorders, three specific medical sleep disorders are sometimes found in patients with insomnia (Byerley and Gillin, 1984). Sleep apnea is characterized by multiple periods of stopping breathing for more than ten seconds while asleep. The resumption of breathing often causes patients to awaken with a start. Complaints of daytime sleepiness are common, and patients' bed partners will describe loud snoring and irregular breathing. Nocturnal myoclonus, characterized by multiple episodes of "jerking" of the legs, may awaken either patients or their bed partners, who may complain of being kicked by these jerks. Restless legs syndrome is the third of the specific sleep disorders. Patients with this disorder describe peculiar feelings in their legs that cause an irresistible need to move around. This often diminishes the sensation. In some ways, it is subjectively similar to akathisia caused by the antipsychotics (see chapter 12).

A minority of patients with persistent insomnia have neither an obvious psychiatric or medical disorder nor do they use substances or medications in a way that explains the sleep problem: in other words, they have primary insomnia. Table 4–7 lists some of the common subtypes of primary insomnia. In psychophysiological insomnia, the disorder is thought to reflect a predominantly conditioned behavior (Mendelson, 1993). It is assumed that a transient stress-related insomnia becomes persistent when patients focus on the problem and "try" to sleep. At that point, the heightened anxiety about the inability to sleep begins to be associated with typical sleep cues such as nighttime or being in bed and these become conditioned stimuli for insomnia. Despite relatively normal functioning in other areas of their lives, these patients become absorbed in the nightly struggle to sleep. It is likely that certain stable personality, temperamental, or psychophysiological traits such as being tense and easily aroused, tending to somatize distress, and possibly being a biologically light sleeper are also more common in this population (Roffwarg and Erman, 1985).

In subjective insomnia, also known as sleep state misperception, patients exhibit normal sleep patterns as documented by EEG, but still complain of poor sleep. Some observers feel that subjective insomnia is a transitional state between normal sleep and objective insomnia (Salin-Pascual, Roehrs, Merlotti, Zorick, and Roth, 1992). Patients with idiopathic insomnia simply do not sleep well (confirmed by EEG) but without the behaviorally linked problems of psychophysiological insomnia. Finally, some patients sleep poorly because they behave in ways that disrupt normal sleep patterns—e.g., working late into the night, keeping irregular sleep patterns, etc.

Certainly, therapists do not need to be able to distinguish among these various disorders. It would be helpful, though, to briefly evaluate a patient for some of the causes of insomnia if complaints of sleep difficulties arise. Are other symptoms of depression, mania, or anxiety present? Is the patient drinking or using drugs or has he recently changed his consumption of these substances? Spending a few minutes probing these few areas may yield a great deal of useful information.

Treatment

Hypnotics, defined as medications causing sleep, are a common treatment for insomnia. Yet their use has declined significantly over the last fifteen years. As an example, only half as many prescriptions for hypnotics were written in 1987 compared to the peak use in 1971 (Mendelson, 1985). Between 1987 and 1991, pharmacological treatments for insomnia, especially sleeping pills, continued to decrease (Walsh and Engelhardt, 1992). Still, the fact that over 4 percent of the entire population each year have been prescribed sleeping pills indicates the magnitude of our societal use of these medications. If one peruses any textbook or review article on the treatment of insomnia, it is clear that hypnotics are recommended only as a small part of the over-all treatment. Why then do so many people take them in real life? The most likely answer is that benzodiazepines, the most common hypnotics prescribed, are predominantly safe and effective. Although a sizeable percent of patients complaining of insomnia could successfully use nonpharmacological remedies, to do so would require more time from the doctor to do a more thorough evaluation and to explain the course of treatment—and more work for the patient. Especially in treating transient insomnia, it is simpler for physicians to prescribe and patients to take a sleeping pill as opposed to using any other method of treatment. A more problematic situation occurs when the hypnotics are refilled on a routine basis without a reevaluation of the ongoing need for them. However, the majority of patients taking hypnotics do so for less than two weeks (Mellinger, Balter, and Uhlenhuth, 1985).

In general, the decision to prescribe hypnotics should depend on the cause of the insomnia. When short-term use is needed—for example, for jet lag or transient stress—benzodiazepines are safe and effective. If the insomnia is due to another psychiatric disorder, such as depression or an anxiety disorder, sleeping pills may be used transiently in the beginning of treatment, but it is even more important that the underlying disorder is treated. Insomnia due to the use of stimulants or alcohol, or to the withdrawal of sedatives/tranquilizers should be treated by addressing the underlying condition. If sleep apnea, nocturnal myoclonus, or restless legs syndrome are suspected, patients should be referred to a sleep expert for evaluation and treatment. Patients with sleep apnea should not take hypnotics because of the risk of increasing the time of not breathing.

The thorniest problem arises with patients who have primary insomnia. (I am excluding those patients who sleep poorly because of inadequate sleep hygiene, for whom the recommended treatment is clear.) Without question, nonpharmacological approaches are best (Morin, Culbert, and Schwartz, 1994). The most important of these is described as good sleep hygiene, characterized by such habits as maintaining regular arousal times, exercising regularly, avoiding hunger at night, and the like (Hauri and Sateia, 1985). Other treatments include relaxation techniques, biofeedback, and other behavioral strategies. For those who do not cooperate with these techniques or for whom these approaches are unsuccessful, hypnotics are inevitably considered. When used in conjunction with nonpharmacological techniques, they can be extremely useful. What is less clear is whether their efficacy continues if taken over months and years (Gillin and Byerley, 1990). My own clinical experience is that some patients with chronic insomnia do maintain a good response to hypnotics over long periods of time.

Table 4–8 lists the classes of hypnotic medications. Overwhelmingly, benzodiazepines are the most commonly prescribed sleeping pills available. Along with zolpidem (Ambien), they are also the most effective. As with treating generalized anxiety, it is likely that all benzodiazepines are helpful as sleeping pills, even though not all agents in the class are officially labeled or FDA indicated as hypnotics. (As discussed in chapter 1, official FDA indications for medications do not always reflect efficacy.) Zolpidem shares some similarities to the benzodiazepines, but because it also has some unique biological effects, is classified separately. Clinically, however, it seems indistinguishable from a short-acting benzodiazepine. (See chapter 11 for more details.) For treating insomnia, the primary consideration is how long the medication lasts. Short-acting benzodiazepines such as triazolam (Halcion) and zolpidem, and intermediate-acting agents such as temazepam (Restoril) and alprazolam (Xanax) cause little hangover in the morning. The major disadvantage to the short-acting medications is the increased risk of causing dependence and precipitating withdrawal symptoms, including rebound insomnia, when they are stopped. The more long-acting benzodiazepines, such as flurazepam (Dalmane), cause more morning hangover but less dependence and fewer withdrawal symptoms when stopped. (See chapter 11 for more details on the different benzodiazepines and withdrawal symptoms.)

As noted earlier in the chapter, although both the barbiturates and the nonbarbiturate sedatives are effective as hypnotics and tranquilizers, they have been appropriately supplanted by the benzodiazepines.

Table 4–8
Pharmacotherapies of Insomnia

Benzodiazepines
Zolpidem
Sedating antidepressants
Sedating neuroleptics
Barbiturates and nonbarbiturate sedatives
Antihistamines
Over-the-counter hypnotics

Because of its reputation (albeit undeserved) as a safe drug, chloral hydrate has survived and is still used occasionally.

Sedating antidepressants are increasingly prescribed as hypnotics. Trazodone (Desyrel) has become the most popular agent used for this purpose because of its relative lack of side effects compared to other sedating antidepressants such as amitriptyline (Elavil) and doxepin (Sinequan). Antidepressants are often prescribed in situations in which the benzodiazepines are either ineffective or contraindicated (e.g., in recovering drug abusers or alcoholics). Sedating neuroleptics are also occasionally prescribed for insomnia. Similar to their use in treating anxiety, this practice is rarely appropriate.

Antihistamines may also be used to treat insomnia because they are sedating and nonaddictive. Their efficacy, however, is somewhat questionable, and they may cause paradoxical responses in some patients, especially the elderly. Over-the-counter hypnotics, generally containing a combination of an antihistamine and a sedating anticholinergic agent, are often taken by patients because they are so easy to obtain. They are only minimally effective and can cause a variety of side effects if taken in large quantities.

In the past, l-tryptophan was a commonly used, safe, nonaddictive, nonprescription hypnotic. Although probably not as effective as the benzodiazepines, it was helpful for mild insomnia. Currently, however, l-tryptophan is available only in low doses as part of multi-amino acid preparations. As a separate compound, it was removed from the market because of over 1,300 cases of allergic reactions, called the eosinophilia-myalgia syndrome, that resulted in at least fifteen deaths. Even though most cases of this allergic reaction were caused by an impurity present in only one manufacturer's batch, tryptophan as a solo agent has still not yet reappeared in health food stores (Belongia et al., 1990).

5

Schizophrenia and Related Disorders

O F ALL PSYCHIATRIC DISORDERS, schizophrenia is the one most synonymous with "mental illness" and "craziness," terms connoting a
severe and disabling disorder that makes other people uncomfortable
and fearful. Other common associations to schizophrenia are an inevitable deteriorating course, homelessness, chronic hospitalizations,
and pharmacological treatment that controls some symptoms but that
causes involuntary movements and is woefully inadequate in allowing
afflicted individuals to live meaningful lives. In some ways, these stereotypes are accurate: schizophrenia *is* the most severe of all psychiatric
disorders, usually characterized by a chronic course and frequently associated with recurrent and sometimes prolonged hospitalizations. No
more than one decade ago, approximately 25 percent of *all*, not just
psychiatric hospital beds in the United States were occupied by schizophrenic patients. (With the recent emphasis on avoiding hospitalizations and marked decreases in the lengths of inpatient stays, the current
figure is unknown.) In 1990, treatment costs of schizophrenia accounted for 2.5 percent of total health care expenditures (Rupp and
Keith, 1993). Between one third and one half of homeless individuals
have schizophrenia (Bachrach, 1992). Furthermore, it is also true that
the hallmark of schizophrenia is the prominence of psychotic or crazy
thinking. (No consensual definition of psychosis exists but as used here
it would include delusions, hallucinations, and/or disorganized speech.)

In many ways, however, these generalizations present too simplistic
a picture of schizophrenia. First, psychosis/craziness and schizophrenia
are far from synonymous; many other disorders—especially mania and
depression—are sometimes characterized by psychotic thinking and
are commonly associated with significant levels of psychosocial dysfunction. Second, the core elements of schizophrenia and the source of
its psychosocial disabilities—include not only psychotic symptoms but
also negative symptoms. With some patients, the psychosis is relatively
mild and is often present intermittently, not continually. Third, the
course of schizophrenia is far more variable than sometimes thought,

with progressive deterioration not a universal outcome. Finally, the pharmacotherapy of schizophrenia is entering a new era: medications available within the last five years and more that will be released in the next decade are qualitatively different—both more effective and with fewer side effects—than those available in the past. Therefore, without minimizing the pain and suffering associated with schizophrenia, there is reason for cautious optimism.

DIAGNOSIS

The overidentification of psychosis with schizophrenia, often expressed as the assumption that all psychotic patients are schizophrenic until proven otherwise—has been one of the most prominent, destructive, and incorrect principles in American psychiatry during the last fifty years. As recently as the early 1970s, medical students (including me) at good medical schools were being taught that "a touch of schizophrenia is schizophrenia"; that any bizarre or psychotic symptom that wasn't absolutely mood congruent and classic for mania or depression should be taken as evidence of schizophrenia regardless of whatever other clinical signs, symptoms, or family history features were also present. Additionally, American psychiatry was swayed by Bleuler's concept of schizophrenia with its emphasis on the "four As": autistic thinking, ambivalence, abnormalities in affect, and disturbed associations. Because this definition de-emphasized overt psychotic thought (such as delusions and hallucinations), it allowed patients to be diagnosed as schizophrenic because of inferred "schizophrenic" thought processes. By blurring the diagnostic boundaries of schizophrenia in these two ways—equating any psychotic thinking with schizophrenia and inferring schizophrenic thinking—American psychiatry broadened the boundaries of the schizophrenic diagnosis to unmanageable proportions. The most telling demonstration of this occurred twenty-five years ago with a study in which diagnostic principles in the United States and Great Britain were compared (Cooper, Kendall, & Kurland, 1972). Using a set of consistent diagnostic criteria and examining a series of consecutive admissions to hospital, the investigators found approximately equal numbers of schizophrenic and manic-depressive patients in Brooklyn and London. In reviewing the local diagnoses of these same patients, the investigators found that London psychiatrists had approximately the same diagnosis as did the study, whereas the Brooklyn psychiatrists had diagnosed schizophrenia *eight* times as often as manic-depressive illness! For mania specifically, of the twenty-two patients diagnosed as manic by the study criteria, twenty-one of them were diagnosed as schizophrenic by the local psychiatrists.

The impact of these inaccurate diagnoses became magnified beginning in the 1950s when medication treatment for different disorders became available. Since a diagnosis of schizophrenia suggested the use of antipsychotics while manic-depressive patients were more appropriately treated with lithium, inaccurate diagnoses led to inaccurate treatment, with a real and potentially tragic impact on prognosis.

Since that time, the diagnostic pendulum has swung again, initially toward narrowing the definition of schizophrenia with an almost exclusive emphasis on psychotic symptoms and now beginning to shift toward a more middle-ground approach in which both psychotic symptoms and negative symptoms are equally considered. As with the other psychiatric disorders in this book, our current diagnostic criteria for schizophrenia are an amalgam of accumulated wisdom, data-based knowledge, and historical trends. As these change, so will our criteria. The current criteria should be considered a guide to diagnosis and *not* the revealed truth.

Unlike mood disorders, in which all patients, by definition, must have a disturbance in mood, schizophrenia has no core identifying characteristic. No symptom is diagnostic of schizophrenia, seen in that disorder and in no other, nor is any symptom common to all schizophrenic patients. The "Schneiderian" symptoms, which are a group of psychotic symptoms thought to be pathognomonic of schizophrenia, have been demonstrated to be present in a variety of other disorders, including mood disorders (Pope and Lipinski, 1978). Similarly, Bleuler's "split" in schizophrenia, which the lay public misidentifies as multiple or split personalities, but which refers to the splitting of "the associative threads that tied together the fabric of thought" (Pfohl and Andreasen, 1986), is too unreliable a description to be used as a diagnostic key. Given its diverse expressions, it is likely that schizophrenia, rather than being one disorder, is a heterogeneous syndrome with a number of disease processes responsible for different symptom clusters (Andreasen and Carpenter, 1993).

The core features of DSM-IV's definition of schizophrenia are a prolonged episode (lasting at least six months) in which (1) prominent psychotic symptoms and/or negative symptoms are present for at least one month, (2) psychosocial functioning is markedly impaired, and (3) a major mood syndrome, if it exists, is relatively brief compared to the schizophrenic symptoms. Typically, there is a prodromal phase and a residual phase during the six-month minimum length of a schizophrenic episode. Table 5–1 shows the DSM-IV criteria for schizophrenia.

The clinical symptoms that may be seen and are consistent with the diagnosis of schizophrenia are varied and include a veritable laundry list of delusions, hallucinations, fractured cognitions, bizarre behaviors, and emotional deficits (negative symptoms). DSM-IV has a particularly succinct and excellent description of these features (American Psychiatric Association, 1994a, pp. 274–280). Any clinician seeing a patient in the active phase of a schizophrenic episode will have no trouble recognizing the profound disturbance of thought. Making the diagnosis during the prodromal phase is much more difficult, especially for those patients who simply withdraw. An 18-year-old who presents with marked social isolation, dropping out of school, and lack of initiative meets three of the nine prodromal symptoms, yet it would be exceedingly difficult to know whether this is prodromal schizophrenia, atypical depression (assuming the classic sleep, appetite, or other symptoms were not present), or some version of adolescent regression secondary to an adjustment disorder or personality disorder. Other prodromal signs such as odd beliefs (e.g., magical thinking), unusually vague or concrete speech, or prominent talking to oneself lead the diagnosis more towards schizophrenia and away from other psychiatric disorders. Nonetheless, it is often only in retrospect that the symptoms are recognized as prodromal signs of schizophrenia. Of course, if a patient has had at least one previous episode, it is important to know his prodromal signs in order to diagnose more accurately the prodromal phase of an episode as early as possible.

In comparison to DSM-III-R, DSM-IV simplified the criteria for schizophrenia while making them more compatible with other international diagnostic systems. The two most important changes in DSM-IV are in placing greater emphasis on negative symptoms while expanding the required duration of active symptoms from one week to one month.

As noted in the DSM-IV criteria, schizophrenic symptoms may be classified as either positive or negative. The current greater emphasis on negative symptoms as core aspects of schizophrenia reflects the rediscovery of a classic observation, noted by Krapelin, Bleuler and others in the nineteenth and early twentieth centuries and then underemphasized in this country for many decades until recently. Positive symptoms are cognitive difficulties and unusual experiences, sensations, or beliefs present in schizophrenia and generally absent in normal functioning. These include hallucinations and delusions. Negative symptoms are those capacities present in normal behavior that are ab-

Table 5–1
Diagnostic Criteria for Schizophrenia

A. *Characteristic symptoms:* Two (or more) of the following, each present for a significant portion of time during a 1-month period (or less if successfully treated):
   (1) delusions
   (2) hallucinations
   (3) disorganized speech (e.g., frequent derailment or incoherence)
   (4) grossly disorganized or catatonic behavior
   (5) negative symptoms, i.e., affective flattening, alogia, or avolition
   Note: Only one Criterion A symptom is required if delusions are bizarre or hallucinations consist of a voice keeping up a running commentary on the person's behavior or thoughts, or two or more voices conversing with each other.

B. *Social/occupational dysfunction:* For a significant portion of the time since the onset of the disturbance, one or more major areas of functioning such as work, interpersonal relations, or self-care are markedly below the level achieved prior to the onset (or when the onset is in childhood or adolescence, failure to achieve expected level of interpersonal, academic, or occupational achievement).

C. *Duration:* Continuous signs of the disturbance persist for at least 6 months. This 6-month period must include at least 1 month of symptoms (or less if successfully treated) that meet Criterion A (i.e., active-phase symptoms) and may include periods of prodromal or residual symptoms. During these prodromal or residual periods, the signs of the disturbance may be manifested by only negative symptoms or two or more symptoms listed in Criterion A present in an attenuated form (e.g., odd beliefs, unusual perceptual experiences).

D. *Schizoaffective and Mood Disorder exclusion:* Schizoaffective Disorder and Mood Disorder With Psychotic Features have been ruled out because either (1) no Major Depressive, Manic, or Mixed Episodes have occurred concurrently with the active-phase symptoms; or (2) if mood episodes have occurred during active-phase symptoms, their total duration has been brief relative to the duration of the active and residual periods.

E. *Substance/general medical condition exclusion:* The disturbance is not due to the direct physiological effects of a substance (e.g., a drug of abuse, a medication) or a general medical condition.

F. *Relationship to a Pervasive Developmental Disorder:* If there is a history of Autistic Disorder or another Pervasive Developmental Disorder, the additional diagnosis of Schizophrenia is made only if prominent delusions or hallucinations are also present for at least a month (or less if successfully treated).

sent or diminished in schizophrenia. These symptoms include lack of motivation (avolition/apathy), affective flattening, lack of social interest and skills (asociality), anhedonia, and poverty of speech. However, many other symptoms are more difficult to classify and are considered either positive or negative, depending on the rating system. Examples of these ambiguous symptoms are thought disorder, bizarre behavior, and inappropriate affect (McGlashan and Fenton, 1992). The distinction between positive and negative symptoms has been used in a proposed scheme for subtyping schizophrenic syndromes (see below).

Although not specifically noted as part of the core criteria for the disorder, depressive symptoms and syndromes are common in schizophrenia. Some depressive syndromes are manifested by the classic symptoms of major depressive episode while others are expressed in self-reported sadness, depressed mood, social withdrawal and suicidal ideation.

Depressive syndromes may be seen in any phase of a schizophrenic disorder. Depressive symptoms are common as part of the prodromal phase of an episode, with overt psychosis emerging later (Green, Nuechterlein, Ventura, and Mintz, 1990). In the midst of a florid psychotic episode, depressive symptoms are prominent, diminishing along with the psychosis (Knights and Hirsch, 1981). A more typical depressive syndrome, with or without the vegetative signs of depression, occurs in up to 25 percent of schizophrenic patients, frequently manifesting itself soon after the resolution of an acute psychotic episode (Siris, 1991; McGlashan and Carpenter, 1976). DSM-IV recognizes this syndrome (in the Appendix as a criteria set provided for further study), calling it the postpsychotic depressive disorder of schizophrenia when the full criteria for major depressive episode are met during the residual phase of the disorder.

The meaning or etiology of the depressive syndromes of schizophrenia has long been debated. It is likely that these syndromes represent a number of different clinical phenomena. These include: a prodromal phase of the disorder, part of an active psychotic phase, side effects from the neuroleptic medication (a.k.a. akinetic depression, or severe akathisia precipitating an intense dysphoric response—see chapter 12 for details), negative symptoms, disappointment/demoralization, a misdiagnosis (e.g., the patient has a mood disorder with psychosis, rather than schizophrenia), or a true depressive syndrome superimposed on schizophrenia. For each patient, the therapeutic plan follows from the conceptualization of the depression. For instance, depressive symptoms as part of a prodromal phase of an acute episode or from the episode itself would be treated by neuroleptics. If the depressive state represents side effects from antipsychotic medication, lowering the dose, adding another medication to decrease the side effect, or switching to a different neuroleptic would be appropriate (see chapter 12). Depressive symptoms, if mild and characterized predominantly by anhedonia and poor motivation, may represent negative symptoms and might be treated by one of the newer neuroleptics or by a structured psychosocial program. Disappointment/demoralization would be best combated by supportive psychotherapy and possibly a more enriched psychosocial program. If the postpsychotic depression is actually a bipolar depression following a psychotic mania in a patient who has been misdiagnosed as schizophrenic, the appropriate maneuver would be to stop the antipsychotic medication and start a mood stabilizer and possibly an antidepressant. A true postpsychotic depression of schizophrenia may be effectively treated by antidepressants (discussed later in this chapter).

Regardless of the way in which depressive symptoms in schizophrenia are conceptualized, it is clear that suicide is a significant risk for patients with the disorder. Approximately 10 percent of schizophrenia patients will ultimately commit suicide (Miles, 1977), and the majority of those who do will have suffered from a depressive syndrome (Roy, 1990). Although suicides may occur at any phase of the illness, most occur during a less active phase of the illness and not during a florid psychotic relapse. The time of highest risk for schizophrenic suicides is after discharge from hospital following an acute psychotic episode and early in the course of illness (Caldwell and Gottesman, 1990). The usual clinical clues—hopelessness, depressive symptoms, communication of suicidal ideation and intent—are somewhat predictive, although schizophrenic suicide may also occur without warning.

Some symptoms, predominantly those described as evidence of a thought disorder or blunted or inappropriate affect, will be apparent in the clinical interview. Other symptoms must be elicited by specific questions. However, patients who have had these symptoms will often deny them because of paranoia or fear of the consequences of admitting to them, or because they hear voices instructing them not to tell anyone about these experiences. Therefore, as with so many other major psychiatric disorders, the use of outside informants, such as husbands, wives, or parents, is sometimes vital in gathering the appropriate information. For instance, despite the patients' denial of hallucinations, their families may describe them as having conversations when no one is present or as seeming to respond to voices not heard by others.

Therapists who do not frequently work with patients who experience the overtly psychotic symptoms seen in schizophrenia may find it difficult to ask specific questions about psychotic thoughts. Sample questions are listed here.

Have you ever felt as if people were trying to harm you? Do you have any idea why they wanted to harm you? (Frequently, probing for the rationale for the paranoia will elicit other psychotic thoughts.)

Does it seem that people are talking about you or making comments about you when you are in public? (A yes answer could indicate either ideas of reference or auditory hallucinations that are being attributed to passersby.)

Do you ever get the feeling that the radio or television is giving you special or specific messages? When you drive, do you ever think that the numbers or letters of the license plates of cars near you have special meaning?

Have you ever heard voices that other people couldn't hear? How often does this occur? What do the voices say? Were they telling you to do things? What were they telling you to do? (If yes, ask specifically whether the command hallucinations suggested potentially violent acts, such as suicide or homicide. Although they are an infrequent precipitant of suicide in schizophrenics, command hallucinations about suicide/homicide, when present, need to be taken seriously.) Did you hear more than one voice? Did they talk to each other about you?

(NOTE: Sometimes, patients will draw a distinction between voices heard inside and outside the head. The meaning of this distinction is unknown. The most important distinction would be between a thought and actually hearing a voice regardless of location. Also, people sometimes describe hearing whispers or hearing someone call their name as they go to sleep. If it only occurs at that time, it does not have major pathological significance.

Visual, tactile [feeling, tingling or crawling], or olfactory [smell] hallucinations also occur in schizophrenia but are less common than auditory hallucinations. The presence of these other types of hallucinations in the absence of auditory hallucinations suggests other diagnoses, such as drug-induced psychoses or some neurological disorders.)

Has it ever seemed that your thoughts were being broadcast out loud so that others could hear them?

Does it ever seem that your thoughts are not your own? Does it ever seem that someone is putting thoughts into your head, or taking them out of your head?

Does it seem as if your body is not your own or that someone else is in control of your body?

(NOTE: My experience of asking these questions is that patients who have never had the symptom in question, especially any of the last few listed above, will frequently not understand the question, since these experiences are somewhat bizarre, and will look at you blankly.)

SUBTYPES OF SCHIZOPHRENIA

With its extraordinary variability of clinical presentation, schizophrenia has traditionally been divided into subtypes. The most common and traditional of these classifications, used in DSM-IV, divides schizophrenia into paranoid, disorganized (formerly hebephrenic), catatonic, undifferentiated, and residual subtypes. The first three subtypes are characterized by symptom patterns that exist during an acute exacerbation of the disorder. The undifferentiated type refers to any patient who is schizophrenic but who does not meet criteria for any of the other subtypes. Residual schizophrenia describes patients who have had at least one schizophrenic episode and are currently mildly symptomatic.

Some consistent differences between the three discrete subtypes exist in age of onset and course of disorder (Fenton and McGlashan, 1991). Paranoid schizophrenics have the latest age of onset and the best outcome while patients with the disorganized subtype tend to manifest an insidious onset of the disorder and the worst prognosis. Despite these generalizations, the clinical utility of subtyping schizophrenia according to these traditional categories is unclear. As an example, a patient with one type may, over time, evolve into another type. Moreover, there is little evidence that treatment considerations differ among the types. Finally, family studies also indicate that the subtypes do not "breed true" within families; that is, in the families of patients with paranoid schizophrenia, there is no higher likelihood of seeing paranoid subtypes than other subtypes (Kendler, McGuire, Gruenberg, and Walsh, 1994). Until more is known, the practice of subtyping according to the traditional scheme is not clinically useful.

Another subtyping scheme makes use of the positive/negative symptom dichotomy. As originally described by Crow (1980), Type 1 and Type 2 schizophrenia are different syndromes, or "dimensions of pathology," which might reflect different underlying pathologies. These were not meant to define two distinct subtypes of the disorder. Some patients may have both types of syndrome, while others may shift from predominantly positive to negative symptoms over time. Type 1 syndrome of schizophrenia is characterized by a good premorbid course, predominantly positive symptoms, acute episodes with good response to antipsychotics, and complete remissions in which a chronic downhill course is not seen. Biologically, Type 1 schizophrenia is thought to reflect normal brain structure and evidence of excessive dopamine activity (explaining these patients' response to antipsychotics/dopamine blockers). Type 2 schizophrenia, on the other hand, is characterized by poor premorbid course, insidious onset, relatively poor response to antipsychotics, and a progressive downhill course with intellectual impairment. It is hypothesized that patients with Type 2 syndrome have a decrease in brain dopamine and would show evidence of brain cell loss (usually described as enlarged ventricles) on neuroimaging studies, such as CT scans or PET scans.

Substantial evidence exists supporting the subtyping of schizophrenic disorders by the predominance of negative symptoms. Earlier studies found some clustering among abnormal CT scans, poor intellectual function, and poor response to medication. Negative symptoms are consistently associated with poor premorbid functioning and poorer long-term outcome and seem to increase over the first decade of the illness. Furthermore, most studies find little to no relationship between positive and negative symptoms, implying that they represent independent processes (McGlashan and Fenton, 1992). However, the results of other studies do not consistently support the Type 1/Type 2 dichotomy according to the criteria described above. A possible explanation for this has been that the concept of negative symptoms was too broad and included both permanent (called primary) and temporary (or secondary) symptoms. Examples of primary, enduring negative symptoms are restricted affect, anhedonia, and diminished social drive.

Secondary negative symptoms appear similar but are caused by treatable factors such as the effects of depression, neuroleptic side effects, social withdrawal due to psychosis, and social deprivation. Using this refinement of the Type 1/Type 2 dichotomy, patients are now described as exhibiting either the deficit (with primary negative symptoms) or nondeficit forms of schizophrenia (Carpenter, Heinrichs, and Wagman, 1988). Patients with deficit schizophrenia are more likely to show neurological impairment, psychophysiological abnormalities, and greater impairment on neuropsychological tests (Buchanan et al., 1994).

A third typology which has gained increasing support recently and is listed in the Appendix of DSM-IV divides the symptoms of schizophrenia into three dimensions: psychotic (delusions and hallucinations), negative (deficit symptoms noted above), and disorganized (disorganized speech, behavior, or inappropriate affect) (Andreasen, Arndt, Alliger, Miller, and Flaum, 1995). The predictive utility of this scheme has yet to be determined.

Over the last fifteen years, it has become increasingly clear that in a subgroup of schizophrenic patients, the disorder arises in the later part of life, typically during the forties, fifties, and sixties. In the past, these late-onset disorders were called paraphrenias; DSM-III labeled them atypical psychoses. However, because the disorder is very similar to classic early-onset schizophrenia, DSM-III-R and DSM-IV no longer describe it as a separate disorder, merely noting that schizophrenia can begin later in life. In comparison to the early-onset disorder, late-onset schizophrenia affects predominantly females and is characterized by increased paranoid symptoms and auditory hallucinations with less inappropriate affect and loose associations. Late onset schizophrenia also has a greater tendency towards chronicity. The psychotic symptoms do respond to antipsychotics, typically at lower doses than are used with younger patients (Jeste, Paulsen, and Harris, 1995). Clinically, the implication is that although a nonmood psychosis (i.e., one that does not occur in the context of a full mood syndrome) arising in early adulthood is still the most common form of schizophrenia, the diagnosis cannot be ruled out because of a late age of onset.

NATURAL HISTORY, EPIDEMIOLOGY, AND GENETICS

Schizophrenia is a disorder that typically first appears in early adult life. It tends to arise a few years later in women than men with an average age of first psychotic episode in the early twenties for men and the mid-twenties for women (Loranger, 1984). Schizophrenia affects from 0.5 to 1.5 percent of the population over a lifetime (American Psychiatric Association, 1994a). Most, but not all, studies find the rate of schizophrenia to be slightly higher among men than women (Lewine, 1988).

The long-term outcome of schizophrenia is a topic that has been investigated repeatedly over the last hundred years. In fact, Kraepelin used a long-term poor prognosis as one of his key diagnostic features to distinguish schizophrenia from manic-depressive illness. As a generalization, chronic illness is the likely outcome in schizophrenia (McGlashan 1988). Yet, the outcome for patients with this disorder that is almost assuredly composed of a number of different subforms is, not surprisingly, heterogeneous. Some studies, evaluating patients over decades, find a substantial subset of patients with the disorder who have a relatively good long-term outcome as defined by work productivity, social functioning, and a lack of symptoms (Harding, Brooks, Ashikaga, Strauss, and Breier, 1987). As a generalization, functional deterioration is maximal during the first five to ten years of the illness, following which there is a plateau or even improvement. Other than primary negative symptoms which predict an overall poor prognosis, the best predictor in any sphere of functioning is the history of premorbid functioning in that area (Strauss and Carpenter, 1974). Thus, a good work history prior to the first schizophrenic episode will predict a good capacity to work after illness onset, but not necessarily a good prognosis for socializing. Cross-sectional psychopathology—that is, the number or severity of symptoms during an acute relapse—is not strongly associated with long-term outcome. Therefore, given the diversity of outcome and our limited ability to predict it with any accuracy, in the initial years of the disorder *no* schizophrenic patient should be treated as an untreatable hopeless case.

Of all the psychiatric disorders, the familial and genetic roots of schizophrenia have been studied the most intensively. There is little doubt that schizophrenia is a familial disorder—that is, there is a significantly higher risk of schizophrenia in the relatives of schizophrenics than in the general population or in the families of patients with other major psychiatric disorders. This increased risk is approximately ten times higher than the risk for the general population (Kendler and Diehl, 1993). Demonstrating that a disorder is familial, however, does not help distinguish between environmental and genetic factors. Studies comparing monozygotic (identical) and dizygotic (fraternal) twins and studies of adopted-away children of schizophrenic parents *do* help make this distinction. The results of these studies give strong evidence that schizophrenia is not only familial but a genetic disorder as well (Kety et al., 1994; Onstad, Skre, Torgersen, and Kringlen, 1991).

Among the schizophrenia spectrum disorders, the evidence is strongest that schizotypal disorder and schizoaffective disorder, depressed type, are genetically linked to schizophrenia, while the evidence for paranoid disorder and atypical psychosis is far weaker (Kendler et al., 1993a; Kendler et al., 1993b).

DISORDERS RELATED TO SCHIZOPHRENIA

Schizophreniform Disorder

DSM-IV uses six months as the minimum time criterion for diagnosing schizophrenia. A disorder characterized by the symptoms of schizophrenia lasting less than six months—including prodromal and residual periods—and that may not necessarily be associated with the same degree of social or occupational impairment is called schizophreniform disorder. When patients with this disorder are followed for longer periods of time, it is clear that schizophreniform disorder is composed of an amalgam of different syndromes (Strakowski, 1994). The majority of schizophreniform patients have schizophrenia that simply has not yet lasted long enough to qualify for the diagnosis. However, other schizophreniform patients probably have a psychotic mood disorder or schizoaffective disorder, while a smaller subgroup have a brief, recurrent good prognosis psychotic disorder. Thus, it should be assumed that the "true" diagnosis for most patients with schizophreniform disorder will became manifest within months to years and, until then, a definitive diagnosis should not be made.

Schizoaffective Disorder

It is difficult to discuss schizoaffective disorder without first noting that the number of different criteria sets used to define the disorder over the last twenty years makes generalizations precarious. In the 1970s, the Research Diagnostic Criteria gave explicit criteria for schizoaffective disorder, dividing it into mainly schizophrenic and mainly affective subtypes (Spitzer, Endicott, and Robins, 1978). DSM-III gave no specific criteria for schizoaffective disorder, in part because of the lack of consensus in the committee studying it. DSM-III-R and now DSM-IV do give defining characteristics, however, and they comprise a reasonable middle ground among the varying definitions. DSM-IV schizoaffective disorder is characterized by an uninterrupted period of illness during which, at the same time: (1) a full manic or depressive syndrome coexists with the psychotic symptoms (the "A" criterion in Table 5–1) of schizophrenia; (2) there has been a period of at least two weeks of hallucinations or delusions in the absence of prominent mood symptoms; and (3) the mood symptoms are present for a substantial portion of the total duration of the illness, including prodromal and residual periods. If the mood syndrome has been manic or mixed, the disorder is called schizoaffective disorder, bipolar type (schizomanic); if depressive, schizoaffective disorder, depressive type (schizodepressive). Thus, a patient with schizoaffective disorder will have an affectively colored psychotic period and a contiguous period of psychosis without mood symptoms with the additional proviso that the purely psychotic symptoms not temporally dominate the overall clinical picture. This last requirement acknowledges that schizophrenic patients can become intermittently depressed without needing to change the diagnosis to schizoaffective disorder.

Barney, now 31 years old, has had psychiatric problems since he was 18. At that time, during his senior year in high school, he started using street drugs. Even when not using drugs, however, he became progressively more emotionally labile and had poor concentration, in marked contrast to his previously excellent school performance. At age 19, he had his first overt psychotic episode, characterized by grandiose, expansive thinking and delusions of grandeur (believing he was the reincarnation of God and was sent here to save the world), along with poor sleep and hyperactivity. Barney was soon hospitalized, during which time he lapsed into a severe depression sleeping fourteen hours nightly, staying in bed, and gaining twenty pounds. He recovered from this episode with medications. From age 21 through 24, Barney had three episodes similar to the first one, except that the psychotic symptoms now occurred during the depressive phases as well as the hyperactive ones. The psychosis also became progressively more bizarre, including somatic delusions and prominent hallucinations. Between episodes, Barney was able to function and showed no evidence of psychosis. He enrolled in college and passed his courses. Yet his capacities seemed less than they had been before his first psychotic episode.

When he was 26, Barney had another psychotic episode, similar to earlier ones. However, after recovery from the depression, he noted that as he drove through the city, license plates held symbolic meanings for him—a license plate with more than one three meant that the holy trinity was watching over him, while the presence of sixes indicated that the devil was after him. He also had frequent feelings that people were commenting on his behavior as he walked through the streets. In class he sometimes would feel that when his classmates shifted in their chairs, their body postures indicated their approval or disapproval of him. Barney was treated with both psychotherapy and a variety of medications including antipsychotics, mood stabilizers, and antidepressants. Although the intensity of symptoms clearly diminished with treatment, Barney continued to experience recurrent psychotic mood episodes with residual psychotic symptoms between episodes.

But what is schizoaffective disorder? Is it a subset of schizophrenia? An unusual looking mood disorder? A separate psychotic disorder? Not surprisingly, the evidence is mixed (Lapensee, 1992a; Levitt and Tsuang, 1988). As a group, schizoaffective patients have family histories with increased genetic loading for both schizophrenia *and* mood disorders. The prognosis for schizoaffective disorder tends to be better than that for schizophrenia and worse than that for mood disorders. Schizoaffective patients respond better to lithium (and probably to other mood stabilizers) than do schizophrenics, but not as well as bipolar patients. Currently, it is most helpful to view schizoaffective disorder as being composed of both schizophrenic and mood-disordered patients, all of whom show atypical symptoms and symptom combinations.

Two subtyping schemes may help distinguish subtypes of schizoaffective disorder with different prognoses and possibly different treatment responses. The first of these schemes divides the disorder into schizomania and schizodepression. Many but not all studies find that schizomania is closer to bipolar disorder than to classic schizophrenia. The family histories of schizomanic patients are generally loaded with mood disorders and not with schizophrenia. They frequently respond to mood stabilizers. Their prognosis is reasonably good—similar to that of bipolar disorder and not to schizophrenia. Schizodepression, on the other hand, is probably closer to classic schizophrenia. Families of patients with schizodepression show significant loading for schizophrenia and not as much for bipolar disorder; generally, these patients respond better to antipsychotics than to mood stabilizers; their prognosis is not as good as that of mood disordered patients and is much closer to that of schizophrenic patients.

The other subtyping scheme divides schizoaffective disorder into chronic and nonchronic forms. For schizomania and schizodepression, patients whose symptoms are more chronic and less episodic have worse prognoses (Coryell, Keller, Lavori, and Endicott 1990a; Coryell, Keller, Lavori, and Endicott, 1990b).

Delusional Disorder

Delusional disorder is DSM-IV's term for what was previously called paranoid disorder. It is characterized by a persistent nonbizarre delusion that is relatively unchanging and not associated with the fragmented thinking or the psychosocial and occupational dysfunction of schizophrenia. There has been astonishingly little research published on the disorder. It has weak genetic links to schizophrenia and may be more related to paranoid personality disorder (Manschreck, 1992). Antipsychotics are generally prescribed since, like delusions of any cause, the delusions in this disorder tend to be refractory to psychotherapeutic intervention. Unfortunately, it is not known how helpful antipsychotics are in treating delusional disorder, because virtually no treatment studies exist and patients with this disorder are rare enough that there is little accumulated clinical wisdom (Kendler, 1980).

> For Erica, the evidence that her husband was having an affair was overwhelming. There was the time he came home with a wrinkle in his pants in a place usually unwrinkled; or the night when he arrived home fifteen minutes later than usual and slightly out of breath. The fact that he had just walked up the two flights of stairs to their apartment was irrelevant to her. She had even hired a detective to follow her husband, but he had found no evidence of an extramarital affair. Her conclusion was that her husband had discovered her plan to hire a private detective, had found this one first, and paid him to lie to her. Occasionally, she would threaten to expose her husband's philandering at his place of work, or to kill him and herself together, but she never made any moves toward carrying out these threats. Divorce was not an option, she said.
>
> Erica's certainty that her husband was having an affair had gradually intensified over the last few years of their ten-year marriage. Yet despite the energy she invested in her belief, Erica held a full-time job at a flower store and kept the house running well. She did not tell her few friends of her belief about her husband. During the one visit she and her husband had with me, she denied hallucinations or more global fears of persecution. At the end of the visit, she made it clear that she had no desire for individual treatment, nor was couples' therapy needed—only that her husband confess his affair and stop. Not surprisingly, they never returned for a second visit.

The somatic subtype of delusional disorder, characterized by a delusional belief in a physical defect, can be considered the psychotic version of body dysmorphic disorder, in which patients are preoccupied with an imagined or slight defect in appearance (Phillips, McElroy, Keck, Pope, and Hudson, 1993). Although DSM-IV classifies body dysmorphic disorder as a somatoform disorder and its delusional equivalent as a psychotic disorder, many observers consider it an obsessive compulsive spectrum disorder (Hollander, Cohen, and Simeon, 1993). The presence of a delusional vs. a nondelusional belief in the physical defect is not associated with differences in other aspects of the disorder such as course, demographics, or treatment response. Consistent with the view that the somatic subtype of delusional disorder is misclassified, body dysmorphic disorder with delusional belief seems to respond relatively well to SSRIs and poorly to antipsychotics (Phillips, McElroy, Keck, Hudson, and Pope, 1994).

Schizotypal Personality Disorder

It is likely that schizotypal personality disorder should be viewed as a schizophrenia spectrum disorder. Because it is classified as a personality disorder in DSM-IV, however, it will be discussed in chapter 7 with the other personality disorders.

MEDICAL DIFFERENTIAL DIAGNOSIS

If we ignore the brief psychoses frequently seen on medical wards due to acute illness, postoperative metabolic imbalance, and so forth (which, presumably, nonmedical psychotherapists almost never see), the list of medical diagnoses that resemble schizophrenia is not very long. This stems not from a lack of possibilities but from the dilemma that what we call schizophrenia is itself probably composed of a variety of neuropsychiatric diseases that, at present, are indistinguishable from each other. The major medical/neuropsychiatric disorders that can present with the psychotic symptom cluster seen in schizophrenia are described in DSM-IV as Psychotic Disorder Due to a General Medical Condition (a.k.a. Organic Mental Disorder in DSM-III-R, a term that has been eliminated because of the etiological connotations). Occasionally, temporal lobe epilepsy and brain tumors may present with schizophrenia-like states. Usually, though, signs of the primary neurological disorder, such as a documented history of seizures or asymmetric weakness, will simultaneously exist. In general, the presence of marked disorientation, confusion, memory impairment, possibly older age of onset (i.e., after age 30), and nonauditory hallucinations as the prominent perceptual symptom are helpful clues that point towards a general medical condition as the etiology of the psychotic state and away from schizophrenia. These signs and symptoms should make the therapist and/or psychiatrist consider a neurological evaluation.

Substance-induced psychotic disorder, delirium, or persistent dementia, those psychotic states caused acutely or chronically by the use of street drugs or alcohol, are the most important group of disorders that may present with schizophrenia-like states. Ongoing use of stimulants, especially amphetamines, can be indistinguishable from acute paranoid schizophrenia. Acute or chronic use of PCP (phencyclidine) or LSD can also precipitate a schizophrenic-like psychosis. Often complicating the clinical picture, schizophrenic patients use street drugs and excessive alcohol at higher rates than the general population. The superimposition of a drug-induced psychosis on schizophrenia will simply present as a very disorganized psychosis, making differentiation of the two conditions virtually impossible. Urine or blood tests are mandatory if drug use is suspected. Obtaining information from the patient's family members or friends can also be helpful.

LABORATORY EVALUATION

There are no tests routinely used in the evaluation of schizophrenia. Typically, the general screening battery of blood tests is obtained more for the sake of completeness than to look for a specific abnormality. If drug use is suspected, blood or urine tests are mandatory. Whether neuroimaging studies such as CT scans or MRI (magnetic resonance imaging) scans should be obtained in patients presenting with their first psychotic episodes is a matter of some controversy. With the current concerns about health care costs, it is likely that most hospitals and psychiatrists do not order these expensive tests in the routine evaluation of first-episode schizophrenia. Of course, with patients who have a well-documented history of classic recurrent or chronic schizophrenia, brain imaging studies are almost never obtained. Similarly, EEGs (electroencephalograms—brain wave tests) are not ordinarily indicated. However, if there is a specific concern, such as a history of epilepsy or epilepsy-like symptoms, or if the course of the disorder or response to treatment is unusual, these tests are obtained.

PSYCHIATRIC DIFFERENTIAL DIAGNOSIS

The distinction between schizophrenia and other psychiatric disorders in which psychotic thinking can occur is vital since the treatment may differ among the disorders. This is especially true in distinguishing between a psychotic mood disorder and schizophrenia. Since the presence of overt psychotic thinking should precipitate a psychiatric consult regardless of diagnosis, it is not vital that psychotherapists know all the nuances of how to distinguish among similar looking psychotic disorders. Nonetheless, a review of DSM-IV definitions of schizophrenia, schizoaffective disorder, and psychotic forms of mania and depression may be helpful. Table 5–2 summarizes the diagnostic distinctions.

Manias and depressions with mood-congruent psychotic features are relatively easy to diagnose. The full mood syndrome is present and the psychotic symptoms are all mood congruent and typical of the classic symptoms that have been described for decades. For depression, these might include depressive themes of poverty or psychotic guilt, of death or sin. For psychotic mania, the themes generally focus on grandiose themes—of special power, achievements, or identity.

Mood syndromes with mood-incongruent psychotic features are more confusing. Patients with this diagnosis will exhibit a full mood syndrome—mania with all its requisite features, or depression with the five of nine criteria listed in Table 3–1. In addition, such patients will exhibit psychotic symptoms that do *not* relate to mood themes but exist coincident with the mood syndrome; that is, the psychotic symptoms are present only when the full syndrome exists. The psychotic symptoms of mood-incongruent syndromes are the schizophrenia-like symptoms such as thought broadcasting, delusions of control, hearing two or more voices talk about the person, and so on.

If the mood-congruent psychotic features are present for two weeks or more in the absence of a full manic or depressive syndrome, then schizoaffective disorder or schizophrenia should be diagnosed. The distinction between these two disorders is based on the relative length of the mood syndrome in comparison to the period of time of psychotic thinking *without* prominent mood symptoms. If the mood syndrome with psychotic symptoms has been brief in comparison to the psychotic syndrome without the mood syndrome, then schizophrenia is diagnosed. If the mood syndrome is present for a substantial amount of the total illness time, then schizoaffective disorder is the appropriate DSM-IV diagnosis.

Table 5–2
Diagnostic Distinctions Among Disorders with Both Mood and Psychotic Symptoms

	Mania or Depression with Mood-Congruent Psychotic Features	Mania or Depression with Mood-Incongruent Psychotic Features	Schizoaffective Disorder	Schizophrenia
Full mood syndrome	Yes	Yes	Yes	Can be present but not for a substantial period of time compared to psychotic symptoms
Timing of psychotic symptoms	Only when manic or depressed	Only when manic or depressed	During mood syndrome plus at least 2 other weeks, mood symptoms present for a substantial portion of total illness time	Dominates clinical picture
Types of psychotic symptoms	Mood-congruent only. Themes of elation, poverty	Not related to mood themes	Not specified	Schizophrenic, not mood related

Without question, these distinctions seem—and are—somewhat arbitrary. They are awkward to describe, difficult to remember, and often not particularly useful when applied to live patients. These distinctions highlight the limits of our diagnostic classification system. Furthermore, since the proportion of psychotic vs. mood symptoms helps distinguish schizoaffective disorder from schizophrenia, the diagnosis may change from the former to the latter if the psychotic symptoms persist in the absence of mood symptoms. Because of these limitations, one can expect that our current classification of disorders that present with some mixture of mood and psychotic symptoms is likely to change over time as we learn more. For now, though, we still need to make "best guess" diagnoses, to distinguish as best we can between these conditions because of the potential treatment implications. As an example, a diagnosis of schizoaffective disorder, bipolar type, would help direct the psychopharmacologist toward a mood stabilizer early on in treatment whereas a diagnosis of schizophrenia would not.

Another important clue that most clinicians utilize to distinguish among similar diagnoses (although it is not used as a diagnostic clue in DSM-IV) is family history. Most psychopharmacologists evaluating a patient with both prominent psychotic thinking and major mood symptoms who did not fit into our neat diagnostic boxes would use the psychiatric family history as an important variable in deciding which medication to prescribe. If the patient had a number of relatives who were chronically psychotic, a diagnosis of schizophrenia would be likely. A family history with a bipolar parent who then stabilized on lithium would tip the diagnosis towards an unusual psychotic mood disorder and the treatment towards lithium or another mood stabilizer.

Ultimately, however, empiricism tends to dominate the best psychopharmacological treatments. For instance, if a patient with prominent mood and psychotic symptoms is provisionally diagnosed as schizophrenic and does not respond adequately to antipsychotic treatment, an antidepressant would inevitably be added. Similarly, if another patient with an admixture of mood and psychotic symptoms was diagnosed as having a primary mood syndrome but relapsed every time the antipsychotic was withdrawn, the neuroleptic would quickly become part of the maintenance treatment regardless of the official diagnosis.

Among the schizophrenia spectrum disorders, schizophreniform disorder is distinguished from schizophrenia by the length of the disorder. If it is less than six months in duration, then schizophreniform disorder is the diagnosis, although, as noted above, the clinical meaning of this distinction is usually dubious. Patients with delusional disorder do not exhibit the other signs of schizophrenia aside from the psychotic thinking; they remain more functional and generally show more fixed delusions than are seen in schizophrenia. Patients with schizotypal disorder (see chapter 7) are distinguished from schizophrenic patients primarily by never having an episode of acute dysfunctional psychosis. When viewed cross-sectionally—that is, without examining the lifetime course of disorder—schizotypal disorder is indistinguishable from residual schizophrenia.

Among the other personality disorders, borderline patients may present with psychotic symptoms. However, their psychotic episodes are far briefer than schizophrenic episodes. Additionally, the characteristic behavior of borderline personalities when the patient is not psychotic helps make the personality diagnosis. Schizoid patients show the interpersonal withdrawal characteristic of schizophrenia, but not the psychosis. Similarly, patients with paranoid personality disorder do not show the overt delusions of paranoid schizophrenia. Occasionally, it may be difficult to make this distinction because these patients are guarded and may not discuss all their symptoms.

Occasionally, obsessions and compulsions may be present as part of the symptom complex of schizophrenia. If the symptoms are first noted after the schizophrenic diagnosis is made, there is little diagnostic confusion. There is a small group of schizophrenic patients, however, during whose prodromal course obsessions and compulsions are prominent. In these patients, one would look for increasing psychotic belief in the meaning of the rituals and, over time, for the more pervasive psychotic thinking and more global dysfunction seen with schizophrenic patients compared to those with obsessive compulsive disorder.

PSYCHOPHARMACOLOGICAL TREATMENT

It is unimaginable for a schizophrenic patient to be diagnosed correctly and to be seen by a mental health professional without the issue of starting antipsychotic treatment being raised immediately as an integral part of the treatment. Antipsychotic medications have revolutionized the treatment of this most severe disorder, helping to turn what was a hospital-based disorder into an outpatient disorder for which, in most cases, the hospital is utilized only intermittently. Yet the use of medications to treat schizophrenia, both acutely and in the maintenance phase of treatment, is not as simple as psychiatrists once thought. The initial dramatic effect of the medication, markedly reducing or eliminating profound psychosis in many individuals, hid a number of the serious limitations of treatment. It soon became apparent that not all the symptoms of schizophrenia responded equally to the medication. Also, a substantial proportion of patients did not respond at all. Furthermore, even though antipsychotics are extraordinarily safe—extremely high doses can be taken without fatal or profoundly dangerous consequences—their potential side effects when prescribed either acutely or chronically can have a negative impact on the patient's well-being. From the 1950s when the first antipsychotic was released until recently, no major breakthroughs occurred in the psychopharmacological treatment of schizophrenia. Although many new medications were released during those years, the efficacy of these agents was identical, their limitations in efficacy considerable, and the profile of side effects seen with their use similar. Thus, the treatment of the most severe of psychiatric disorders required the prescription of medications that were indispensable, difficult for many patients to tolerate, and typically inadequate in their beneficial effects.

With the release of clozapine in 1990, risperidone in 1994, and a number of other medications likely to be released over the next few years, however, a new era of pharmacotherapy for schizophrenia has begun. At least one agent, clozapine, has now been well documented as more effective than other antipsychotics. The biological profile, probable mechanism of action, and side effect profile of many of these newer agents differ considerably from those of the older antipsychotics. Although the exact place of these newer agents in treating schizophrenia is not yet clear and many of their limitations are probably still unknown, for the first time, there is the promise of real choices for patients and psychopharmacologists alike in treating schizophrenia.

Unlike other disorders such as depression or panic disorder, in which a number of different medication classes can be beneficial (discussed in chapters 3 and 4 respectively), psychopharmacological treatment of schizophrenia virtually begins and ends with the antipsychotics. Although other biological treatments (discussed later in this chapter) may be considered if the disorder is refractory to antipsychotics, significant evidence of efficacy for these other medications in treating the typical schizophrenic patient is lacking. This is equally true for acute and maintenance treatment. Therefore, this section will focus primarily on the use of antipsychotics in the various phases of treatment.

Before the role of antipsychotics in treating schizophrenia is discussed in detail, a definition of this medication class is necessary. The antipsychotics, or neuroleptics as they are often called, are a class of medications, all of which have potent effects in decreasing both psychotic thinking and the agitation associated with psychosis, regardless of the diagnosis in which the psychosis occurs. Thus, these medications are used in a variety of disorders in which psychotic thinking is seen. Antipsychotics are also sometimes called dopamine blockers, since all currently available antipsychotics block the effect of the neurotransmitter dopamine. However, this term is used less now since the newer antipsychotics and many that will be released over the next few years have multiple mechanisms of action aside from dopamine blockade. Further information on antipsychotics, including their use in disorders other than schizophrenia as well as the names, doses, and side effects of the individual medications, is found in chapter 12.

Psychopharmacological Treatment of Acute Schizophrenia

The efficacy of antipsychotics in treating acute schizophrenia is so clear and well established that it would be unethical to conduct further drug/placebo trials with any of the standard antipsychotics. In the classic study published twenty-five years ago (Cole, Goldberg, and Klerman, 1964; Goldberg, Klerman, and Cole, 1965), 75 percent of patients on antipsychotics improved markedly, with no patients deteriorating compared to 25 percent of patients on placebo who improved while 50 percent of patients got worse. Despite these impressive differences, it must also be admitted that the efficacy of pharmacological treatment of acute schizophrenia is often less than adequate. Estimates of nonresponders to antipsychotics range between 10 and 30 percent. Even among those patients who are classified as responders, many show only partial benefit with residual symptoms being the rule rather than the exception.

Given the variety of symptoms and the frequency of partial treatment responses in schizophrenia, it is relevant to ask whether all psychopathology improves en masse with treatment or whether different symptoms show a differential response to antipsychotics. It is generally thought that negative symptoms are less responsive to antipsychotic medications than are positive symptoms such as delusions and hallucinations. This question is more important for maintenance treatment since it is difficult and probably irrelevant to evaluate negative symptoms during an acute frenzied psychosis. For acute schizophrenia, it is reasonable to assume that the more disruptive aspects of the disorder, however classified, are equally responsive to treatment.

Although some improvement is often seen quickly after antipsychotic medications are begun, the full therapeutic effects of antipsychotics in acute schizophrenia occur gradually over many weeks. Typically, psychotic agitation, sleep disturbance, and/or catatonic withdrawal begins to improve within days while the major effect on psychotic thinking occurs more slowly over many weeks. Although this sequence of response is not universal, the important issue clinically is to be aware that a patient who is still symptomatic after four weeks but has been gradually improving may not need higher doses of medication but rather a longer time on the same dose.

The first choice to be made in treating acute schizophrenia is that of a specific antipsychotic agent. Since 1952, when chlorpromazine (Thorazine) was first noted to have an extraordinary capacity to reduce psychosis, no new antipsychotic with the exception of clozapine has been shown to be more effective. However, since clozapine is never prescribed as a first-line agent because of its capacity to cause dangerous side effects (see below and chapter 12), it is not an option for treatment of typical acute schizophrenic episodes and will be considered separately. All other currently available antipsychotics are equally effective in groups of patients. Therefore, comparative efficacy cannot be utilized to choose a specific antipsychotic. As with many other psychopharmacological decisions, this is both bad news and good news. On one hand, there is no "best" antipsychotic. On the other hand, there is a good chance that if a patient cannot tolerate one antipsychotic, a different one may have fewer or different side effects with just as much chance of being clinically effective. In fact, the initial subjective response to an antipsychotic may be very important since an initial dysphoric response to a specific antipsychotic ("I hate this medication. It makes me feel terrible") may predict a poor response to the medication at the end of hospitalization (Van Putten and May, 1978). Whether this dysphoric response reflects side effects or other factors is unknown. Therefore, the decision to pick a specific antipsychotic should rest on two considerations—past response and side effects. If there is a history of past hospitalizations, or past medication treatment, it is important for the psychopharmacologist to obtain any available information from the patient or, if possible, from family members or past therapists. If no past medication history exists, then side effect considerations are paramount.

In choosing a specific antipsychotic for treating acute schizophrenia, the current options are either conventional agents (which include all medications released prior to 1990) or atypical or novel agents of which risperidone (Risperdal) is the only currently available medication. All new antipsychotics likely to be released in the near future will belong to the class of atypical agents. Conventional antipsychotics can then be divided into two groups: the low-potency antipsychotics (low potency does not imply low efficacy, just that a greater number of milligrams are needed for a therapeutic dose) are more sedating, cause more anticholinergic side effects such as dry mouth and constipation, and more postural hypotension (dizziness upon standing up) but fewer neurological side effects, called extrapyramidal symptoms (EPS). (See chapter 12 for details on side effects.) Medications such as chlorpromazine (Thorazine) and thioridazine (Mellaril) are representative of this group. The high-potency antipsychotics cause less sedation, anticholinergic, and postural hypotensive effects but cause far more EPS. Haloperidol (Haldol) and fluphenazine (Prolixin) are the prototypical high-potency antipsychotics. Of course, some conventional antipsychotics are midway between these two extremes, causing some sedation and some EPS. Trifluoperazine (Stelazine) and thiothixene (Navane) are examples. When conventional agents are prescribed for treating schizophrenia, many clinicians prefer prescribing the less sedating antipsychotics whenever possible, since sedation can be a significant problem with the low-potency medications, especially after the patient begins to improve. There is no evidence for the myth that sedating antipsychotics are better for agitated schizophrenics while nonsedating medications are more helpful for withdrawn patients.

In deciding between a conventional neuroleptic and risperidone, the latter is associated with fewer extrapyramidal side effects such as akinesia or akathisia when compared to high-potency neuroleptics such as haloperidol (Haldol) (Marder and Meibach, 1994). However, risperidone is markedly more expensive than conventional agents and not all patients respond equally well to either type of medication. Therefore, if a patient has previously done well on a conventional neuroleptic, it should be prescribed. For those patients who have shown either an inadequate response (in positive and/or negative symptoms) or troublesome side effects, switching to risperidone is a reasonable choice.

Once a specific medication is chosen, the method of administering the medication—as a pill, a liquid, or an injection—must be made. Without question, oral medication is preferable to injectable *if* the patient complies with treatment. This sounds reasonably straightforward but, as any clinician who has worked on an inpatient unit knows, some patients are astonishingly creative in finding ways of surreptitiously not taking their medications. The most common way is "cheeking" the medication: keeping the pill between the teeth and the inside of the cheek, swallowing the water, walking away from the nurses' station, and spitting the pill out. The use of liquid medication obviates this possibility. Short-acting injectable antipsychotics are generally reserved for involuntary patients who refuse oral medication.

Another important choice is how to manage acutely fragmented, agitated, paranoid, psychotic patients soon after they are admitted to hospital. Patients like this are extremely frightening to themselves, to other patients, and to the staff, and all concerns are focused on how to decrease the risk of violence. A common choice is to use repeated doses—perhaps every hour—of high-potency neuroleptics until the patient is calmed. Because of the inherent safety of the antipsychotics, extraordinarily high doses are sometimes used in this approach. Unfortunately, there is little evidence that this high-dose treatment, called "rapid neuroleptization," is more effective than giving moderate doses (Baldessarini, Cohen, and Teicher, 1988). It is probably used as much to treat the psychiatrist's and the staff's need to do *something*—and quickly—as it is for the patient. Another strategy, one that may be preferable, is to give a benzodiazepine tranquilizer in addition to a moderate dose of the antipsychotic. The major advantage of this approach is that by avoiding high doses of neuroleptics, the risks of more severe neuroleptic-induced side effects such as akinesia and akathisia (see chapter 12 for details) are minimized. The subjective discomfort associated with severe neuroleptic-induced side effects often results in the patient disliking the medication, causing current or future noncompliance. The typical side effects seen with the benzodiazepine tranquilizers are sedation and occasional poor balance, both of which are quickly reversible upon dose reduction and generally less subjectively distressing compared to neuroleptic side effects. The third possible strategy is physical restraint of the patient. Although this may sound primitive and even cruel to those without experience on inpatient wards, it can be effective and safe when done on modern wards with frequent observation. In fact, when treating an acutely frenzied, psychotic patient, all three of the above approaches are variants of restraint. The difference is simply that two are chemical and one is physical.

The trial of an antipsychotic to treat acute schizophrenia should last from four to six weeks. Of course, if a patient cannot tolerate a reasonable dose of one particular antipsychotic, another one that causes less of the offending side effect should be substituted.

Consensus strategies for patients who are unresponsive to a full trial of a single neuroleptic have yet to be established. Common approaches include waiting longer on the same dose, increasing to very high doses of the same antipsychotic, or switching to a different neuroleptic. In a recent study comparing these three commonly used strategies, none was shown to be consistently effective (Kinon et al.,

1993). Of course, a small percent of patients are likely to respond to high-dose antipsychotics but this is uncommon. When patients fail to respond to a conventional neuroleptic, it is not yet clear whether switching to risperidone or another of the newer agents to be released in the near future is more likely to be effective than switching to another of the older medications.

In contrast to the overall similar efficacy seen with the other antipsychotics, clozapine (Clozaril) is, without question, a more effective agent for treating schizophrenia. For patients who have failed to respond to other antipsychotics, switching to clozapine is significantly more likely to be helpful than switching to any other agent or adding any other adjunctive agent (Kane, Honigfeld, Singer, Meltzer, and the Clozaril Collaborative Study Group, 1988). Most but not all observers feel that clozapine is more effective in treating negative symptoms independent of its effects on decreasing positive symptoms. Whether clozapine is more effective than other neuroleptics for patients who are *not* treatment-resistant—that is, those who have not failed to respond adequately to other antipsychotics—is unknown. In contrast to other neuroleptics, an adequate trial of clozapine requires twelve to twenty-four weeks, with gradually increasing efficacy often seen continuing up to one year after initiating treatment (Lieberman et al., 1994).

Clozapine also has a completely different side effect profile from all other currently available antipsychotics and has been prescribed successfully for patients who are intolerant of other neuroleptics (Lieberman et al., 1994). (See chapter 12 for details of side effects of clozapine and other antipsychotics.) Despite the clear evidence of its superior efficacy, clozapine is never prescribed as a first-line agent in treating schizophrenia because of its capacity to cause potentially fatal agranulocytosis, a condition in which the bone marrow stops making white blood cells, thereby making the person vulnerable to overwhelming infection. Because clozapine-induced agranulocytosis occurs in just under 1 percent of treated patients, weekly blood counts are mandatory aspects of treatment for all patients, thereby demanding meticulous compliance and incurring an extraordinary financial expense which, without medical insurance, is prohibitively expensive for many patients.

Alternative Treatments of Acute Schizophrenia

In considering alternative treatments, it is clear that despite decades of exploration, no alternative treatment has arisen to rival antipsychotics in efficacy or safety in treating schizophrenia. Thus, most of the interest and hope in treating those patients who have not responded to currently available neuroleptics is centered around the medications to be released in the near future with the hope that they will be more effective agents with fewer side effects and better patient acceptance. Nonetheless, a variety of secondary approaches are available for use in conjunction with antipsychotics, or as single agents when patients are unresponsive to antipsychotics (Christison, Kirch, and Wyatt, 1991). Table 5–3 lists these alternative or adjunctive treatments.

Because of its pronounced effect in treating manic states and because of the difficulty in distinguishing between psychotic mood disorders and schizophrenia, it is not surprising that lithium has been explored as an alternative treatment for schizophrenia. Lithium is likely to be effective in only a minority of schizophrenic patients when prescribed alone or, as is more common, when given in combination with an antipsychotic (Delva and Letemendia, 1982). The extent of the improvement, when seen, is variable. Although the presence of affective symptoms may predict a somewhat better response to lithium, a positive response does not require the presence of these features. Lithium should be tried in treatment-resistant schizophrenia, but the likelihood of a marked clinical effect is small.

Another alternative treatment is high-dose propranolol (Inderal), a beta-adrenergic blocker, commonly used to treat angina, high blood pressure, tremors, migraine headaches, and other medical conditions. Over the last decade, a number of studies have demonstrated that high-dose propranolol can be helpful to some patients when added to a neuroleptic. However, raising the dose of propranolol too quickly is associated with a host of difficult side effects. Because of this, high doses may take more than one month to achieve. Propranolol should therefore be considered a medication to be used for schizophrenia only after most other strategies have failed.

Table 5–3
Alternative or Adjunctive Treatments of Acute Schizophrenia

Lithium
Propranolol
Benzodiazepines
Antidepressants
Electroconvulsive therapy (ECT)

Benzodiazepines, the most common class of tranquilizers (see chapter 11), have also been used to treat schizophrenia. When prescribed alone (i.e., not in conjunction with antipsychotics) in extraordinarily high doses, these medications are occasionally effective (Lingjaerde, 1991). More consistently, moderate doses of benzodiazepines are associated with clinical improvement when added to neuroleptics (Wolkowitz and Pickar, 1991). This strategy may result in an improvement of clinical symptoms and may make it possible to decrease the dose of antipsychotics needed, thereby diminishing the risk of side effects.

Although antidepressants have an unquestionable place in the treatment of depressive syndromes in schizophrenia (discussed below), there is also intriguing preliminary evidence on the efficacy of antidepressants in treating other aspects of schizophrenic symptomatology. Fluoxetine (Prozac), the SSRI antidepressant (see chapter 9), has been shown to benefit some schizophrenic patients in broad-based ways when added to neuroleptics (Goff, Brotman, Waites, and McCormick, 1990). For those schizophrenic patients with prominent obsessions and compulsions, clomipramine (or other antidepressants useful in treating obsessive compulsive disorder—see chapter 4) may be beneficial (Zohar, Kaplan, and Benjamin, 1993).

Although electroconvulsive therapy has been used rarely in the last decade within the United States, there is a substantial literature from Great Britain on its use in treating schizophrenia. It does seem that ECT can be effective in treating acute schizophrenia, especially in those cases where catatonic or affective symptoms are prominent (Sackeim, Devanand, and Nobler, 1995). There is also some evidence that ECT plus antipsychotics may be more effective than neuroleptics alone in treating schizophrenia. ECT is not effective in chronic psychotic states.

Acute Treatment of Schizoaffective Disorder

There are very few consistent generalizations that can be made about the pharmacotherapy of schizoaffective disorder. This reflects both the diagnostic uncertainty surrounding these patients, the heterogeneity of the disorder (see above), and the simple lack of studies examining the issue (Lapensee, 1992b). For treating schizoaffective disorder, bipolar subtype (schizomania), the three most common first-line treatments are mood stabilizers, mood stabilizers plus antipsychotics, and antipsychotics alone. Among these three options, a mood stabilizer alone may be least likely to be effective.

Schizodepressive patients, probably because their disorder is closer to pure schizophrenia, seem to require antipsychotic medications prescribed either alone or in combination with antidepressants and/or mood stabilizers. For those schizoaffective patients with either subtype who have not responded to more conventional treatment, clozapine may be beneficial (Frankenburg and Zanarini, 1994).

Continuation Treatment of Acute Schizophrenia

Once remission of the acute psychotic symptoms occurs, how long should the patient continue on medication if maintenance treatment is deemed inappropriate? The figures in the psychiatric literature vary enormously, from a few months to five years. The wide range is due both to the different goals of the continuation period and to a lack of a clear demarcation between continuation and maintenance phases for schizophrenia. (See chapter 1 for further discussion of phases of treatment.) As an example, should the continuation period be used for simple symptom stabilization? Should a deeper exploration of family interactions or vocational rehabilitation occur then? Is this the time for social skills training? Clearly, the more ambitious the goals of the stabilization period, the longer continuation treatment will need to be.

Maintenance Treatment of Schizophrenia

Since in most cases schizophrenia is a chronic disorder characterized by intermittent relapses, the question of prescribing maintenance medication treatment as a means of preventing or forestalling relapse inevitably arises. It has been definitively shown that, compared to placebo, maintenance treatment is more effective in preventing schizophrenic relapses. The rates of relapse on active medication in contrast to placebo in different studies are extremely varied due to differences in patient selection and the length of follow-up. Overall, the best summary statistics are that, when schizophrenic patients are followed for just under one year, the relapse rate when antipsychotics are withdrawn is 53 percent vs. 16 percent when the medication is continued (Gilbert, Harris, McAdams, and Jeste, 1995).

A cursory glance at these numbers would make most observers conclude that maintenance antipsychotics are virtually always indicated in treating schizophrenia. Yet scratching below the surface of this issue yields a much more complicated clinical decision. First, as previously noted, schizophrenia is an extremely heterogeneous disorder with widely varying outcome. Most patients assuredly need long-term antipsychotics, while others might do well without them. The need for neuroleptics may also change over time since, as noted above, the illness seems most virulent in the first decade with stability or even improvement occurring afterwards. Second, neuroleptics are far from benign medications with side effects ranging from a subtle sense of dullness and weight gain to tardive dyskinesia, a potentially irreversible movement disorder. (See chapter 12 for more details.) Because of these side effects along with other factors, compliance with long-term antipsychotics is exceedingly difficult. In many cases, the issue of whether the patient should be on maintenance neuroleptics is decided by the patient—who refuses. Third, generalizations tell us little about specific subpopulations. For instance, only two of the sixty-six published studies on neuroleptic discontinuation have evaluated patients early in their illness. How then does one respond to a 22-year-old schizophrenic patient who has been well stabilized on antipsychotic medications for eighteen months following only one psychotic episode and who asks whether he needs to be on this medication without interruption for the rest of his life, having had no chance to try being medication-free?

It would be extremely helpful to have well-documented predictors of those who are most likely to respond to medication but, even more, those who will do well off medication. Unfortunately, no such predictors are currently available.

Even though maintenance neuroleptics unquestionably decrease relapse rates, they do not seem to alter some of the most fundamental psychopathology of the disorder. Although some schizophrenic patients behave, function, and feel normal when they are not in an overt psychotic state, more of them will exhibit clear signs of the disorder even when not in acute relapse. The negative symptoms—the lack of motivation, the relative social isolation, the poor social skills, the nonintegration with the world—continue even with optimal medication treatment. What this implies is the inadequacy of defining clinical outcome only by symptoms or rehospitalization rates for a disorder that affects so many different aspects of functioning. Patients on medication who are not psychotic or hospitalized over one year will be classified as "successes" in a research study. Yet they may spend their time in a board and care facility, smoking cigarettes, doing little of meaning or satisfaction for weeks, months, or years. Antipsychotics may be mandatory to keep schizophrenic patients from being frequently or chronically hospitalized—but too often they are not enough.

It is also relevant and important to examine the potential cost of maintenance medication, especially in terms of side effects. Through a series of elegant studies it has become clear that medium doses of antipsychotics are more effective than low doses in preventing psychotic symptoms. However, the cost of the higher dose is increased side effects that are frequently unrecognizable, subjectively distressing, and affect psychosocial functioning (Marder et al., 1984; Marder et al., 1987; Hogarty et al., 1988). In these studies, low-dose patients had psychotic exacerbations more frequently (as defined by an increase in psychotic symptoms) but these were well handled by simply increasing the medication dose without need for hospitalization. However, the low-dose patients were less physically slowed down, less tense, and exhibited less emotional withdrawal, implying that these symptoms were unrecognizable subtle side effects of higher-dose antipsychotics.

These studies highlight the complex question of risk versus benefit of different doses of antipsychotics in schizophrenia. Is it worth some mild sluggishness in order to avoid times of mild auditory hallucinations or mild ideas of reference? How bad are the psychotic symptoms? How quickly do they evolve from mild to severe? How much do they affect the person's job or relationships? How sluggish is the patient on medication? Frequently, these questions can take years to answer fully for any individual, assuming different doses and a period off medication are tried. It is in this most delicate area—constructing risk/benefit ratios with side effects being such an important factor—that the novel antipsychotics such as risperidone and those to be released in the near future may play vital roles. Even if the newer medications show no greater efficacy compared to the older agents, if they cause fewer side effects and patients are more likely to be compliant with their use, then they will provide important advantages, especially as a maintenance treatment.

The most well-known complication of long-term use of antipsychotics is tardive dyskinesia (TD). Although details on tardive dyskinesia will be presented in chapter 12, no discussion on the risks and benefits of maintenance antipsychotics would be complete without addressing the concern about using a medication that can cause an irreversible side effect. It is clear that TD is a potential risk in any patient treated with any currently available antipsychotic (with the possible exception of clozapine) over an extended period of time. Furthermore, the risk for developing TD gradually increases over at least the first five years of antipsychotic treatment. Surprisingly, the long-term course of TD is variable; some patients show stabilization or worsening of the involuntary movements, while in others the movements may even diminish.

There is little doubt that the most logical strategy in a patient who has already developed tardive dyskinesia would be to stop the antipsychotic. Yet, as already noted, most schizophrenic patients need and benefit from maintenance neuroleptics and would suffer relapses if the medication were withdrawn. Therefore, because most cases of TD are mild and the course of the movements is variable even when the neuroleptic is continued, the most common strategy in treating a patient with TD is to attempt to reduce the antipsychotic to its lowest effective dose. For those patients whose tardive dyskinesia is marked or socially disabling, switching to clozapine is a very reasonable strategy since it rarely causes TD and is consistently associated with a decrease in abnormal movements (Tamminga, Thaker, Moran, Kakigi, and Gao, 1994).

Even those patients who have demonstrated benefit from maintenance neuroleptics frequently have breakthrough psychotic symptoms. Although In this situation these patients are almost always treated with supplemental doses of their antipsychotic medication, it is still unclear whether this approach is consistently effective, compared to psychosocial intervention such as simple hospitalization without a change in medication dose (Steingard, Allen, and Schooler, 1994).

Because of the many difficulties inherent in maintenance neuroleptics, not the least of which is that of patient refusal, the strategy of intermittent or targeted medication has been explored. The intermittent medication approach is predicated on the observation that many, if not most, schizophrenic patients are only intermittently psychotic and may not need medication on a continual basis. If clinical exacerbation/relapse can be anticipated or treated when the symptoms first become apparent, patients might be well treated with far less cumulative exposure to the medication, thereby minimizing both acute side effects and possibly tardive dyskinesia. Intermittent pharmacotherapy, however, depends heavily on patient/family/therapist insight, support, and cooperation as well as an appreciation of the nature of the patient's prodromal signs. Overall, this strategy has not been shown to be particularly effective (Herz et al., 1991; Carpenter et al., 1990). Patients treated with intermittent pharmacotherapy use less total medication but show higher rates of exacerbation, relapse, and hospitalization. Additionally, although side effects may be diminished using intermittent pharmacotherapy, there is no evidence that rates of tardive dyskinesia are altered by this approach. Thus, intermittent medication should be considered only for a small subset of schizophrenic patients such as those whose episodes emerge slowly, where insight is retained and drug refusal is rare.

For those patients who experience frequent relapses despite a maintenance regimen of a conventional neuroleptic, consideration should be given to switching to one of the novel antipsychotics. As with treating acute schizophrenia, it is not yet clear whether risperidone is more effective as a maintenance antipsychotic (as opposed to more easily tolerated) compared to conventional agents. It is clear, however, that clozapine is more effective. Therefore, any patient who has recurrent psychotic episodes despite maintenance neuroleptic treatment at reasonable dose should be strongly considered for a clozapine trial.

Probably the most difficult decision for psychopharmacologists working with schizophrenic patients is how to treat a patient who exhibits chronic or frequently profound psychotic symptoms while on medications (including clozapine) with little or no evidence of antipsychotic efficacy. Typically, this type of patient will be treated with higher and higher doses of antipsychotics each time an exacerbation or relapse occurs, despite the evidence that higher doses have not been effective and may even make the patient worse. If the psychopharmacologist then begins to lower the dose, the patient is likely to relapse—since relapse is probable in any case. This will be incorrectly interpreted by psychiatrist, therapist, patient, and/or family as evidence that the dose is too low and the escalation to higher doses then resumes. Most relatively treatment-resistant schizophrenic patients are on excessive doses of medication for these reasons and can safely have their doses lowered slowly and cautiously (Inderbitzin et al., 1994). Some of these patients may even show mild improvement with lower doses, presumably due to a decrease in unrecognized side effects from the high antipsychotic doses. For patients whose episodes are not prevented at all by a maintenance treatment of antipsychotics, the intermittent pharmacotherapy approach outlined above should be considered.

An important technical consideration in maintenance treatment of schizophrenia is whether to use oral or long-acting injectable antipsychotics. Currently, two injectable antipsychotics are available which last two to four weeks. The medication is mixed with an oil-based preparation such that after the injection into either fat or muscle (typically into the buttocks or the arm), it is released gradually over many days. The obvious advantage is that the daily struggle for compliance is avoided. Since relapses rarely occur soon after medication withdrawal, patients on oral medication who miss one day's dose or two may find they feel, if anything, slightly better. They then stop the medication entirely, convinced that they no longer need it, only to relapse months later since the effect of maintenance treatment is primarily preventive. With the use of long-acting injectable antipsychotics, the patient must comply only once every two to four weeks. Also, if the patient becomes more symptomatic, the always present problem of ascertaining whether noncompliance with medication helped precipitate the relapse is avoided. There is no evidence that long-acting injectable antipsychotics are more effective, only that compliance is better controlled. The primary consideration in the decision to use injectable antipsychotics, therefore, should be the individual patient's capacity to comply with medication treatment.

Maintenance Treatment of Schizoaffective Disorder

The maintenance treatment of schizoaffective disorder, either bipolar or depressed type, is decided on purely empirical grounds. For schizomania, the most common maintenance treatment is probably a combination of a mood stabilizer along with an antipsychotic. Schizodepressive patients are frequently treated with a maintenance regimen of either antipsychotics alone (reflecting their closeness to pure schizophrenia) or a combination of an antidepressant plus an antipsychotic. Occasionally, a schizodepressive patient will do best on a mood stabilizer, an antidepressant, and an antipsychotic.

Treatment of Depression in Schizophrenia

Until recently, it was generally assumed that antidepressants were difficult to use in schizophrenic patients, conferring the risk of exacerbating psychosis and being unlikely to be very effective in most cases. These assumptions were, in part, related to: (1) the difficulty in distinguishing between a true depressive syndrome and other dysphoric states such as those caused by drug-induced akinesia, the psychosis itself, and so on; and (2) the possibility of differing effects if antidepressants are added during an acute psychotic phase of illness vs. during a more stable and less psychotic outpatient phase. Now, after a decade of more sophisticated studies examining the use of antidepressants for schizophrenic patients, different conclusions apply: First, antidepressants can clearly be helpful if prescribed for schizophrenic patients who have a clear depressive syndrome (and not just a sad mood), who are not in the midst of an acute psychotic relapse, and whose akinetic side effects—which can mimic a depressive syndrome—have been adequately treated (Plasky, 1991). Second, schizophrenic patients at highest risk for psychotic exacerbation from antidepressants are those who are treated in the midst of a psychotic relapse (Kramer et al., 1989). Third, the response to antidepressants may be substantial and many of these patients may need to continue the adjunctive antidepressants for an extended period of time—possibly years—with relapses common if the antidepressants are withdrawn (Siris, Morgan, Fagerstrom, Rifkin, and Cooper, 1987; Siris, Bermanzohn, Mason, and Shuwall, 1994). There are no guidelines to help in the selection of a specific antidepressant for schizophrenic patients except that bupropion might not be a wise first choice because of its effect on dopamine and the possibility of provoking a psychotic exacerbation.

6

Disorders of Impulse Control

Eating Disorders, Drug and Alcohol Abuse, and Adult Attention Deficit/Hyperactivity Disorder (ADHD)

D IFFICULTIES IN IMPULSE CONTROL are seen in a variety of psychiatric and psychological disorders. In a few of these, such as eating disorders and drug and alcohol abuse, these problems are central aspects of the pathology. In others, such as attention deficit/hyperactivity disorder, the problems surrounding impulse control may not be as central but nonetheless are common and are frequently the clinical features that bring the patient to the attention of mental health professionals. Compared with previous chapters, less detail will be provided here on the disorders themselves, because medication is generally not a primary treatment for some eating disorders (specifically, anorexia nervosa) and drug abuse, and because less is known about adult attention deficit/hyperactivity disorder.

EATING DISORDERS

Both anorexia nervosa and bulimia nervosa, as they are called in DSM-IV, are characterized by a preoccupation with food and weight. Although separated into two disorders, there is clear and consistent overlap between them. As an example, up to 50 percent of anorexic patients develop bulimic symptoms; in DSM-IV, these patients are described as having anorexia nervosa with binge-eating/purging subtype. Some patients with anorexia nervosa may alternate between restricting and bulimic subtypes (American Psychiatric Association, 1993a). Similarly, significant numbers of bulimic patients develop anorexic symptoms. Other common features between the two include a propensity for compulsive exercising, bizarre food preferences, social isolation, and depressive symptoms. Despite the many similarities between the two disorders, the place of pharmacotherapy in their treatment differs. Medications are infrequently prescribed for anorexia nervosa while antidepressants are consistently effective and used frequently in treating bulimia nervosa.

Anorexia Nervosa

In anorexia nervosa, there is an obsession with and a distortion of body image with an intense fear of gaining weight and/or becoming fat. Abnormal behaviors seen in anorexia nervosa are related to regulating this distorted self-image. In DSM-IV, patients with anorexia nervosa are subtyped into either the restricting or binge-eating/purging subtype. Restrictors do not binge or purge, but control their weight by dieting, fasting, or excessive exercise. Those with the binge-eating/purging subtype, despite similar preoccupation with body image and weight, manifest cycles of losing control by binges and the restoration of control by purging or misuse of laxatives, enemas, or diuretics.

Conceptually, medications could be used either in the acute treatment phase, or as part of a longer-term maintenance program. The vast majority of studies examining the efficacy of medications have focused on the initial phase of short-term treatment, typically in inpatient settings, during which time the goal is above all weight gain. In contrast to bulimia nervosa, few well-controlled studies have even examined the role of pharmacotherapy in treating acute anorexia nervosa.

Pharmacological approaches during the early phase of treatment for patients with anorexia nervosa are complicated by a number of factors. First, anorexic patients, especially in the early stages of treatment when their weight is very low, are at high risk to have a variety of metabolic and other biological disturbances from the self-induced starvation. Because of this, there is an increased danger in using any medication. Second, patients with anorexia nervosa are exceedingly sensitive to and intolerant of nondangerous medication side effects, both from the starvation effects and from their own sensitivity to unwanted feelings or changes in their bodies. Third, these patients often equate taking medication with losing control, further increasing the resistance to taking them.

Conceptually, medications might be helpful in the treatment of anorexia nervosa in a number of ways: by stimulating appetite and/or promoting weight gain, by decreasing depression, by decreasing anxiety, and by diminishing obsessional thinking. All medications occasionally used for anorexia nervosa have one or more of these effects. However, since some of these symptoms—most notably, the obsessionality and the depression—are likely to be effects of starvation and not the cause, bringing about weight gain and better nutrition by any means will effectively treat these symptoms too.

Medications explored have included the more sedating tricyclic antidepressants, fluoxetine, antipsychotics, lithium, and cyproheptadine, an antiserotonergic antihistamine (American Psychiatric Association, 1993a). Although many anecdotal reports have demonstrated the success of one treatment or another, and in some controlled studies medications have shown modest efficacy (e.g., cyproheptadine), the consensus in the field is that no one particular type of medication is consistently helpful in the acute weight restoration phase.

Antidepressants are often considered as adjunctive treatments for acute anorexia nervosa. Initially a part of this rationale stemmed from the prominence of depressive symptoms in patients with anorexia nervosa. However, depression in anorexia nervosa is difficult to interpret because of the effects of starvation in causing dysphoric mood, apathy, and irritability, symptoms that then remit upon weight gain (Strober and Katz, 1986). Although well-controlled trials have not shown positive results, the antidepressants used in those studies were the most sedating and hypotensive ones which probably contributed to their poor outcome. Less sedating antidepressants are more easily tolerated and might be more helpful. The SSRIs might show an advantage over the tricyclics because they are not associated with rapid weight gain and because of their potential antiobsessional effects. Anecdotally, fluoxetine has been helpful for treatment-resistant patients with anorexia nervosa (Gwirtsman, Guze, Yager, and Gainsley, 1990).

With the lack of evidence pointing to any one medication type as effective in treating acute anorexia nervosa, clinical decisions are generally made on an empirical basis. As examples, antidepressants should be considered for patients with persistent depressive symptoms, especially in those who have gained weight and in whom the starvation effects have therefore been minimized. Patients with marked obsessionality (even beyond what is typical for patients with anorexia nervosa) should be considered for SSRIs, while psychotic-like thinking might suggest the use of low-dose neuroleptics. Marked anticipatory anxiety before meals might be aided by low doses of antianxiety agents.

Because of the consistent evidence that anorexia nervosa is a chronic disorder, recent attention has increasingly focused on the potential use of medications in the maintenance phase of treatment. At this point, patients have regained sufficient weight to be out of hospital and are not suffering the psychiatric and physical effects of acute starvation. The goal of the maintenance phase is weight maintenance, restoration of more normal eating and exercise patterns, diminished preoccupation with food, and prevention of relapse. Although very few studies have examined the efficacy of medications in this phase, pharmacotherapy might have more of a role here (albeit still limited) compared to the acute treatment phase. The anecdotal evidence has been most encouraging for SSRIs, primarily fluoxetine (Prozac). Anecdotally, restrictors may respond better than do those with binge/purge symptoms (Kaye, Weltzin, Hsu, and Bulik, 1991). As with their potential use in the acute phase of anorexia nervosa, it has been hypothesized that SSRIs might help in the maintenance phase by diminishing anxiety, depression, or obsessionality. The possibility that SSRIs might diminish the obsessionality around food is especially intriguing given the effects of these medications in treating classic obsessive compulsive disorder. If SSRIs continue to be demonstrated as effective, this would be consistent with the proposal of anorexia nervosa as an obsessive compulsive spectrum disorder (see chapter 5). However, no well-controlled studies have yet been published indicating the efficacy of SSRIs for maintenance treatment. Currently, then, SSRIs should generally be considered as a potential adjunctive treatment to other more primary modalities. There is no evidence whatsoever that medications alter the long-term outcome of anorexia nervosa.

Bulimia Nervosa

Those with bulimia nervosa share with anorexic patients the overconcern with body shape and size. The hallmark of bulimia nervosa, however, is the repetitive cycle of out-of-control binge eating alternating with a variety of behaviors that attempt to undo the effects of the binging, such as self-induced vomiting, laxative abuse, fasting, or vigorous exercising. Although a number of patients exhibit core features of both anorexia nervosa and bulimia nervosa, the majority of patients who present for treatment have normal-weight bulimia.

In contrast to anorexia nervosa, medications—specifically antidepressants—have documented efficacy in decreasing the binge-purge cycle in short-term treatment studies. Compared to those treated with placebo, bulimic patients on antidepressants will show a greater decrease in binge frequency, with that decrease averaging 70 percent across studies (Walsh and Devlin, 1995). All antidepressants seem to have potential efficacy in reducing bulimic behavior. Those formally evaluated in double-blind studies have ranged across the antidepressant classes and have included tricyclic antidepressants, MAO inhibitors, trazodone (with which the effects may be weaker), SSRIs (specifically fluoxetine), and bupropion (Wellbutrin). Therefore, any one of these with the exception of bupropion are appropriate choices for treating bulimia nervosa. (Bupropion is contraindicated for bulimia nervosa because of the evidence that it confers an unusually high risk for grand mal seizures in this population [Horne et al., 1988]. Presumably, this reflects the interaction of the medication's effects with the electrolyte imbalance and shifts commonly seen in bulimic patients.) However, the efficacy of antidepressants alone in treating bulimia nervosa is typically far from complete, with remission rates (complete cessation of binging and purging) ranging between 20 and 35 percent.

With no substantive evidence that one antidepressant has significantly greater efficacy than the others, how does a psychopharmacologist pick a specific agent? The same factors used in choosing an antidepressant for depression (see chapter 3) also apply for bulimia nervosa. In the majority of cases, this translates clinically into suggesting an SSRI first for side effect and patient acceptance reasons (especially the lack of weight gain with these medications). In one of the best double-blind studies yet published, fluoxetine (Prozac) was clearly effective in reducing bulimic behavior, with daily doses of 60 mg more effective than 20 mg (Fluoxetine Bulimia Nervosa Collaborative Study Group, 1992). The efficacy of the other SSRIs, although not as extensively evaluated in formal studies, is likely to be similar.

Often, when one antidepressant is ineffective, a different agent will work, so that several trials are warranted in the patient who fails to respond to the first medication prescribed (Mitchell et al., 1989). Given the lack of adequate response to a single agent, bulimic patients are often treated with medication combinations, similar to treating depression. Antidepressant doses in treating bulimia nervosa are the same as those for depression, except for fluoxetine and possibly the other SSRIs as noted above. (See chapter 9 for details of other antidepressant doses.) The time course to response—up to six weeks for a maximum response—is also similar.

A number of studies have also evaluated whether antidepressants add to the outcome of patients treated with structured short-term psychotherapies, especially cognitive behavioral therapy. The results of these studies are somewhat inconsistent, with some showing no additional benefit from antidepressants over that seen from psychotherapy while additive effects have also been reported (Mitchell et al., 1990; Agras et al., 1992).

Compared to the short-term treatment studies, longer-term follow-ups of bulimic patients treated with antidepressants present a more negative view. Patients often relapse despite continued antidepressant treatment, necessitating medication switches, additions, and the like (Walsh, Hadigan, Devlin, Gladis, and Roose, 1991). Similarly, side effects often become more subjectively troublesome over time, culminating in noncompliance and drug refusal. Bulimic patients who discontinue antidepressants after a successful outcome are also at high risk for subsequent relapse (Walsh and Devlin, 1995).

Although initially the efficacy of antidepressants in treating bulimia nervosa was considered possible evidence that this disorder was a depressive equivalent, further work (and thought) has made this idea untenable. As noted in chapter 9, it is clear that antidepressants, especially the SSRIs, are broad-spectrum medications with documented efficacy in a variety of disparate disorders that are unlikely to all be manifestations of the same core pathology. It is unquestionably true that bulimic patients commonly suffer from comorbid depression (Brewerton et al., 1995). Yet the presence of depression in bulimic patients does not predict a better response to antidepressants in controlling binge frequency. Depression and bulimia, when they coexist, do not necessarily remit together. At times, the binging may respond to treatment while the depression continues; at other times the reverse sequence is seen. Overall, then, conceptualizing bulimia and depression as a single disorder with multiple manifestations seems inaccurate. What is more likely is that the two disorders are commonly occurring comorbid conditions; that is, that the presence of one condition (bulimia nervosa) makes the presence of the other (depression) more likely, analogous to the frequent co-occurrence of depression and borderline personality disorder (Strober and Katz, 1987). Additionally, sources of dysphoria in bulimic patients are multiple: depression is mixed with dysphoric mood stemming from poor self-esteem and shame due to the bulimia along with other characterological sources of depressed mood.

Other than antidepressants, medications for treating bulimia nervosa are generally ineffective. These have included lithium, carbamazepine, fenfluramine (Pondimin—a serotonergically active weight loss agent), and naltrexone (Trexan or ReVia, an opiate antagonist) (Walsh and Devlin, 1995).

Given the information just reviewed, what guidelines should a therapist use in considering the referral of a bulimic patient for possible antidepressant treatment? With the consistent evidence for the efficacy of both psychotherapies and antidepressants and the possibility of greater effect when the two modalities are combined, many viable options are available. Clearly, patients differ in their individual needs and preferences. For many bulimic patients who want to avoid medications, it is reasonable to start with one of the structured psychotherapeutic approaches, using antidepressants only if the patient is unresponsive to psychological approaches. For others, antidepressants will be viewed positively, may accelerate treatment response, diminish treatment costs, and should be started early in therapy. In general, antidepressants should not be used as the sole initial treatment for treating bulimia nervosa.

If antidepressants are considered, a clinician must first pay attention to the possible fears and resistances involved. Since issues of control are so central to bulimia, patients often are frightened of being addicted to medications and are concerned that taking medication is an indication of lack of self-control. Bulimic patients also fear that the medications will make them fat. Once the implications of using medications as a part of the treatment have been explored, therapists should consider a psychopharmacological consultation.

Table 6–1 presents the factors to be used in considering medications for treating bulimia nervosa. Other than patient preference, prime considerations include the presence of other comorbid disorders, and a nonresponse to other treatment modalities. Although the presence of depression does not predict a better antibulimic response to antidepressants, the medications may nonetheless successfully treat an associated depression, if present. The alleviation of the depression is likely to help the patient work more productively in any other treatment modality by increasing concentration and energy and by combating pessimism, negative expectation, and helplessness while promoting a general sense of well-being. Since, as mentioned above, the multiple sources of depressive symptoms in bulimic patients sometimes blur the

Table 6–1
Guidelines for Considering Medications
in Treating Bulimia Nervosa

Patient desires medication as adjunctive treatment
Patient has moderate to severe current major depressive disorder
History of recurrent depression when *not* bulimic
Presence of other comorbid disorders (especially anxiety disorders)
Patient has not improved from a well designed treatment program not involving pharmacotherapy

distinctions among these overlapping diagnoses, a history of depression when the patient was *not* bulimic suggests that she is at high risk for a difficult-to-recognize major depressive episode which may then complicate the treatment of the bulimia. Aside from depression, bulimic patients are also at high risk to have comorbid anxiety disorders, such as social phobia, panic disorder, or generalized anxiety disorder (Brewerton et al., 1995). When present, medications appropriate for treating these disorders (see chapter 4) should be strongly considered. Finally, since there are no established predictors for response to any treatment for bulimia, the last guideline stresses the empirical nature of treatment planning. If the patient continues to binge and purge despite active participation in a multimodal treatment program, the addition of antidepressants may be very helpful.

A more recently delineated variant of bulimia nervosa is called binge-eating disorder. Classified in DSM-IV in the Appendix as a criteria set provided for further study, it is characterized by the same binges as seen in bulimia nervosa but without the compensatory behaviors to maintain weight control, such as purging, fasting, excessive exercise, and so on. Not surprisingly, most patients with binge-eating disorder are significantly overweight. The few studies so far published and open clinical experience have suggested that, compared to treating bulimia nervosa, antidepressants are less consistently effective in treating binge-eating disorder (Walsh and Devlin, 1995).

ADULT ATTENTION DEFICIT/HYPERACTIVITY DISORDER

Little doubt remains that attention deficit/hyperactivity disorder (ADHD) exists as an adult psychopathological entity (Spencer, Biederman, Wilens, and Faraone, 1994). Yet adult ADHD remains undiagnosed and therefore untreated in many affected individuals. Equally true, however, is the recent tendency in the mid-1990s to make the diagnosis reflexively in a number of individuals who have poor occupational outcome (i.e., perceive themselves as underachievers) and low self-esteem, but without real evidence of any of the core features of ADHD. Thus, adult ADHD has simultaneously become an underdiagnosed and overdiagnosed disorder. A significant part of the difficulty in diagnosing ADHD has been the lack of consistent attention (pun unintended) in developing diagnostic criteria that are appropriate for adults. Without clearly delineated diagnostic criteria, core issues about the disorder—including how best to define it—remain unclear. In contrast to prior DSMs, DSM-IV has rectified this situation, but only somewhat. Many of the DSM-IV criteria (described in more detail in chapter 8) are more applicable to adults. In addition, patients who once met the full criteria but are now only partially symptomatic (as often occurs in adults) can be given the diagnosis and described as being in partial remission. The more prominent place of inattention in making the diagnosis, as opposed to the excessive focus on hyperactivity in previous DSMs, also helps promote the diagnosis in those adults who are no longer hyperactive or never were. Despite this, the DSM-IV criteria for ADHD still contain a number of items that are difficult to apply in adult patients, such as "often leaves seat in classroom or in other situations in which remaining seated is expected."

The core features of DSM-IV ADHD are a variety of inattention symptoms and/or hyperactivity-impulsivity symptoms, or both, beginning before age 7. A major problem in making the diagnosis in adults then, is ascertaining the presence of core diagnostic features decades later. ADHD children grown up show relatively high rates of forgetting childhood symptoms (Mannuzza, Klein, Bessler, Malloy, and La-Padula, 1993). Further confusing the history, the desire for a biological explanation for adult failure may cause an exaggeration of symptoms, resulting in false-positive diagnoses. Having parents describe how their adult children behaved when they were children may be beneficial since these descriptions often differ from those of the patients (Wender, Reimherr, and Wood, 1981). Unfortunately, it is often difficult to obtain parents' evaluation in adult patients. Even if parents are not available, if adult ADHD is suspected, an attempt should be made to meet with the patient's significant other for at least an observer's description of the adult behavior. A final complication in making the diagnosis in adults is the frequent presence of comorbid disorders, such as drug and alcohol abuse, anxiety, and mood disorders.

Aside from the DSM-IV criteria, the other commonly used diagnostic criteria for adult ADHD are known as the Utah criteria (Wender, Wood, and Reimherr, 1985). Patients diagnosed as adult ADHD by the Utah criteria must have demonstrated symptoms consistent with attention deficit/hyperactivity disorder when they were children, but as adults also exhibit two core symptoms and other associated ones. The core adult symptoms are persistent motor activity—characterized by restlessness and difficulty settling down—and attention deficits such as distractability, wandering off while doing tasks, and forgetting or misplacing things. Additionally, these patients must exhibit two of the five following characteristics: (1) affective lability—a lifetime of moodiness, sometimes in response to life events and other times spontaneously, with both dysphoria and periods of excitement that last from hours to days; (2) inability to complete tasks, disorganized ways of approaching a series of tasks, and leaving things unfinished while switching to another task; (3) a hot temper, with short-lived outbursts that may be frightening to both patients and others; (4) impulsivity in decisions involving both work and relationships with potential inappropriate risk-taking behavior; and (5) stress intolerance, as manifested by excessive emotional reactions to everyday life stresses.

Regardless of the specific criteria used, adults with ADHD generally resemble children with ADHD (Biederman et al., 1993). ADHD adults are typically described by others as moody, restless, unpredictable, and "all over the place," who just can't ever seem to stick to anything for very long and who tend to be underachievers. They change jobs frequently, citing restlessness, boredom, and difficulty getting along with supervisors. Because of these traits, adults with ADHD often gravitate towards independent positions such as owning their own businesses in which they can be active and are less likely to be required to keep rigidly defined schedules.

Those patients whose symptoms are primarily related to inattention with no or minimal hyperactivity/impulsivity and who are not moody, are more easily missed. Their childhood histories are less remarkable since they do not exhibit the kinds of disruptive behaviors that draw the attention of teachers or parents. Among children (and possibly among adults), girls with ADHD are overly represented among the inattentive subtypes compared to the hyperactive/impulsive types (Lahey et al., 1994). These patients may be even more difficult to diagnose as adults since their impaired concentration, although chronic, is frequently less than global. Many adult ADHD patients may be able to focus well on certain tasks of particular interest but not on other tasks, in contrast to the attentional problems of depression, in which the concentrating deficit is more global.

In its classic form, adult ADHD can be a very easy diagnosis to make (assuming the clinician considers it in the first place). In many other cases, however, distinguishing adult ADHD from other disorders is more difficult. One common and important diagnostic distinction is between adult ADHD and the milder bipolar disorders, such as cyclothymia. Adult ADHD shares a number of features with mild bipolar disorders such as impulsiveness, irritability, and most importantly, mood lability (criterion #1 in the Utah criteria listed above). Typically, ADHD patients misdiagnosed as cyclothymic are given lithium with no benefit. Childhood histories virtually always reveal evidence of ADHD, an uncommon finding in bipolar patients. It is also vital to remember that, despite the simplistic stories in the lay press, attention deficits and poor achievement are seen in a variety of other psychiatric disorders such as dysthymia, personality disorders, or primary drug or alcohol abuse. Given the lack of good studies examining optimal ways of distinguishing between many of these disorders, a careful history, thoughtful skepticism, and interviewing patients' significant others is the best current course.

By definition, adults with ADHD had evidence of the disorder (whether the diagnosis was made or not) as children. The converse of this relationship—the percent of children with ADHD who still show evidence of the disorder as adults—is still unclear, but estimates range between 10 and 50 percent (Cantwell, 1985; Mannuzza et al., 1993). The implications of these estimates are that ADHD symptoms diminish and disappear during adolescence and early adulthood in a substantial portion of children with the disorder. Those who continue to show ADHD symptoms are at high risk to have antisocial behavior, drug and alcohol abuse, or both (Mannuzza et al., 1993). This triad of adult ADHD, antisocial behavior, and drug/alcohol abuse is commonly seen among this population.

The likelihood of ADHD adults suffering from comorbid psychiatric disorders other than antisocial behavior and drug/alcohol abuse is in some dispute. One prominent long-term study found little evidence of mood or anxiety disorders in a group of ADHD adults in their twenties who had been followed since childhood (Mannuzza et al., 1993). In contrast, other studies examining adults with ADHD have found high rates of a variety of anxiety disorders, major depression, and dysthymic disorder (Biederman et al., 1993; Wender, Reimherr, and Wood, 1981).

Psychopharmacological Treatment

The list of potentially effective medications for treating adult ADHD overlaps substantially with agents used for treating children with ADHD. Partly, this reflects the notion that the childhood and adult disorders are the same, and therefore likely respond to similar treatments. Another reason, however, is that with the paucity of pharmacological treatment studies of adult ADHD, the list is drawn heavily from child and adolescent studies with little documentation of the efficacy of many of these medications in adults. Until more is known, however, drawing on the more extensive childhood studies is necessary.

As with children, medications with stimulant properties are the mainstay of treatment for adult ADHD. These include those that cause heightened arousal as their primary effect—called stimulants (see chapter 13)—as well as certain antidepressants with analogous stimulating properties. Table 6–2 lists the medications that have been reported as effective in adults with ADHD (Wilens, Biederman, Spencer, and Prince, 1995).

Often, it is difficult to accurately gauge response to treatment for adult ADHD. One reason for this is that stimulants have nonspecific effects on most people who take them, not just those with ADHD. A single dose of oral d-amphetamine will cause surprisingly similar effects in normal adults and children compared to children with ADHD, with all three groups describing increased vigilance, increased learning, and decreased motor activity (Rapoport, et al., 1980). Because of this, many patients with nonspecific attentional problems who are given stimulants will show increased energy and concentration that will do little to aid in diagnosis. Finally, the ego-syntonic nature of the ADHD may make it difficult for patients to self-evaluate accurately. Since so many of the manifestations of the disorder are behavioral, they are frequently

Table 6–2
Medications for Attention Deficit/Hyperactivity Disorder in Adults

First-Line

Stimulants
  Methylphenidate (Ritalin, Ritalin-SR)
  d-Amphetamine (Dexedrine, Dexedrine spansules)
  Pemoline (Cylert)

Second-Line

Antidepressants
  Bupropion (Wellbutrin)
  Tricyclic antidepressants: desipramine (Norpramin), nortriptyline (Aventyl, Pamelor)
  Venlafaxine (Effexor)
  Monamine oxidase inhibitors: tranylcypromine (Parnate), selegiline (Eldepryl)

Other Agents

  Fluoxetine (Prozac) and other SSRIs?
  Clonidine (Catapres)?

easier to observe by others than by patients themselves. Therefore, as with making the diagnosis, it is vital to involve significant others in treatment evaluation.

Stimulants—primarily methylphenidate (Ritalin) and d-amphetamine (Dexedrine)—are the most commonly used treatments for adult ADHD, as they are for children ADHD. However, the documentation of their efficacy with adults in well-controlled studies is far smaller than that for children. Part of the reason for this is the previously alluded to lack of consensus on how to select the appropriate patients to be treated. Because, as noted above, many patients with impulsivity, irritability, and self-reported concentration problems have diagnoses other than ADHD, treating a group of patients with a variety of disorders will predictably yield mixed results. Nonetheless, there is clear evidence that stimulants are helpful for ADHD adults: Patients show improvement in global functioning, increased attention, decreased motor activity, more mood stability and diminished impulsivity (Wender, Reimherr, Wood, and Ward, 1985; Spencer et al., 1995). As with ADHD children, stimulants are thought to work with adult ADHD patients by increasing their level of alertness and capacity to attend, correcting a postulated poor attentional capacity with secondary effects on hyperactivity and distractability. The positive effects of both methylphenidate and d-amphetamine begin quickly, within hours to days of reaching the correct dose. As with children, tolerance to the medication effects generally does not occur.

Stimulants do have drawbacks, though. First, their clinical effects last only two to five hours, necessitating three to four doses daily. Sustained release preparations of both methylphenidate and d-amphetamine exist but they are not always absorbed as gradually as one would want. Second, since a significant percentage of adult ADHD patients have a history of drug abuse, it is tricky at best to give them an abusable drug. Furthermore, because some of these patients also engage in criminal behavior and stimulants have potential street value, the possibility that these medications will ultimately be ingested by persons other than those for whom they were prescribed is significant. Side effects seen with stimulants include irritability, anxiety, and insomnia in some patients, while others complain of excessive sedation or feeling like a zombie.

Pemoline (Cylert) is another stimulant whose advantages and disadvantages differ from those of methylphenidate and d-amphetamine. Overall, it is probably not as effective in treating ADHD, although some patients respond extremely well (see the case presented below).

However, in marked contrast to the other stimulants, it is virtually nonabusable, producing little or no euphoria and having no street value. The corollary to this is that, as opposed to the rapid effect of methylphenidate and d-amphetamine, pemoline's effects are seen gradually over many weeks. It is also long lasting so that it needs to be taken only once daily. Unfortunately, this makes pemoline more likely than the other stimulants to cause insomnia. Finally, because it causes liver inflammation in a small percentage of those treated, patients taking pemoline need to have regular blood tests, a procedure to which many patients object.

The second-line medications to consider for adult ADHD are bupropion, desipramine, and nortriptyline, antidepressants with the strongest effects on norepinephrine and dopamine, similar to the effect of stimulants. Although no double-blind studies have yet been published on its effects in adults, bupropion has been shown to be effective in an open study in which more than half the patients treated chose to continue bupropion rather than switch back to their stimulant medication (Wender and Reimherr, 1990). Desipramine and nortriptyline, two tricyclic antidepressants, have also been shown to be anecdotally helpful for ADHD at typical antidepressant doses (see chapter 9 for details). Similarly, venlafaxine, the novel antidepressant with biological effects on norepinephrine as well as on serotonin, may be occasionally helpful. Like pemoline, antidepressants are not abusable, although their positive effects in ADHD may be seen very quickly in contrast to their longer latency of action in treating depression. The use of MAO inhibitors, however, is complicated by two clinical problems. First, tolerance to their effects in treating ADHD is common. Second, because of the dietary restrictions inherent in their use (see chapter 9), these are not medications ideally suited to treat a population of impulsive patients with tendencies toward drug abuse.

Other second-line treatments for adult ADHD listed in Table 6–2 can be recommended purely on the basis of experience with children. No case reports even exist supporting the use of fluoxetine, other SSRIs, or clonidine for adults with ADHD. Clonidine's hypotensive and sedative properties make it a difficult drug to use in adults.

On what basis, then, might a psychopharmacologist choose a specific medication to treat adult ADHD? Without question, if the patient is cooperative and has no history of either drug abuse or significant criminal behavior, methylphenidate or d-amphetamine are the treatments of choice. If these medications are ineffective or cause intolerable side effects, or if the patient has a recent or current history of drug abuse or criminal behavior, then pemoline, bupropion, or a tricyclic antidepressant would be appropriate first choices. With patients who have read a story in the lay press and are adamant about the diagnosis of ADHD despite a paucity of evidence, using pemoline or bupropion first often tests the patient's commitment to treatment while giving the clinician a chance to further evaluate the patient during the medication trial.

Madeline was 26 years old and had lived a chaotic life since childhood. As a child, she had always been a behavior problem—demanding, moody, and angry at home and rebellious if disciplined at school, complaining of feeling constantly bored there. She would talk continuously in class and would not stop for more than short periods of time when disciplined. Sitting down and doing homework seemed impossible for her despite a remarkable variety of enticements, rewards, and punishments by her parents. If she was very interested in something, such as certain television shows, Madeline was able to sit for hours and watch them. Although no one thought of her as a "bad kid," Madeline seemed unwilling—or unable—to deal with her age-appropriate tasks. Her moods fluctuated enormously; she was mostly irritable and dysphoric, especially when pushed, but could also be playful, charming, and filled with grand and even grandiose plans at times. Because of her superior intelligence, Madeline was able to graduate from high school despite her behavioral problems. Following graduation, she lived in five cities in the next eight years. In each city, she would get low-paying jobs easily which would never last more than four months, because of poor attendance (explained by boredom according to her), fighting with her boss, and sullen behavior. After each move, Madeline quickly made friends and created good social supports. However, after a few months to years, she would feel increasingly restless and move somewhere else where the cycle would repeat. She had tried every possible street drug but used only marijuana on a regular basis and intermittently drank alcohol to excess.

Madeline came from a middle-class family in which there were two paternal uncles and a first cousin with alcoholism. Her father was a businessman who had had learning difficulties as a child but had never been evaluated or treated psychiatrically.

Surprisingly, Madeline had had little contact with the mental health field. She had seen a few therapists for no more than one or two visits each in high school. At age 14, she was given methylphenidate (Ritalin) for a number of weeks. She remembered no response at all and had discontinued the medication quickly.

Because of a growing frustration with her inability to create a successful career—which, being ambitious, she very much wanted—Madeline sought therapy. After eliciting the above history, her therapist recommended a psychopharmacological consultation, suspecting ADHD. When Madeline's parents confirmed the history, she was given methylphenidate which caused marked dysphoria, even at low dose. It was discontinued and pemoline (Cylert) was begun. After a few weeks, she became more settled. Her moodiness, irritability, and occasional impulsive behavior were still present but in greatly diminished proportion. More important, she was able to stay in her psychotherapy for the next two years, dealing with her issues of self-esteem and inconsistency in relationships. She eventually stopped using marijuana regularly. Recently, she has been training as an assistant in film production, a field she has now worked in for over one year. She continues in psychotherapy, making steady progress.

Systematic long-term studies of adult ADHD—following these patients into their thirties, forties, and fifties—do not exist. As noted above, a substantial number of patients with childhood ADHD seem to "outgrow" the disorder by the time they are young adults. Would a similar proportion of young adults with adult ADHD show similar natural improvement by the time they are in their thirties? Without this information, it is impossible to make recommendations regarding long-term medication treatment for adult ADHD. For now, then, the best recommendation might be to taper and withdraw the medication periodically (e.g., every few years) in order to reassess the continuing need for it. When this is done, it should ideally be with the knowledge of significant others, since ADHD patients do not always recognize the changes in mood and behavior that might ensue following medication discontinuation.

Additionally, my own clinical experience is that those patients with adult ADHD who seek treatment virtually always need psychotherapy. Even if they have avoided substance abuse and are not particularly antisocial, they have grown up labeled as bad kids, underachievers, unable to accomplish as much as peers with similar intelligence. The effects on self-esteem (as exemplified by Madeline) are pervasive, appropriate social skills are often lacking, and patients frequently gravitate towards inappropriate peer groups. Once a good effect from medication has been achieved, long-term psychological work can be both productive and rewarding.

ALCOHOL AND DRUG ABUSE

It may seem paradoxical, at best, to consider prescribing medications in the treatment of patients who have problems modulating their use of drugs since medications, after all, are simply prescribed drugs. Because of this paradox, of all the disorders discussed in this book, drug and alcohol abuse present the most difficult challenges. Psychopharmacologists treating substance abusers should therefore have intensive experience in prescribing medications *for these specific disorders.* In fact, there are some situations in which medications are mandated by law to be administered only by those facilities and practitioners specifically set up to treat the drug abuse—methadone treatment for heroin users, for instance. Even in other situations, however, the problems of drug and alcohol abuse require a unique combination of individual and group treatments without which any medication treatment will be worthless.

For both therapist and psychopharmacologist, the difficulties inherent in treating these patients are heightened by the potential consequences of inappropriate management. For instance, some substances such as cocaine can be stopped suddenly without significant risk to the patient; but abruptly stopping short-acting benzodiazepines that have been taken for a long time at high dose can cause significant withdrawal symptoms, including, rarely, grand mal seizures, and stopping high-dose barbiturates after prolonged use can be life-threatening.

Moreover, accurately diagnosing other psychiatric disorders in the presence of significant drug and alcohol abuse hovers between difficult and impossible. To thoughtfully evaluate an alcohol-abusing patient for a major depression, for instance, almost always requires at least three weeks of sobriety, which the patient usually resists, insisting the alcohol is being used to treat an underlying depression (see below). It is in these types of clinical dilemmas that programs designed to work with alcoholics who may have other disorders (dual diagnosis programs) can be extremely helpful.

Nonetheless, although they never play more than an adjunctive or transient role in overall treatment, medications can be helpful in four possible situations in treating drug and alcohol abuse: (1) in making detoxification safer, simpler, and less painful; (2) in diminishing craving for the abused substance; (3) in diminishing relapse; and (4) by treating coexisting disorders. In this section, I will review the use of medications for all four purposes, with a focus on outpatient treatment of drug and alcohol abuse rather than issues such as inpatient detoxification protocols. Table 6–3 lists the medications considered in the treatment of drug and alcohol abuse, divided by the phase of treatment in which they are used.

Table 6–3
Medication Strategies for Drug/Alcohol Abuse

Drug of Abuse/Phase of Treatment	Medication	Efficacy Rating
Alcohol		
Detoxification	Benzodiazepines	+++
	Anticonvulsants	++
	Beta-blockers	+
	Clonidine	+
Maintenance	Naltrexone	++
	SSRIs	+
	Disulfiram	+
Cocaine		
Detoxification/maintenance	Amantadine	+
	Bromocriptine	+
	Other dopamine agonists	+
	Desipramine	+
	SSRIs	+
Opiates		
Detoxification	Naltrexone/clonidine	+++
	Methadone	+++
Maintenance	Methadone	+++
	LAAM	+++

+++ = Definite efficacy
 ++ = Probable efficacy
  + = Possible efficacy

Alcohol Abuse

Since alcohol abuse is the most common substance abuse disorder, affecting over 13 percent of the American population over a lifetime (with even higher rates among those who have other types of psychopathology), the issue of recognizing and treating it is vital—and difficult (Regier et al., 1988). The problem is complicated by the availability of alcohol and its sanctioned status as a legal and acceptable drug in our society. In my experience, alcoholism is the most commonly missed diagnosis by mental health professionals, including myself.

Traditionally, medications have been considered to play a small role at best in treating alcoholism. In managing acute alcohol withdrawal, there are a number of important variables to be considered: inpatient vs. outpatient status, whether to use adjunctive medications, and if so, which one. Additionally, there is a significant risk of a variety of medical problems when patients stop drinking after long periods of alcohol use, especially if consumed in significant quantities. Therefore, it is often helpful to obtain a consultation from someone expert in this particular area before the detoxification occurs. This is especially true with those patients who have had major problems during previous withdrawals, those with serious medical illnesses, or those with multiple substance abuses who are likely to have a more complicated withdrawal.

A variety of medications listed in Table 6–3 are used to diminish the symptoms inherent in the acute detoxification process (Bohn, 1993). These have included benzodiazepines, anticonvulsants, beta-blockers, and possibly clonidine. Benzodiazepines are the most commonly used, since they are cross-tolerant to alcohol, block the withdrawal symptoms, and diminish the seizure risk during acute withdrawal. Both older long-acting preparations such as chlordiazepoxide (Librium) and shorter-acting agents that are safer for those with liver disease commonly seen in alcoholics—oxazepam (Serax) or lorazepam (Ativan)—are commonly prescribed. Anticonvulsants such as carbamazepine (Tegretol) also seem to block the withdrawal symptoms and reduce seizure risk. Beta-blockers and clonidine may diminish some withdrawal symptoms but do nothing to decrease the risk of withdrawal seizures.

Over the last few years, increased attention has focused on a potential role for medications during the maintenance treatment phase of those with alcohol abuse where the goals are to decrease craving and alcohol consumption. The two agents most promising in this regard are naltrexone, an opiate antagonist, and the SSRI antidepressants.

Although it may seem counterintuitive that an opiate antagonist would aid in treating alcoholism, there are many links between alcohol and opiate effects (O'Brien, Eckardt, and Linnoila, 1995). As examples, alcohol increases endorphins while low doses of morphine increase alcohol consumption in animals. Naltrexone (now marketed as ReVia but previously known as Trexan when it was used solely in the treatment of opiate abuse) may be useful in maintaining abstinence among alcoholics. In two double-blind studies, naltrexone decreased alcohol craving, number of drinking days, and relapse to heavy drinking (Volpicelli, Alterman, Hayashida, and O'Brien, 1992; O'Malley, et al., 1992). Naltrexone may also diminish the alcohol-induced "high" that reinforces alcohol abuse (Volpicelli, Watson, King, Sherman, and O'Brien, 1995). However, it is as yet unclear how helpful naltrexone will be with alcoholics in clinical, nonresearch settings. For the vast majority of alcoholics, naltrexone should not be considered as an effective treatment when prescribed alone, but as a useful adjunct to rehabilitative programs. The usual dose of naltrexone is 50 mg daily. Nausea and headache are the most common side effects.

Less definitively, there may also be a place for the SSRIs in the maintenance treatment phase of alcohol abuse. Overall, SSRIs seem to reduce alcohol consumption in half the alcoholic patients treated in short-term studies (O'Brien, Ekardt and Linnoila, 1995). This effect, in contrast to its antidepressant effects, occurs within the first dose of the SSRI. However, longer clinical trials (i.e., 12 weeks) have not shown consistently positive results (Kranzler et al., 1995). For now, the use of SSRIs to aid in relapse prevention for alcohol abuse should be considered an intriguing possible option and not a routine treatment.

Another common use of medication in the maintenance/prevention phase of alcoholism is to cause an unpleasant reaction if the person does drink, thereby promoting a negative consequence to alcohol use. Disulfiram (Antabuse) is prescribed for this purpose. It works by blocking an intermediate step in the metabolism of alcohol, causing a marked increase in the blood level of acetaldehyde. Usually occurring from one-half hour to a few hours after ingesting alcohol, common symptoms from drinking while taking disulfiram are flushing, sweating, a throbbing headache, nausea, vomiting, chest pain, palpitations, and extraordinary malaise. In unusual circumstances, the reaction may be life-threatening. Disulfiram may serve primarily as a test of motivation or as a mild reinforcer for already motivated patients. Studies documenting its efficacy are few (Kranzler and Orrok, 1989). Patients taking disulfiram who want to drink will simply stop it for a number of days and then drink. Unfortunately, the amount of time needed off disulfiram to avoid a negative reaction with alcohol varies a great deal, thereby putting the patient at risk to have a reaction if he drinks. Reactions may also occasionally occur with disguised forms of alcohol such as cough syrup or aftershave lotion that is absorbed through the skin. Even without alcohol, disulfiram can cause side effects such as fatigue, restlessness, and an unpleasant taste. Overall, then, disulfiram cannot be considered a useful treatment for the majority of alcoholics. Its best use is in aiding those patients who are reasonably motivated but need help resisting the impulse to drink. By itself, disulfiram will *not* keep patients from drinking.

The trickiest and most common clinical dilemma regarding medications in treating alcoholics focuses on diagnosing and treating other coexistent psychiatric disorders or, as it is often framed, finding the underlying problem that "causes" the patient to drink. (It must be understood that little evidence supports such "causative" hypotheses.) A remarkable number of alcoholics also have other psychiatric disorders with estimates ranging up to 75 percent (Ross, Glaser, and Germanson, 1988). With the exception of other substance abuse disorders, the most common coexistent psychiatric disorders among alcoholics are major depression, anxiety disorders, and antisocial personality. Compounding the problem even further is the fact that persistent drinking can cause a great number of the symptoms—such as depression, anxiety, confusion, or psychosis—that are seen in these other disorders (Schuckit, 1983).

Diagnosis of some psychiatric disorders—schizophrenia or mania as examples—can be made with some confidence even in the face of excessive alcohol use. If accurately diagnosed, they can then be treated even while alcohol detoxification is proceeding. Distinguishing between alcohol abuse and depression, however, is a more difficult diagnostic dilemma, since alcohol is a depressant, causing a variety of symptoms also seen in primary depression. Furthermore, many of the secondary effects of alcoholism, including the use of other drugs, psychological responses to life havoc induced by alcohol, and loss of social supports, may exacerbate the depressed mood. Therefore, depending on when the patient is interviewed and how the diagnosis of depression is made, estimates of depression in alcoholics have ranged from 3 to 98 percent! (Keeler, Taylor, and Miller, 1979). The most important consideration in evaluating an independent depressive disorder in alcoholics with prominent depressive features is to establish a clear history of significant mood symptoms prior to the onset of substance abuse (Renner and Ciraulo, 1994). This sequence, however, can be exceedingly difficult to establish due to unreliable histories, cognitive impairment from alcohol, and denial. Information from significant others in this circumstance may be very useful. The best estimate is that for 90 percent of those with both alcoholism and depression together, the primary diagnosis is alcoholism, not depression (Schuckit, 1986).

In general, therefore, the only reliable method of establishing the primary etiology of depressive symptoms in those with alcohol abuse is to evaluate the patient after abstinence has been achieved. A minimum of three weeks of abstinence is required for alcohol-related depressive symptoms to remit (Brown et al., 1995). However, some experts—especially those strongly committed to twelve-step programs—suggest that waiting a number of months is better, since continued mood swings are often seen in abstinent alcoholics for months following sobriety. Whatever the appropriate time frame, it is clear that prescribing antidepressants to heavy drinkers or to those who have been sober for only a few days is generally neither clinically warranted nor wise. Only in the small percent of alcoholics who show evidence of primary depression should there be any consideration of antidepressants until sobriety has been achieved (Nunes et al., 1993).

Similar considerations apply in evaluating anxiety symptoms in alcoholics, although less research has been done in this area. Given alcohol's powerful acute effect in diminishing anxiety, it is not surprising that comorbidity between alcohol abuse and anxiety disorders is high, although as with depression, the effect of alcohol in causing anxiety symptoms complicates the picture (Regier et al., 1990; Schuckit and Hesselbrock, 1994). Therefore, establishing the temporal sequence between alcohol abuse and anxiety symptoms is similarly important—and just as difficult. As in evaluating depressive symptoms in alcoholics, a period of at least a number of weeks of abstinence is required for meaningful evaluation of anxiety symptoms (Frances and Borg, 1993).

In considering pharmacotherapies for patients with alcohol abuse and comorbid anxiety disorders, an important consideration is the cross-tolerance between alcohol and benzodiazepines, the most commonly prescribed class of antianxiety agents. Abstinent alcoholics may experience more euphoria from benzodiazepines than do nonalcoholics, further enhancing the risk of excessive use (Ciraulo et al., 1989). Because of this, other pharmacological agents useful in treating the various anxiety disorders (see chapter 4) should generally be considered first. Buspirone (Buspar) (see chapter 11), which is neither cross-tolerant with alcohol nor associated with physical dependence, may be particularly helpful in treating anxious abstinent alcoholics and may decrease the risk of returning to alcohol abuse (Kranzler et al., 1994).

Finally, when both alcoholism and another primary Axis I disorder coexist, there is a tendency, usually reinforced by the patient, to assume that treatment of the nonalcohol disorder will, by itself, treat the alcoholism. In general, this simply is not true. When two disorders coexist, they must both be treated independently and vigorously.

Cocaine Abuse

Cocaine use in our society mushroomed in the late 1970s and 1980s. With the availability of more dangerous and self-reinforcing preparations—free-base and crack that are smoked rather than insufflated (snorted)—the addictive and dangerous properties of cocaine have been more appreciated, resulting in enhanced public education about the drug. By the early 1990s, therefore, the number of people using cocaine on an occasional basis had decreased. However, during the same period, the number of people using the drug on a regular basis continued on a relatively constant basis (Johanson and Schuster, 1995). Because of this, in conjunction with an increased understanding of the biology of cocaine, a substantial amount of research has explored the use of pharmacological aids to stop cocaine craving and/or to block the effects of the drug. Overall, however, as with alcohol abuse, pharmacotherapy plays a secondary role in the current treatment of cocaine abusers. Nonpharmacological treatments, such as specialized psychotherapies and twelve-step programs, should still be considered the most important factors in diminishing cocaine use and maintaining abstinence.

Potential pharmacological strategies for decreasing cocaine craving have evolved from our knowledge of the biological effects of the drug. Although it has effects on multiple neurotransmitters, cocaine's effects are primarily due to its ability to enhance dopamine activity in the brain. The primary but not exclusive mechanism by which cocaine raises dopamine activity is by reuptake blockade, thereby allowing more of the dopamine to activate the postsynaptic receptors, especially in the mesolimbic and mesocortical pathways in the brain (see chapter 2) (Withers, Pulvirenti, Koob, and Gillin, 1995). Enhancing dopamine activity causes both acute stimulation and euphoria. It also causes paranoia, analogous to the hypothesized dopamine overactivity seen in other paranoid states, such as schizophrenia (which is treated by dopamine blockers). Cocaine craving and withdrawal symptoms probably represent dopamine depletion. Cocaine also blocks the reuptake of other neurotransmitters such as norepinephrine and serotonin, effects that may also help explain its addictive properties (and suggest potential pharmacological treatment strategies) (Hyman and Nestler, 1993). Understanding the longer-term effects of cocaine and the biology of cocaine craving weeks and months after drug discontinuation is complicated by a variety of cellular adaptations that occur after chronic exposure to cocaine's effects (Nestler, Fitzgerald, and Self, 1995).

In contrast to other drugs (such as alcohol), it is difficult conceptually to separate the use of medications to treat acute cocaine withdrawal from those that prevent relapse (Kosten and McCance-Katz, 1995). Since acute cocaine withdrawal is uncomfortable but never medically dangerous, no specific medications need be considered at that time. Typically, when medications are used, they are started soon after drug use ceases and continued into the longer relapse prevention phase.

Strategies for treating cocaine users initially focused on increasing brain dopamine in the acute withdrawal and post-withdrawal period in an attempt to diminish the dopamine depletion and cocaine craving. However, since cocaine also enhances norepinephrine and serotonin function, more recent strategies have explored pharmacotherapeutic approaches affecting these neurotransmitters. Table 6–3 lists the medications used for cocaine abuse.

Dopamine-enhancing medications used to treat cocaine abusers have included amantadine (Symmetrel), bromocriptine (Parlodel), methylphenidate (Ritalin), bupropion (Wellbutrin), and l-dopa (the central ingredient in Sinemet used for treating Parkinson's disease). Although some initial studies have indicated some utility for all of these agents, none has shown consistent efficacy in reducing cocaine abuse. Nonetheless, each of these medications may have some beneficial effect in some patients.

Desipramine (Norpramin, Pertofrane), the tricyclic antidepressant, has been the subject of the most extensive evaluation as a pharmacological treatment for cocaine abuse. The rationale for despramine's use has been its capacity to decrease dopamine receptor sensitivity, thereby reversing the supersensitivity caused by chronic cocaine use. Early studies showed a positive effect of desipramine in diminishing craving and enhancing abstinence (Gawin et al., 1989). Unfortunately, more recent studies have shown less positive results (Carroll et al., 1994). Doses of desipramine prescribed are comparable to those used to combat depression.

Because of cocaine's effects on serotonin, serotonergic antidepressants have been evaluated for treating cocaine abusers. Acutely, fluoxetine (Prozac), the SSRI antidepressant, may diminish the euphoric effect of cocaine (Walsh, Preston, Sullivan, Fromme, and Bigelow, 1994). Unfortunately, fluoxetine's capacity to diminish cocaine use on a longer-term basis is much less clear (Grabowski et al., 1995).

A number of other medications have also been explored for treating cocaine abusers (Kosten and McCance-Katz, 1995). These have included carbamazepine (Tegretol, an anticonvulsant), naltrexone (ReVia, the opiate antagonist), and disulfiram (Antabuse). Currently, none can be recommended as specifically effective.

Just as in evaluating alcoholics for other psychiatric disorders, it is useless to attempt to diagnose an underlying depression or bipolar disorder while a patient is either using cocaine or in the first few weeks of abstinence, since the symptoms seen at that time are more likely secondary to the drug's effects than to a coexisting disorder. Cocaine abusers, however, are at high risk to abuse other substances, typically alcohol or tranquilizers, in order to modulate the cocaine-induced stimulation. This is especially relevant since those patients who abruptly stop benzodiazepines along with cocaine may have simultaneous withdrawal syndromes, one producing depression and the other, irritability and anxiety.

Opiate Abuse (Heroin and Narcotic Analgesics)

Opiates are the most effective and most powerful painkillers available. Heroin is not legal in the United States, while morphine, meperidine (Demerol), hydromorphone (Dilaudid), oxycodone (Percodan), codeine, and propoxyphene (Darvon) are prescribed medications. Since the treatment of opiate abuse virtually always takes place in specialized facilities, the most important recommendation that can be made is that neither therapists nor general psychiatrists should treat serious opiate abuse in a solo practice setting. Table 6–3 lists the medications used in treating opiate abuse.

Aside from the treatment of acute opiate overdose, for which naloxone (a narcotic antagonist which reverses the effects of the drug) is very effective, medications are used to aid opiate detoxification and prevent relapse. For detoxification, a commonly considered approach is the use of naltrexone, the opiate antagonist, along with clonidine, which effectively blocks both the objective and, to a lesser extent, subjective effects of opiate withdrawal. Although side effects such as sedation and dizziness often complicate its use, clonidine is completely nonaddictive. By combining clonidine with an opiate antagonist, relatively quick detoxification can be accomplished (Bigelow and Preston, 1995). Another common approach for detoxification is prescribing methadone for a few days and then tapering it over one to two weeks.

During the ongoing maintenance program of opiate addiction, for those patients who seem to be unable to remain drug-free, methadone, naltrexone, and LAAM may be useful. Methadone, a long-acting oral opiate, can be used as a long-term substitution drug that is prescribed under careful supervision or can be thought of as a transitional treatment with the long-term goal of complete abstinence.

Naltrexone is an opiate antagonist similar, in some ways, to naloxone (see above). It therefore blocks the effect if illegal narcotics are taken. As might be expected, its acceptance among addicts has not been high. It may be most helpful as an aid to those who have good social supports and are already well motivated.

LAAM, approved in 1993, is the most recently approved maintenance medication for opiate abusers. It is chemically related to methadone but is even longer-acting, thereby allowing dosing on a less than daily regimen (typically three times weekly). Similarly, buprenorphine (Buprenex), an opiate partial agonist has been used recently in maintenance treatment of opiate abuse. Because it is a partial agonist, it may be associated with less abuse liability (but still some) compared to methadone and LAAM.

Other Drugs

In the treatment of drug abuse involving other drugs, medications play very little to no role, except in treating acute toxic reactions, a situation that is generally confined to emergency rooms. The only other use of medications is in detoxifying patients who take high doses of short-acting sedatives (such as barbiturates). In these cases, a common strategy is to substitute a long-acting barbiturate, such as phenobarbital in equivalent doses, and then gradually taper it over seven to ten days. Since blood levels of long-acting medications decrease gradually when tapered, withdrawal symptoms are minimized. A similar approach is sometimes used to withdraw a patient from short-acting benzodiazepines, in which a longer-acting tranquilizer, such as clonazepam, is substituted and then tapered.

7

Personality Disorders

WITHOUT QUESTION, the use of medications to treat personality disorders and traits is the most interesting, exciting, and frustrating area in all of psychopharmacology. All aspects of clinical importance—how to diagnose personality disorders, when to consider medications, which medications to consider, how long to continue them—are mired in a conceptual muddle. Compounding the confusion, in no other area of psychopharmacology is there such clinical interest, regular prescription of medications—and an astounding lack of studies to guide treatment. This unstable mix of interest and ignorance has been heightened by the controversy surrounding *Listening to Prozac* (Kramer, 1993). Editorials are written complaining about "cosmetic psychopharmacology" and the overuse of medications in treating normal human suffering and angst. At the same time, many individuals quietly call their internists or therapists after reading *Listening to Prozac* and ask about trying Prozac, hoping to obtain the types of "transformations" described in the book. All of this hoopla unfortunately distracts from the central issue: do psychotropic medications effectively treat personality disorders and, if so, how can they be utilized most thoughtfully?

DIAGNOSIS

The notion of describing or diagnosing personality types or disorders is not new. From the ancient Greeks who suggested that the balance of the bodily humors determined personality types to the nineteenth-century term "constitutional psychopathic insanity" describing what we now call antisocial personality, there has always been interest in categorizing the patterns of behavior subsumed under the current use of the word personality. DSM-IV, like its predecessors, uses a categorical scheme in which disorders are judged to be present or absent and in which there is a defined demarcation between having the personality disorder and not having it. With little empirical basis for most of its per-

211

sonality disorder categories, DSM-IV seems—and to a large degree is—arbitrary. An alternative approach to classifying personality traits/ disorders uses a dimensional approach in which patients are described along a continuum of traits analogous to the measurement of intelligence. Dimensional approaches themselves differ greatly, with the number of personality dimensions ranging between two and forty. A well-known and validated example of a dimensional approach to personality description is that of Eysenck and Eysenck (1964).

Even if we accept the categorical approach of DSM-IV in defining personality disorders, the problem of overlap among the disorders makes diagnosis and treatment planning confusing. Most patients with one personality disorder will meet criteria for at least one other (and frequently more) (Widiger and Rogers, 1989). This overlap may be charitably described as comorbidity (the occurrence of two or more discrete disorders) but typically reflects the overlap in the diagnostic criteria, with the patient having one set of traits that fit into two (or more) of our diagnostic boxes. In order partially to address this problem, DSM-IV describes personality disorder clusters in which a group of disorders that overlap the most in their diagnostic criteria can be considered as related entities. (By defining personality disorder clusters, DSM-IV acknowledges the fluid boundaries of personality disorder categories, and creates a crudely dimensional view of personality dysfunction.) Cluster A comprises the odd or eccentric personality disorders. Within this group are the paranoid, schizoid, and schizotypal disorders. Cluster B, characterized by intense, chaotic emotionality, includes antisocial, borderline, histrionic, and narcissistic disorders. Cluster C, consisting of those disorders primarily manifested by anxiety or fear, is composed of avoidant, dependent, and obsessive compulsive disorders.

Inherent in the notion of personality is that the described traits are relatively constant over time and do not change markedly over weeks or months as might, for instance, symptoms of Axis I disorders. Therefore, in the definition of personality disorders, DSM-IV requires that the personality traits used for making diagnoses be inflexible, pervasive, and enduring over time and across a broad range of personal and social situations. Furthermore, consistent with DSM-IV definitions of Axis I disorders, personality disorders lead to significant impairment and distress in social, occupational, or other areas of functioning.

Given the central notion of personality traits and disorders as stable and enduring, inferring the presence of these traits in the midst of a moderate to severe Axis I disorder is fraught with difficulties (Hirschfeld et al., 1983). As an example, dependency traits measured during a major depression may reflect either a true personality trait or depressive symptoms that will remit along with the depression. Similarly, manipulative, antisocial, and passive-aggressive traits seen during a manic or hypomanic episode may be due to either the mood disorder or a personality disorder. Certainly, not all manifestations of personality will change during an episode of mania, depression, or other Axis I disorder but enough do to suggest caution. It makes more sense simply to wait until the patient has emerged from the acute episode before making a personality diagnosis.

Even after cautious evaluation, symptom-based Axis I disorders and personality disorders frequently coexist. A number of models have been proposed to explain the possible relationship between these two types of disorders (Docherty et al., 1986). The classical psychodynamic model is that the personality disorder predisposes the individual to the Axis I disorder, typically depression. Thus, a narcissistic or dependent patient who relies on external objects to achieve a stable sense of self will be greatly affected by the loss of a relationship such that a depression might ensue. Another possibility is that the personality disorder is simply an attenuated version of the Axis I disorder. In many ways, this model describes a dimensional approach, considering personality traits and symptoms as representing similar clinical phenomena. (This approach is frequently used in considering psychopharmacological approaches for personality disorders and is discussed more below.) In many cases, DSM-IV defines the disorders in a manner consistent with this approach. As an example, some characteristics of DSM-IV borderline personality disorder—impulsivity, affective instability, intense anger—utilize the language of Axis I mood disorders. A third possibility is that the personality disorder is a result—or complication—of the syndromal disorder. Patients with panic disorder who are also dependent and avoidant would be conceptualized as first having had the panic disorder which then led to the personality disorder because of the fearfulness and helplessness that is a characteristic result of panic attacks. The fourth model postulates that the two coexisting disorders stem from the same causative factors. A combination of genetic predisposition and poor early environment would then result, for instance, in both depression and narcissistic personality disorder.

Of course, the models just presented are simplifications that allow us to begin to consider these complex relationships among disorders. For any individual patient, one model (or more than one) will fit the clinical picture better than others. Sometimes, a combination of models fits best. In the case of John (described in chapter 3), his narcissistic personality (a predisposing cause) may have contributed to his cocaine abuse which then precipitated his bipolar disorder which, in combination with his personality disorder, culminated in a demoralization state (as a complication).

Just as an Axis I disorder may mimic symptoms of a personality disorder, the presence of a severe personality disorder may mask the onset of an incipient Axis I disorder. Two of the more common situations of this type are: (1) when a patient who is chronically dysphoric as part of a personality disorder has the new onset of a major depression, and (2) during the ongoing treatment of a borderline or narcissistic patient whose life is filled with constant crises and who begins to have bipolar/cyclothymic mood swings that are superimposed upon the person's life-event-driven chaos (as shown in the case of Donna in chapter 14). In these cases, the key to accurate diagnosis is to ask the right questions. If a patient with a personality disorder appears to get worse during ongoing treatment, asking the questions needed to make the diagnoses of mania and/or depression (see chapter 3) will often help clarify the clinical situation.

SUBTYPES

Cluster A: Odd or Eccentric Personality Disorders

Cluster A disorders encompass paranoid, schizoid, and schizotypal types. Patients with these personality disorders have the core characteristics of being interpersonally distant, emotionally constricted, and, in paranoid and schizotypal disorders, interpreting events in unusual ways. Historically, these disorders have generally been linked with schizophrenia, despite a lack of consistent evidence justifying this link for other than schizotypal disorder (Kendler, Gruenberg, and Kinney, 1994). No significant changes in the diagnostic criteria for Cluster A personality disorders have been made in DSM-IV.

Paranoid patients are characterized simply by pervasive paranoid feelings and behaviors—expectations of being slighted, hypervigilance for subtle negative cues, excessive suspiciousness, mistrust without cause, and so on. Virtually no research exists on paranoid personalities. Aside from the other disorders in this cluster, these characteristics are frequently seen in borderline or antisocial personalities.

Schizoid personalities are distant, removed people, having few (or no) friends, experiencing few (or no) intense emotions, and seeming indifferent to praise or criticism. Many of these patients could also be diagnosed as avoidant personalities because of the overlap in the diagnostic criteria. However, the hallmark of schizoid patients is that they do not miss having emotions and relationships, whereas avoidant patients are (allegedly) too pained to be with others but would like to be.

Schizotypal patients show the interpersonal constriction and emotional flatness of schizoid and paranoid patients but also exhibit a variety of odd cognitive and perceptual behavioral symptoms such as ideas of reference, odd beliefs (e.g., telepathy), magical thinking, unusual perceptual experiences, and nonlinear speech (e.g., vague, circumstantial, or overly metaphorical). It is likely that many of these patients are misclassified as having personality disorders and should be more correctly thought of as having a schizophrenia spectrum disorder (Siever, Kalus, and Keefe, 1993). Other schizotypal patients will also be diagnosed as borderline.

> Denise came to the clinic to be evaluated because of an inner sense that something was wrong, although she couldn't quite describe what it was. Talking about her feelings in a disjointed, hard-to-follow manner, she described how she lived by herself in a small house in a canyon outside Los Angeles with her six cats, three dogs, and many rabbits. Denise had no friends, explaining that she felt pressure when she was with people and a sense that they disliked her and were mocking her. Her communication with her animals was more satisfying. Furthermore, when people had visited her in the past, it annoyed her that they always commented on her collection of used aluminum foil which she kept in piles in the living room. At times, during smoggy days, she was sure she could feel an evil spirit pervading the atmosphere which promised the destruction of the city, an experience she related without any particular concern. She denied true hallucinations or well-formed delusions. When the interviewer expressed interest in Denise's sense of "something wrong" and offered to see her again, she compliantly agreed but didn't keep the appointment. Since Denise had no telephone in her house, the therapist wrote a letter to which there was no response.

Cluster B: Emotional or Chaotic Personality Disorders

Antisocial, borderline, histrionic, and narcissistic types are included in this group. These patients are characterized by their chaotic lives and, with the possible exception of antisocial personality, chaotic emotions and relationships. The presence of intense emotionality in these patients superficially links Cluster B disorders and Axis I mood disorders. However, as will be discussed more below, Cluster B personality disorders include a combination of affective and impulsive/aggressive traits.

The core feature of antisocial personality disorder is a pervasive pattern of disregard for, and violating the rights of others. These features must be present since age 15, thereby ruling out the disorder in a patient who exhibits new-onset criminal behavior in his twenties or thirties. Thus, antisocial personality describes traits similar to those of child/adolescent conduct disorder that have continued into adulthood. Antisocial traits include repeated illegal acts, lying, aggressive behavior usually resulting in fights or assaultiveness, irresponsibility, and lack of remorse. Compared to prior manuals, the criteria for antisocial personality have been simplified considerably in DSM-IV, although the core descriptive features are consistent.

Borderline personality disorder is characterized by emotional, intrapersonal, and interpersonal chaos. The choice of the term "borderline" is unfortunate since it implies that these patients are on the edge of another disorder. Historically, the term originally referred to borderline schizophrenia, but it is clear that using our current definitions, the vast majority of borderline patients have a disorder that is unrelated to schizophrenia. DSM-IV borderline personality disorder shares some similarities with, but is far from identical to, the psychoanalytic term borderline personality organization.

The DSM-IV criteria for borderline personality disorder, shown in Table 7–1, describe a diverse group of behaviors and characteristics including unstable relationships, intense affects, self-image problems, and impulsivity. DSM-IV also added a new criterion describing the tendency of borderline patients to have stress-related psychotic or dissociative symptoms.

Partly because the features defining the disorder cut across a wide variety of domains, patients with borderline personality disorder vary enormously in their clinical presentation. Thus a number of subtyping schemes for borderline personality have been proposed, with the hope that these subgroups will describe a more unitary disorder for which specific treatment responses (including those to medications) can be predicted. The most intriguing of these subtyping schemes divides the symptoms of borderline patients into four patterns: hysteroid dysphoric, schizotypal, observed affective (empty), and impulsive (Soloff, 1989). Hysteroid dysphoric patients (this unfortunate name is derived from an older concept taken from mood disorder subtypes—see chapter 3) show prominent mood lability, rejection sensitivity, and atypical

Table 7–1
Diagnostic Criteria for Borderline Personality Disorder

A pervasive pattern of instability of interpersonal relationships, self-image, and affects, and marked impulsivity beginning by early adulthood and present in a variety of contexts, as indicated by five (or more) of the following:

(1) frantic efforts to avoid real or imagined abandonment. **Note:** Do not include suicidal or self-mutilating behavior covered in Criterion 5.

(2) a pattern of unstable and intense interpersonal relationships characterized by alternating between extremes of idealization and devaluation

(3) identity disturbance: markedly and persistently unstable self-image or sense of self

(4) impulsivity in at least two areas that are potentially self-damaging (e.g., spending, sex, substance abuse, reckless driving, binge eating). **Note:** Do not include suicidal or self-mutilating behavior covered in Criterion 5.

(5) recurrent suicidal behavior, gestures, or threats, or self-mutilating behavior

(6) affective instability due to a marked reactivity of mood (e.g., intense episodic dysphoria, irritability, or anxiety usually lasting a few hours and only rarely more than a few days)

(7) chronic feelings of emptiness

(8) inappropriate, intense anger or difficulty controlling anger (e.g., frequent displays of temper, constant anger, recurrent physical fights)

(9) transient, stress-related paranoid ideation or severe dissociative symptoms

Reprinted with permission from the *Diagnostic and Statistical Manual of Mental Disorders, Fourth Edition.* Copyright 1994 American Psychiatric Association.

depressive features. Borderline patients with the schizotypal pattern show prominent psychotic features and cognitive/perceptual distortions, such as depersonalization, derealization, magical thinking, and transient psychotic symptoms. Patients with prominent "empty" symptoms typically exhibit pervasive depressive mood, apathy, endless neediness, and dependency. Those with predominantly impulsive/aggressive features exhibit prominent reactive acting-out behavior, including drug and alcohol use, promiscuous sexuality, self-mutilation, and overdoses. Although conceptually useful, the validity of subtyping schemes has yet to be demonstrated.

Histrionic personalities are primarily characterized by excessive emotionality and attention-seeking behavior. Dramatic and exaggerated responses to everyday situations are typical, as are unusually sexually seductive qualities. Histrionic patients are easily influenced by others. They often consider relationships to be closer than they actually are, creating a pattern of pseudo-intimate friendships.

Narcissistic personality is defined by behaviors and feelings that are midway between the profound chaos of borderline personalities and the less destructive features of histrionic patients. Narcissistic patients are characterized by preoccupation with self-aggrandizement and grandiosity with a striking lack of empathy for others. The only change in the DSM-IV criteria has been to highlight the arrogant behaviors and attitudes of narcissistic individuals.

Cluster C: Anxious or Fearful Personality Disorders

This group comprises avoidant, dependent, and obsessive compulsive types. Patients with these disorders are characterized by constricting behaviors (similar to agoraphobia) that seem designed to limit risks. Thus, avoidant patients simply avoid interpersonal situations, dependent personalities avoid being personally responsible for decisions, and obsessive compulsive patients use overly rigid rules that preclude new behaviors or situations. The major change in DSM-IV Cluster C personality disorders has been the deletion of passive-aggressive personality disorder, which is now found in the Appendix as a criteria set provided for further study. The DSM-III-R definition of passive-aggressive personality disorder was too narrow in its scope, and its diagnostic criteria were too redundant to justify its inclusion as an enduring, pervasive personality disorder.

Patients with avoidant personality disorder manifest a pervasive pattern of social inhibition, hypersensitivity to being evaluated by others, and a preoccupation with feelings of social inadequacy. Because of these feelings, they tend to be viewed by others as shy and emotionally inhibited. In contrast to schizoid individuals, avoidant patients desire more and better relationships.

Dependent personality disorder is characterized by a pervasive need for being taken care of by others and fear of separation. This leads to a pattern of submissive and clinging behavior within relationships. Often, dependent individuals will submit to inappropriate demands or abusive behavior in order to continue the dependent relationship.

The core characteristic of obsessive compulsive personality disorder is a preoccupation with orderliness, perfectionism, and control. When present to a lesser degree and when they do not dominate the personality structure, these same traits may be adaptive. The rigidity, focus on details, and preoccupation with work seen in obsessive compulsive individuals typically erode their interpersonal relationships. It is these difficulties—especially in romantic relationships—that usually bring the obsessive compulsive individual into treatment.

NATURAL HISTORY, EPIDEMIOLOGY, AND GENETICS

By definition, personality disorders are chronic and enduring. However, the natural history of personality disorders has infrequently been studied empirically. Cluster B disorders, especially antisocial and borderline personalities, seem to show gradual improvement during middle age (Robins, 1987; Tyrer, Casey, and Ferguson, 1991). Other personality disorders are less likely to show natural improvement over the years.

Personality disorders are relatively common in the general population, with estimates ranging between 10 to 13 percent (Gunderson and Phillips, 1995). For specific personality disorders, epidemiological estimates are most well documented for antisocial personality disorder which is found in 3 percent of the population (Robins et al., 1984). Paranoid, narcissistic, obsessive compulsive, and antisocial personalities are more common in men, while borderline, histrionic, and dependent personalities are more common in women.

The genetic links for personality disorders and for their relationships to Axis I disorders have been inconsistently studied. Among the Cluster A disorders, schizotypal personality disorder is linked to schizophrenia (Kendler, Gruenberg, and Kinney, 1994). Paranoid and schizoid personality disorders bear a more uncertain relationship to schizophrenia. Paranoid personality disorder, however, may be genetically linked to delusional disorder (Bernstein, Useda, and Siever, 1993). For Cluster B disorders, antisocial patients have increased rates of alcoholism and somatization disorders in their families as well as high rates of other family members with antisocial personalities (Guze, 1976). The familial increase in rates of antisocial personalities is seen even in adopted-away offspring, implying that the link is at least partially genetic (Crowe, 1974). Borderline personality disorder probably runs in families, although it is not clear how much of this link is genetic (Siever, Steinberg, Trestman, and Intrator, 1994). More consistently, certain personality traits, such as impulsivity and affective instability seem genetically transmitted, possibly providing vulnerability factors for the development of Cluster B disorders under certain environmental (e.g., familial) conditions. Borderline personalities show high rates of depression in their families, although this is seen only in the families of borderline patients who are themselves depressed (Gunderson and Phillips, 1991). Among Cluster C disorders, avoidant and dependent personality traits seem familial (Reich, 1989).

PSYCHOPHARMACOLOGICAL TREATMENT OF PERSONALITY DISORDERS

In the treatment of many patients with personality disorders, especially milder ones, the issue of using medications as an adjunct to psychotherapy will never arise—nor should it. However, patients with the more difficult personality disorders, especially those with borderline personality, are at best difficult to treat and at times unmanageable. Behavioral outbursts, impulsive suicide attempts and gestures, intense overwhelming affects, marked reactive mood changes, occasional odd perceptual and cognitive experiences such as depersonalized states often leave both therapist and patient wondering whether medication might be of any help. As a generalization, the more severe the personality disorder, the more reasonable it is to pursue psychopharmacological consultation. This usually means borderline, schizotypal, severe narcissistic and avoidant personalities. Not coincidentally, the description of a personality disorder as more severe often refers to the presence of associated symptoms, such as those seen in Axis I disorders. As an example, a dependent patient may have a clear pattern of interpersonal maladaptive behaviors but a paucity of clearly describable psychiatric symptoms. A borderline patient, on the other hand, will have both abnormal interpersonal relationships along with clear symptoms such as affective lability and impulsive behaviors. The more a patient's difficulties can be described in symptom terms—as opposed to intrapsychic or interpersonal pattern terms—the more likely it is that medication may be somewhat helpful.

Conceptual Models of Pharmacotherapy: What Are We Treating?

Three models have been suggested to explain what we are treating when medications are prescribed for personality disorders: (1) treating the personality disorder itself; (2) treating symptom clusters within or across disorders; and (3) treating associated Axis I disorders (Gitlin, 1993b).

The first model, that medications can treat the personality disorder itself rests on two assumptions: (1) that at least some personality disorders as defined by the DSMs are discrete diagnostic entities for which specific treatments can be delineated; and (2) that at least *some* aspects of personality are derived from biological factors. The first of these assumptions is unlikely to be valid since, as noted previously, there is so much evident overlap between personality disorders. As currently defined, personality disorders cannot be considered clearly demarcated entities with specific treatments that reduce or eradicate their symptoms. Therefore, even if it can be shown that a medication can reduce the symptoms of a personality disorder (e.g., SSRIs for borderline personality), it seems inaccurate to conceptualize the disorder itself as being successfully treated.

Evidence for the second assumption, that some of what is defined as personality is biologically determined, is increasingly compelling. Animal breeding represents one of the clearest examples of this. In dogs, for instance, breeds differ by personality attributes such as aggressiveness or sociability, nervousness and timidity (McGuffin and Thapar, 1992). In humans, genetic influences in normal personality traits vary, with most traits, including well-defined constructs such as neuroticism and extraversion, showing 40 to 60 percent heritability (Gitlin, 1995a). Consistent with these observations, monozygotic twins raised apart have shown comparable personality similarities compared to monozygotic twins raised together (Bouchard, Lykken, McGue, Segal, and Tellegan, 1990). Overall, then, some of the traits subsumed in the term personality can be considered biological in origin. Given this conclusion, it is possible that medications could alter these traits with an overall change in personality functioning.

The second model, that medications are effective in treating personality disorders by ameliorating symptom clusters, is predicated on a dimensional model. Using this model, pharmacological approaches would be constructed based on postulated dimensions or symptom clusters. The most commonly proposed scheme, delineating four basic dimensions of psychopathology is shown in Table 7–2 (Siever and Davis, 1991). Using this approach, a clinician would target specific characteristic traits/symptoms for pharmacotherapy. One would then conceptualize using medications to treat, for instance, affective instability, regardless of whether the disorder being treated was a personality disorder, such as narcissistic, borderline, or histrionic types, or an Axis I disorder such as atypical depression (as described in chapter 3).

Another example of the symptom cluster approach to pharmacotherapy for personality disorders is that delineated in *Listening to Prozac*, which describes psychopathological dimensions such as rejec-

Table 7–2
Proposed Psychopathological Dimensions/Symptom Clusters

Dimension	Axis II Disorders	Characteristic Traits	Axis I Disorder
Cognitive/ perceptual organization	Cluster A disorders	Disorganization psychotic-like symptoms	Schizophrenia
Impulsivity/ aggression	Borderline and antisocial disorders	Readiness to action, irritability/aggression	Impulse control disorders, mood disorders
Affective instability	Cluster B disorders especially borderline and possibly histrionic disorder	Environmentally responsive, transient affective shifts	Mood disorders
Anxiety/ Inhibition	Cluster C disorders	Autonomic arousal, fearfulness, inhibition	Anxiety disorders

Adapted from *American Journal of Psychiatry*, Vol. 148, p. 1649, 1991. Copyright 1991 the American Psychiatric Association. Reprinted by permission.

tion sensitivity, rigidity/compulsivity, inhibited temperament/risk avoidance, and low self-esteem (Kramer, 1993). All these dimensions are postulated as being responsive to selective serotonin reuptake inhibitors (SSRIs).

In many ways, the biological aspects of model 1 and the dimensional aspects of model 2 reflect a similar notion: that medications can treat those aspects of personality that are biologically determined. Insofar as the symptoms of a specific personality disorder reflect these temperamental aspects of personality, medications could be useful. Those personality disorders that are predominantly defined by nonbiologically derived traits would theoretically be less amenable to pharmacotherapy.

The third model, that medications are effective in treating personality disorders by treating comorbid Axis I disorders that may be hidden by the prominent personality features, highlights Axis I/Axis II comorbidity. Using this model, the efficacy of an antidepressant in treating borderline personality disorder would be understood as treating an underlying depression. This model may be occasionally valid since the treatment of a comorbid depression in a borderline personality would, for instance, be associated with a global clinical improvement. Yet, for a variety of reasons, model 3 is not likely to explain the efficacy of medications for most patients with personality disorders. As an example, the response of borderline patients to an antidepressant is independent of the presence of a comorbid major depression (Soloff et al., 1989). Additionally, the depressive quality of borderline patients may differ from that associated with classic Axis I depressive disorders (Rogers, Widiger, and Krupp, 1995).

Currently, conceptualizing medications as treating the components of personality disorder that reflect biological, temperamental aspects of personality seems the most reasonable. Clinically, the most practical use of this conclusion would be to consider patients with personality disorders for pharmacological intervention if they exhibit one or more of the symptom clusters/dimensions shown in Table 7–2. At the same time, however, it must be acknowledged that no study has yet demonstrated that identifying a symptom dimension for targeted treatment has helped predict which patients with personality disorders will improve from specific pharmacotherapies. Therefore, this scheme should be considered conceptually useful but not necessarily practical.

PSYCHOPHARMACOLOGICAL TREATMENT OF SPECIFIC PERSONALITY DISORDERS

This section follows the DSM-IV clusters and disorders since these are the terms and categories most familiar to clinicians. At the same time, however, many clinical decisions are based upon dimensional thinking, such as treating affective lability, regardless of whether the patient has a borderline or narcissistic personality. Table 7–3 shows the medications to consider in treating patients with personality disorders. In keeping with the above discussion, the table is organized by DSM-IV clusters, dimensions/symptom clusters, and specific disorders.

Cluster A: Odd or Eccentric Personality Types

The symptom cluster associated with Cluster A personality disorder is that of cognitive/perceptual abnormalities. Not surprisingly, therefore, the antipsychotics are the medications most commonly considered to treat patients with these disorders. Unfortunately, because both para-

Table 7–3
Medication Strategies for Personality Disorders

Disorder	Symptom Cluster/ Dimension	Medications	Efficacy[a]
Cluster A Paranoid Schizoid	Cognitive/perceptual	Antipsychotics	+
Schizotypal		Antipsychotics	+
Cluster B	Affective instability	SSRIs, MAO inhibitors, neuroleptics, beta blockers, lithium	
	Impulsivity/aggression	SSRIs, carbamazepine	
Antisocial Borderline		Neuroleptics	++
		SSRIs	++
		MAOIs	+
		Carbamazepine	+
Histrionic/ narcissistic	SSRIs	++	
		MAOIs	++
Cluster C	Anxiety/inhibition	Benzodiazepines, antidepressants	
Avoidant Dependent Obsessive compulsive		SSRIs, MAOIs	++

+++ = Definite efficacy
 ++ = Probable efficacy
  + = Possible efficacy
[a] Either for the disorder or for associated symptom clusters commonly seen in the disorder

noia and lack of insight are so common in these disorders, few of these patients, especially those with paranoid and schizoid personalities, will enter treatment and even fewer will take medication. No studies on treating either paranoid or schizoid patients with medication exist.

There is some evidence, on the other hand, for the efficacy of low-dose antipsychotics in the treatment of schizotypal personalities (Gitlin, 1995a). Many of the patients treated in these studies were both schizotypal and borderline, however, thereby making it more difficult to ascertain therapeutic effects for pure schizotypal patients. Nonetheless, some schizotypal patients show improvement on a variety of symptoms including ideas of reference and odd communication but also in social isolation and phobic anxiety. The magnitude of the therapeutic effect tends to be modest, suggesting that although the medications help, they rarely make a dramatic difference in patients' symptoms or psychological functioning (Soloff et al., 1986b). Generally, the higher-potency neuroleptics have been used and at lower doses than are typically prescribed for schizophrenic patients. At this point, it seems that antipsychotics have a limited role in the treatment of schizotypal patients, although when patients respond to the medications, it is likely to be in a broad-based manner.

Cluster B: Emotional or Chaotic Personality Types

The vast majority of interest, clinical work, and research in the pharmacotherapy of personality disorders has centered on Cluster B disorders—antisocial, borderline, histrionic, and narcissistic personalities—with the bulk of the interest focused on borderline patients. Because of their intensity and the prominent biological "feel" they exhibit, such as affective lability or recurrent decompensations under stress, these patients are commonly considered for pharmacological treatment. Cluster B personality disorders are dominated by symptoms in the affective instability and impulsivity/aggression dimensions. These two psychopathological dimensions have been demonstrated to be associated with both characteristic biological abnormalities and to have genetic roots (Coccaro and Siever, 1995; Siever, Steinberg, Trestmen, and Intrator, 1994). The most consistent finding has been the association between low serotonin metabolites and impulsive aggressive personality traits, whether directed against self (self-mutilation, suicide attempts) or others (violent aggressive or antisocial acts). Although the implication of these findings would be the use of serotonergic medications for patients with these characteristics, and this clinical strategy is common, few studies have yet validated this approach.

Patients with Cluster B personality disorders are at high risk to have an associated mood disorder. Atypical depression characterized by mood reactivity is specifically seen in patients with Cluster B disorders (see chapter 3 and below).

There is no evidence that antisocial personality responds in any way to medications. Many of these patients, however, show the types of impulsive aggressive traits that might respond to some medications. Carbamazepine (Tegretol), lithium, and propranolol (Inderal) have all shown some efficacy in diminishing explosive outbursts (Gitlin, 1995a). Unfortunately, the efficacy of SSRIs for antisocial personality patients with explosive outbursts has yet to be explored. Other antisocial patients may also have attention deficit/hyperactivity disorder (ADHD), which can be treated by stimulants or similar agents. However, because amphetamine-like stimulants have clear street value, they must be prescribed with extreme caution to antisocial patients who have ADHD (see chapter 6). Prescribing stimulants for antisocial patients without substantial clinical evidence for associated ADHD is an invitation to therapeutic disaster.

As befits a disorder that is broad in its manifestations and difficult in its treatment, borderline personality disorder has been treated with virtually every type of medication prescribed by psychiatrists. Often, they are prescribed out of the therapeutic desperation engendered during the tumultuous treatment. Complicating the picture is the remarkable clinical diversity of borderline patients, as exemplified by the subtyping scheme described earlier in the chapter. Despite these attempts at creating order out of the chaos of these patients' symptoms, pharmacotherapeutic strategies still rely heavily on an empirical "shotgun approach." As shown in Table 7–3, a variety of medications seem to be helpful for at least some borderline patients.

The most well-documented observation is that some borderline patients show a clear, albeit limited response to low-dose antipsychotics (Gitlin, 1995a). All neuroleptics are likely to be effective, with the choice of a specific agent made by side effect profiles (see chapter 12 for details). Most of the research studies on this topic have focused on the more severe borderline patients who are hospitalized. It is likely that less disturbed patients will both derive less benefit and be more intolerant of neuroleptic side effects (Soloff et al., 1993). When neuroleptics are beneficial, the therapeutic effects may be broad-based with improvements seen in anxiety, depression, feelings of self-control, and paranoia. Less improvement tends to be seen with the more intrapsychic and interpersonal symptoms. Clinically, my experience with borderline patients who are not in hospital is that those who are in crisis and show fragmented thinking and overwhelming anxiety respond best to low-dose antipsychotics, frequently averting either hospitalization or significant acting out. Rarely, a severely ill borderline patient with prominent psychotic symptoms (but far less severe than would be seen in schizophrenia) will respond to clozapine (Frankenburg and Zanarini, 1993).

A variety of antidepressants are used to treat borderline patients. As noted above, the presence of a comorbid major depression does not enhance the likelihood of a response. Most likely to be effective are SSRIs and MAO inhibitors, presumably because of their serotonergic effects. In contrast, cyclic antidepressants seem to have little positive effect in treating borderline personality disorder. Both SSRIs and MAO inhibitors consistently reduce irritability, mood lability, and anger outbursts (Cowdry and Gardner, 1988; Salzman et al., 1995). At the same time, strong recommendations for these medications must be tempered by the more modest effects seen in research studies for MAO inhibitors and the paucity of studies using SSRIs. However, anecdotal studies and general clinical experience (including my own) indicate that borderline patients often show clear improvement when treated with SSRIs. When effective, they allow excessively mood-reactive and irritable patients to become far more able to tolerate the interpersonal stresses that are part of personal and therapeutic relationships. Self-destructive behavior resulting from the intense inner tension so common in these patients also diminishes.

Despite the affective lability of borderline patients, mood stabilizers have been infrequently studied as a pharmacological option. Lithium has no documented efficacy. Carbamazepine (Tegretol) may be effective specifically in those patients with frequent behavioral outbursts, such as wrist cutting, head banging, and so on (Cowdry and Gardner, 1988). Valproate (Depakote) has not been systematically examined for treating borderline patients but is occasionally used successfully in clinical practice.

Benzodiazepines, such as alprazolam (Xanax), and tricyclic antidepressants, such as amitriptyline (Elavil) can sometimes cause a paradoxical effect in borderline patients, precipitating an increase in behavioral dyscontrol; this would suggest caution in their use (Soloff, George, Nathan, Schuz, and Perel, 1986; Cowdry and Gardner, 1988).

Given the range of pharmacotherapeutic options for treating borderline patients, it would be helpful to have a logical treatment algorithm. As noted above, the symptom cluster/dimensional grouping, although helpful conceptually, has not been shown to predict treatment response. Similarly, the borderline subtyping scheme which divides the disorder into hysteroid dysphoric, schizotypal, empty, and impulsive/aggressive subtypes does not successfully predict response to specific medication treatments. Most observers still assume that these subtyping schemes do have merit and will predict treatment once the subgroups are better delineated and we have a keener knowledge of our medications. Until then, however, an empirical approach still holds sway: if an appropriate treatment seems not to be effective, working with another agent from a different class (e.g., switching from an SSRI to a neuroleptic) would be appropriate.

Little is known about the optimal time frame of pharmacotherapy for those borderline patients who have benefited from the medications. In general, because of the risk of tardive dyskinesia with prolonged use (see chapter 12), antipsychotics should be prescribed for as short a period of time as is clinically appropriate. Those patients with predominant symptoms of mood lability and/or acting-out behavior who have benefited from SSRIs or MAO inhibitors might be considered for a one- to two-year medication trial. If at that time the patient is doing well, it would be reasonable to consider slowly withdrawing the medication. My experience, however, is that most of these patients relapse after medication withdrawal.

> Ann, 32 years old, has been in a very unstable marriage and has a 4-year-old child. She has had a long history of short stormy relationships, frequently with inappropriate partners. During her past relationships as well as during her current marriage, intense verbal screaming matches were common. She has never made a suicide attempt, although when feeling trapped, she has fantasized about it often. Chronic feelings of life dissatisfaction without a sense of how to improve things have been prominent during her adult years, as have feelings of emptiness.
>
> Because of her commitment to her child, Ann has stayed in her poor marriage. Fights were becoming more frequent, during which she recently began throwing plates and dishes. After the fights, she would feel numb, spending up to days in a blank, depersonalized state in which she would be unable to care for her son or do household chores. Despite ongoing twice weekly psychotherapy, both individual and marital, these episodes continued and became more frequent. A trial of MAO inhibitors resulted in unacceptable postural hypotension. The antipsychotic thiothixene (Navane) was then prescribed, starting at 2 mg daily and then increasing to 4 mg at night, and had the effect of markedly diminishing the rage and the subsequent withdrawal. Because of this, Ann and her husband were better able to effectively discuss and resolve some issues without the constant threat of marital dissolution, an improvement that also allowed her to feel more competent. Although the thiothixene continued to be effective when taken during times of crisis, Ann's core feelings of emptiness and much of her mood lability continued. Eventually, Ann consented to a trial of fluoxetine. At the relatively low dose of 10 mg daily, she noted a clear decrease in her irritability and inappropriate anger and a consistent increase in her capacity to tolerate stresses. This effect

was apparent in her marriage, her ability to deal with her child, and in dealing with interpersonal conflicts at work. She discontinued the thiothixene. Life (and her therapy) continued to be a struggle but at a far more manageable level. Over the years, Ann has attempted to discontinue the fluoxetine three different times. Each time the dose has been lowered, she noticed an increase in her mood reactivity and marital conflict after which she reluctantly raised the dose with the return of the therapeutic effect.

Borderline patients often have other psychiatric disorders as well which may be hidden by the chaos of the personality disorder. Treatment of these associated states often results in somewhat more manageable psychotherapy. Most common among these are mood disorders, with a lifetime history of major depression seen in approximately half of all borderline patients (Gunderson and Elliott, 1985). However, these depressions may not be as responsive to antidepressants as are depressions in the absence of severe personality pathology. Borderline patients are at high risk to manifest atypical depressions, which typically respond to MAO inhibitors and probably SSRIs (Parsons et al., 1989). Cyclothymia may also be more common among borderline patients, although the possibility of a simple misdiagnosis between two disorders, each of which is characterized by mood lability, may explain this association (Levitt, Joffe, Ennis, MacDonald, and Kutcher, 1990). Borderline patients are at high risk to abuse drugs and alcohol. The diagnosis of the comorbid substance abuse is not always easy since patients are frequently less than straightforward about their drug use.

To summarize the psychopharmacological treatment of borderline personalities: (1) Despite the inherent merit of subtyping schemes, no consistent predictors of medication responsiveness currently exist. (2) Although low-dose neuroleptics are the most well-documented treatments, they may be more effective and better tolerated in the more severely ill patients. (3) SSRIs and MAO inhibitors may be very useful in diminishing the irritability, anger, and affective lability of borderline patients. (4) Carbamazepine may help the smaller subgroup of patients with explosive outbursts directed to self or others. (5) Despite the occasional extraordinary response to SSRIs, more typically, medication effects are modest-moderate.

Treating either histrionic or narcissistic personality disorders with medications has not been systematically explored. However, since affective lability and rejection sensitivity are common in histrionic, narcissistic, as well as borderline personality disorders, MAO inhibitors and SSRIs would be appropriate pharmacological considerations.

> Harry was a successful screenwriter who was known among his friends and family as the "moody artiste" type. He seemed absorbed in his own work and reputation, consistently angry at others who were more successful, and demanding to those around him. Even though he worked in a field in which emotional outbursts were relatively common, Harry was notorious for his intolerance of rejection. If a screenplay was not sold or if his work was severely criticized, Harry would respond in one of two ways—either by overwhelming rage, during which times he would scream and belittle everyone around him, get into physical fights, and be incredibly obnoxious, or by disappearing from sight for one day to two weeks. During these withdrawals, he would stay in his house, refuse to talk to anyone on the phone, feel apathetic, and sleep up to fourteen hours daily. He had been in psychotherapy for over ten years with two different therapists. During this time, his sense of entitlement, demandingness, and envy had diminished to manageable proportions, but his response to rejection was unchanged. Tranylcypromine (Parnate) was prescribed in increasing doses up to 40 mg daily. The effect was dramatic: He was able to stay in meetings in which his work was being criticized without exploding or leaving. When his work was rejected, he felt very upset but was able to function. Because of sexual side effects, he ultimately decreased the dose to 20 mg daily which was less effective but still afforded him some significant benefit.

When Bipolar II disorder or cyclothymia coexists with narcissistic personality, mood stabilizers can be helpful. Distinguishing between "biological" and "psychological" mood swings is difficult, especially when they coexist. (The case history of Donna in chapter 14 exemplifies this difficulty.) The best clues to the presence of true bipolar mood swings in narcissistic patients are behavioral manifestations of the hypomanias: The person not only feels grandiose and euphoric but exhibits behavioral changes associated with these feelings such as sleeping less, talking more, spending more money, making more long distance phone calls, or other typical signs of mania (Akiskal, Khani, and Scott-Strauss, 1979).

Cluster C: Anxious or Fearful Types

Cluster C personality disorders—avoidant, dependent, and obsessive compulsive types—are conceptually linked with the symptom cluster of anxiety/inhibition. In contrast to clusters A and B, however, almost no biological research or psychopharmacological treatment studies have evaluated Cluster C personality disorders. The only meaningful link suggesting the dimensional quality of Cluster C disorders has been the observation that anxiety disorders in adults (especially panic disorder) and behavioral inhibition in children (defined by a withdrawal or anxiety response in response to novel situations) are frequently seen in the same families (Rosenbaum et al., 1988; Rosenbaum et al., 1991).

Patients with Cluster C personality disorders are generally thought to be at high risk for anxiety disorders. As an example, comorbidity between avoidant personality disorder and social phobia has been noted to be as high as 90 percent (Schneier, Spitzer, Gibbon, Fyer, and Liebowitz, 1991). Yet this is probably due to the marked overlapping definitions of the two disorders in DSM-III-R/DSM-IV as opposed to the presence of two discrete disorders. Other than definitional overlap, there may be a stronger link between anxious personality disorders and vulnerability to depressive disorders than to Axis I anxiety disorders (Shea, Glass, Pilkonis, Watkins, and Docherty, 1987).

No studies have specifically examined the response of Cluster C personality disorders to pharmacotherapy. In considering medications for avoidant personality disorder, since many of those patients have social phobic symptoms, treating the latter disorder—for example with MAO inhibitors, SSRIs, or benzodiazepines (see chapter 4)—is likely to improve some of the avoidant traits as well (see the case of Bob in chapter 4) (Reich, Noyes, and Yates, 1989). Whether medications would be helpful for avoidant patients without social phobia is not known.

Treating dependent personalities or traits with medications seems unlikely to be of benefit. Dependent people, however, are at risk to become depressed if the objects of their dependency reject or leave them. In these situations, treating the coexistent depression may provide some relief acutely, although it is unlikely to cause significant change in the personality disorder itself. Among panic disorder patients, there is a link between the presence of phobic avoidance or agoraphobia and dependent personality traits (Reich, Noyes, and Troughton, 1987). In treating patients with both disorders, it is probably more helpful to treat the anxiety disorder first, since without the capacity to go out into the world without having a panic attack, trying to decrease dependency seems fruitless.

Given the similarity in names, obsessive compulsive personality disorder (OCPD) and obsessive compulsive disorder (OCD) are often assumed to be related and, therefore, to respond to similar treatments.

However, OCPD is present in only a minority (less than 10 percent in some studies) of patients with OCD, with other personality disorders more common in these patients (Baer et al., 1990). The responsivity of obsessive compulsive personality disorder without OCD to the serotonergic antidepressants that are well documented as effective in OCD is unknown. However, when patients with both OCPD and OCD are successfully treated for OCD, personality symptoms—including those of OCPD—tend to improve (Ricciardi et al., 1992).

Depressive Spectrum Personality Disorders

Although not officially designated as a personality disorder in DSM-IV, depressive personality disorder is listed in the Appendix as a criteria set provided for further study. Depressive personality disorder is defined by a group of symptoms such as low mood, poor self-esteem, being self-blaming and critical, a tendency to brood, being negativistic, judgmental, pessimistic, and prone to guilt. It differs from dysthymic disorder (defined as a DSM-IV mood disorder and discussed in chapter 3) by its lack of a time frame (as befits a personality disorder) and a lack of vegetative features in its diagnostic criteria. Consistent with the definitional differences, many individuals with depressive personality do not meet the criteria for dysthymic disorder and vice versa (Gitlin, 1995a). The majority of individuals with depressive personality who present for treatment, however, also have a strong history of more severe mood syndromes such as major depression (Hirschfeld and Holzer, 1994).

Unfortunately, no study has examined the pharmacological treatment responses of depressive personality patients. Yet many individuals with these characteristics have been clinically treated with SSRIs by psychiatrists or primary care physicians. Anecdotally, many of these patients respond robustly with a decrease in brooding and critical irritability and an increase in joyful capacities.

A related group of individuals often considered among the depressive spectrum personality types are those who describe excessive anxiety, mood lability, and exquisite rejection sensitivity without becoming so depressed as to be described as depression with atypical features. Similar to depressive personalities, no pharmacological treatment studies exist but anecdotally, SSRIs seem consistently effective.

As with borderline personality disorder, the appropriate length of pharmacotherapy for patients with depressive personality syndromes has not been established. The usual recommendation of a six-month continuation treatment for major depressive episode is not applicable to these chronic pervasive syndromes that last for years to a lifetime. Anecdotal experience with mild chronic depressive syndromes is mixed: some patients seem to do well after withdrawal from medications while more often, depressive symptoms return quickly, requiring the reinstatement of medications. No predictors currently exist to help ascertain which depressive personality patients need long-term maintenance medication. For now, then, a reasonable guideline would be the same as for borderline patients: following one to two years of good medication response the possibility of a trial off medication should at least be discussed. Many patients, however, will politely and firmly decline a trial off medication, in which case continuing the treatment is reasonable.

MANAGEMENT ISSUES

Because of the interpersonal and intrapsychic manifestations of personality disorders, especially Cluster B types, optimal pharmacotherapy of these patients requires a great deal of attention to management issues. Some of these issues apply to all patients, while others are specific to patients with specific personality clusters (Gitlin, 1995a).

One important area requiring attention reflects the need to frame appropriate expectations from the pharmacotherapy. With the plethora of recent articles and books describing the "transformations" that can occur with pharmacotherapy for personality traits and disorders, many patients approach the use of medication with inappropriate expectations and wildly unrealistic fantasies. Therefore, before medication is prescribed, both psychopharmacologist and therapist must help shape realistic expectations. Although extraordinary personality changes may occur with pharmacotherapy, patients should be aware that the improvements are typically more modest, especially in severe Cluster B personality disorders such as borderline patients. Unrealistic expectations lead to incorrect evaluation of the treatment's efficacy with attendant disappointment and then noncompliance. Similarly, clear guidelines must be set forth as to how the treatment's efficacy will be evaluated because, with expectations of complete personality change, patients (especially Cluster B patients) may not perceive the diminished amplitude of their mood swings, rage, and acting out since they are still dysphoric, have a poor primary relationship, and so on.

Before treatment begins, it is also helpful to acknowledge that despite the field's growing knowledge in this area, optimal pharmacotherapy contains some (albeit educated) trial and error. Whether it is choosing a specific SSRI for a particular patient or deciding whether a low-dose neuroleptic or an SSRI will be the appropriate first choice for borderline personality, patients should be prepared to work collaboratively in an endeavor that is frequently more difficult than they expect. Similarly, the shifting clinical needs of borderline patients over time imply that the pharmacotherapy is unlikely to remain static either. Adjunctive treatments used in times of crisis that are then withdrawn weeks later should be anticipated as the expected course of treatment, not as evidence of the failure of the maintenance medication.

Another set of difficulties in managing the pharmacotherapy with personality disordered patients reflects the effect of some patients' demandingness and manipulativeness on the pharmacotherapist. To best manage these complexities, collaboration between pharmacotherapist and psychotherapist is vital. Cluster B patients often demand medication stridently, insisting on a pill to cure every dysphoric affect. An optimally modulated response to these demands is difficult; pharmacotherapists must resist the tendency to overtreat the patient by yielding to inappropriate requests while also ensuring that appropriate medications are not withheld in a defensive response to the patient's demanding, obnoxious tone. Therapists must simultaneously work with the patient to be able to accept the continued presence of unpleasant affects and disappointments that are not amenable to pharmacotherapy.

Conversely, patients who have chronic suicidal ideation and/or a history of prior overdoses can provoke an overly cautious attitude from a potential prescriber. If an overdose is a potential risk, less potentially lethal medications may be prescribed (e.g., SSRIs vs. tricyclics). Alternatively, the medication may be held by the therapist and given out one week at a time. With reasonable safeguards, most acting-out patients can be safely treated. If the medications are effective, the risk of overdosing will diminish.

As previously noted, patients with personality disorders are at high risk for other comorbid disorders. Of paramount importance is alcohol/substance abuse, which is common in these patients, may not always be readily described by them, and will undermine the most thoughtful of pharmacological strategies. When present, the substance abuse must be addressed and almost always treated before medications should be prescribed. Additional attention must also be paid to the potential for underlying Bipolar II disorder in patients who present with Cluster B mood swings.

Finally, compliance is always a struggle in psychopharmacological treatments but especially when treating patients with Cluster B personality disorders. (See chapter 14 for more details.) Patients with chaotic personalities and lives often take prescribed medication in random patterns, alternating excessive and inadequate doses. Those with a history of substance abuse may be at highest risk to control their own medication intake in accordance with previously established patterns. Additionally, transference feelings may affect compliance. Anger at the prescribing physician—whether due to side effects or an interpersonal interaction—is often followed by a discontinuation of the medication with subsequent symptomatic regression and demands to be rescued. Often, the therapist will be more aware of these struggles than will the pharmacotherapist.

8

Treatment of Special Populations

Children/Adolescents, the Elderly, and Women

T HE VAST MAJORITY of the accumulated experience in psychopharmacology has been derived from treating nonpregnant patients in
the middle of their lives, in the age range of 20 through 60. This is even
more true with new treatments or experimental uses of already established medications. Certainly, it makes good sense to avoid unproven
treatments in the young, the old, or pregnant women. Elderly patients,
who are more likely to suffer from concomitant medical disorders, are
at higher risk to develop potentially harmful side effects. In children
and adolescents, biological and psychological development might be
adversely affected by psychopharmacological agents at such a sensitive
time. Yet both young and old suffer from psychiatric disorders, some of
which are unique to their age groups while others are common to all
age ranges. Even with disorders that are seen in all age groups, such
as depression or anxiety, special considerations apply in using medications with younger and older patients.

The possibility of using medications around the time of pregnancy
presents a unique set of circumstances. Pregnancy typically occurs at a
time of life when major psychiatric disorders such as mania, depression, schizophrenia, and panic disorder are either already present or are
most likely to emerge for the first time. In treating pregnant women,
questions about medication effects reflect concern for both mother and
developing fetus. This dual set of concerns then continues into the
postpartum period with issues around breastfeeding at a time when
mother-infant bonding is so vital. Although the topic is somewhat simpler when a fetus/infant is not involved, pregnancy-related concerns
form a segment of the larger topic worthy of review—the use of medications for female-specific issues and disorders.

In this chapter, we focus first on the use of medications in treating
disorders of childhood and adolescence, and then turn to some special
concerns about elderly patients. The final section will address issues of

pharmacotherapy applicable only to women—during pregnancy, post-partum periods (including breastfeeding), menopause, and for pre-menstrual syndrome.

CHILD AND ADOLESCENT DISORDERS

Aside from the potential for long-term effects noted above, there are good reasons why mental health professionals have traditionally been reluctant to treat children with medications. First, good research on the validity and reliability of psychiatric diagnoses in childhood is a very recent phenomenon, far more recent than even that of adult diagnoses. Without established ways of making diagnoses, medications could hardly be considered as appropriate for specific disorders or even specific behaviors within disorders, a situation that raised concerns about a "shotgun" approach to treatment. Moreover, the shifting nature of age-appropriate behavior in children and adolescents makes diagnosis more difficult. Fortunately, over the last fifteen years, there has been a concerted effort to clarify the nature of childhood disorders. These studies have demonstrated that disorders such as depression can be reliably diagnosed in children and adolescents. Second, the dependent relationships that children have with adults, both parents and mental health professionals, make the cooperative venture that is characteristic of good psychopharmacology more difficult and allow for possible abuse of medications as a coercive form of behavioral control without clear guidelines. Third, studies documenting the efficacy of medications to treat child and adolescent disorders are remarkably few in number. Attention deficit/hyperactivity disorder, which has been treated with medications for over fifty years, is the only childhood disorder with any significant history. Only in the last fifteen years, as our ability to diagnose childhood disorders has improved, has pharmacotherapy been investigated in a more thoughtful manner than previously. Finally, there are concerns that taking medications, especially over an extended period of time, will leave a serious, potentially permanent scar on children's and adolescents' sense of themselves and may plant the seeds of chronic self-esteem problems.

Each of these concerns is individually valid. Yet similar to adult psychiatry, the purpose of diagnosis and pharmacotherapy in children is to alleviate the suffering and dysfunctions from disorders that diminish the quality of their lives. It would certainly be better if we had a more well-validated diagnostic system and more documentation for the efficacy and safety of medications (or for any of our treatments) in children. Until this information is available, however, we must still treat our young patients as best we can with currently available modalities, knowing that as we learn more, our diagnostic and treatment strategies will change.

Children's capacities to express subjective feelings and voice concerns differ from those of older adolescents or adults. Evaluating symptoms, therefore, is more difficult, typically requiring multiple observers from a variety of settings and often repeated visits with the child (Towbin, 1995). Similarly, a child's concerns about the meaning of taking medication, its possible effects, and/or side effects should be sensitively addressed even though the child may not express these concerns as clearly as might adults.

Of most importance, medications should be considered only to treat patients—both children and adults—who are suffering from psychiatric/psychological problems of sufficient severity to interfere significantly with their lives. It is appropriate to worry about the effect of lithium on a 14-year-old's cognitive function and school performance. This risk, though, must be weighed against the psychological effect of the manic episode for which the lithium is being prescribed and *its* effect on self-esteem, peer relations, and school performance. Just as with adults, decisions on using medications in children need to be examined using a risk/benefit approach. The individual issues may differ but the method of making good judgments in treating youngsters with medications is the same as with adults. And, of course, considering the use of medications never negates the use of other types of treatments. In virtually all cases, a child or adolescent for whom medications are prescribed will need other types of therapy.

Table 8-1 lists the childhood disorders for which medications are often prescribed. Overall, principles used for prescribing medications for children and adolescents and deciding on doses are similar to those used for adults, with two exceptions: First, for smaller children, doses are sometimes recommended based on a ratio of milligrams of drug per kilogram (2.2 lbs) of the patient's weight, written as mg/kg. Thus, d-amphetamine might be prescribed in 0.5 mg/kg dosage. For a 65-pound child, which would translate to 30 kilograms, the daily dose would be $0.5 \times 30 = 15$ milligrams daily. Second, compared to older adolescents and adults, children and early adolescents require larger weight-adjusted doses because they metabolize and excrete medications more efficiently. The ability to metabolize medications gradually declines to adult values by age 15 (Clein and Riddle, 1995). With the

Table 8–1
Commonly Used Medications in Child and Adolescent Psychiatry

Disorder	Medication Class (or Medication)	Efficacy Rating
Major depression	Antidepressants	+ to ++
Bipolar disorder	Lithium	++
Schizophrenia	Antipsychotics	++
Autistic disorders	Antipsychotics	+
	Serotonergic antidepressants	+
Obsessive compulsive disorder	Clomipramine, SSRIs	+++
Separation anxiety disorder	Imipramine	+
	Benzodiazepines	+
Attention deficit/hyperactivity disorder	See Table 8-3	
Night terrors	Benzodiazepines	+++
	Tricyclics	+++
Sleepwalking disorders	Benzodiazepines	+++
	Tricyclics	+++
Enuresis	Tricyclics	+
Conduct disorder	Lithium, neuroleptics	+
	Anticonvulsants, beta-blockers, clonidine	+
	Serotonergic antidepressants	+
Self-injurious behavior	Antipsychotics	+
	Opiate antagonists	+
	SSRIs	+
Tourette's disorder	Haloperidol, pimozide	++
	Clonidine	++

+++ = Definite efficacy
 ++ = Probable efficacy
  + = Possible efficacy

higher doses prescribed for children, however, plasma levels of the medications are comparable to those seen with adults.

Similar to trends in adult psychopharmacology, medication combinations are increasingly prescribed for children and adolescents (Wilens, Spencer, Biederman, Wozniak, and Connor, 1995). The reasons for multiple simultaneous medications are the same as those for adults (see chapter 1): inadequate response to single agents, treating comorbid disorders, treating side effects, and so on. In general, medication combinations should be considered to represent a reasonable treatment approach—assuming the rationale for any pharmacotherapy is correct—but they need to be managed carefully by a skilled practitioner.

Mood Disorders

Diagnosis

Among the key findings of the last decade of research in child psychiatry has been the consistent documentation of clearly recognizable depressions and manias in children and adolescents. Prior to 1975, studies of mood disorders were hampered by a number of traditions: the notion that children did not possess the intrapsychic maturity to have states such as depression or mania, both of which theoretically required a well-developed superego; the idea that normal adolescence was filled with turmoil, a point of view that discouraged searching for specific psychopathological syndromes in this age group; the quick acceptance of "masked depression" or "depressive equivalents" as ways that a mood syndrome would present; and the problem of distinguishing a true depressive disorder—major depression or dysthymia—characterized by a group of signs and symptoms as well as a mood component (see chapter 3 for details), from other types of depressive pathology. Especially notable among childhood depressive states that may resemble depressive disorders is the chronic demoralization seen in children who live in chaotic or nonnurturing environments and which is characterized by apathy, anhedonia, and dysphoric mood, but without other depressive symptoms.

Major depression, using virtually the same criteria as used for adults, is unquestionably diagnosable in both children and adolescents (Carlson and Cantwell, 1980). To do so, clinicians must elicit the appropriate information from *both* parents and child, asking the questions about depressive symptoms directly but using language tailored to the patient's age and linguistic maturity, especially with prepubescent children. Children do not generally spontaneously report symptoms but will respond if asked directly in language they understand. For instance, a 7-year-old may not complain about depressed mood, and may deny it when asked, but may respond positively using different words, such as "blue" or "feeling bad inside myself."

Some few age-specific differences do exist between adult and childhood mood disorders, more in children than adolescents. Depressed children are more likely to look depressed, complain of somatic symptoms, show separation anxiety, and experience hallucinations (but not delusions) (Ryan et al., 1987). Children may express weight loss by simply not gaining the expected weight. Suicidal ideation is common in the depressions of both children and adolescents, though the former are less likely to act on these feelings, presumably because of cognitive difficulty in formulating and acting out an attempt.

Other psychiatric disorders are often seen concomitantly with depression. In children, separation anxiety, other anxiety disorders, attention deficit/hyperactivity disorder and conduct disorder are common; in adolescents, drug and alcohol abuse are often seen.

Both major depression and dysthmia in children and adolescents are associated with high rates of recurrence, chronicity, and psychosocial dysfunction (Rao et al., 1995; Kovacs, Akiskal, Gatsonis, and Parrone, 1994). This risk seems to continue into adulthood, further strengthening the link between child and adult depressive disorders (Harrington, Fudge, Rutter, Pickles, and Hill, 1990).

Even more than depressive disorders, mania/hypomania is commonly missed in youngsters, especially prepubertal children (Bowring and Kovacs, 1992). One reason for this is that mania in prepubertal children may present with atypical features such as prominent irritability and other mixed manic/depressive features, a less cyclical and more chronic course, and prominent features consistent with comorbid attention deficit/hyperactivity disorder (Wozniak et al., 1995). Bipolar adolescents, on the other hand, are far from rare and look similar to adult presentations with the possible exception of increased mood-incongruent psychotic features. Adolescents with classic melancholic features, strong genetic loading, and depressive delusions are at high risk to become bipolar over the next few years (Strober and Carlson, 1982).

Pharmacotherapy

Conclusive evidence of the efficacy of antidepressants in treating child and adolescent depression is currently lacking. Anecdotes and open studies suggest that, like adults, many young patients respond to these medications. However, relatively few double-blind studies on the use of antidepressants in this population exist and these do not consistently demonstrate a difference between medication and placebo (Steingard, De Maso, Goldman, Shorrock, and Bucci, 1995). The reason for the marked difference between child/adolescent antidepressant studies and adult studies is not yet clear but may reflect a number of factors, including higher placebo response rates in child/adolescent depression studies, higher comorbidity in depressed youngsters, and differences between adults and children/adolescents in the biology of depression (Kye and Ryan, 1995). Using plasma levels of tricyclic antidepressants to regulate doses may help improve response rates.

Since almost all controlled studies have utilized tricyclic antidepressants, the efficacy of the newer antidepressants (SSRIs, bupropion, venlafaxine—see chapter 9) should be considered predominantly untested. (A recent double-blind study presented at conference but not yet published, however, demonstrated the efficacy of fluoxetine over placebo.) Those agents requiring divided doses, such as bupropion (Wellbutrin) and venlafaxine (Effexor) may be associated with lower compliance. MAO inhibitors are rarely prescribed for children and adolescents, given the cumbersomeness of the dietary restrictions (see chapter 9).

The above statements imply that, until more evidence has been gathered, prescribing antidepressants for children or young adolescents with depression should not be considered as routinely as with adults. The exact circumstances in which antidepressants should be instituted is, as yet, unclear, but a reasonable approach would be to consider them when other interventions have been unsuccessful or not possible and the child shows functional impairment.

Especially in view of the rather negative studies with tricyclic antidepressants and because of their relatively benign side effect profiles, SSRIs are viewed by many experienced clinicians as first line antidepressant agents for children and adolescents. If the antidepressant is ineffective, the relative utility of augmentation agents (e.g., lithium, T_3—see chapter 9) vs. switching to a different antidepressant in this population is unknown.

Antidepressant doses used depend on the child's age. For children, SSRI doses are approximately half those used for adults, while for those in late latency and adolescence, adult doses are typical. Tricyclic antidepressants are usually started at low dose—0.5 mg/kg/day (typically translating to 10–20 mg daily) and gradually increased to 3 mg/kg/day (or 1.5 mg/kg/day for nortriptyline) with antidepressant plasma levels obtained at these doses to ensure that the dose is not excessive. (See chapter 9 for a discussion on plasma levels.) Higher doses of up to 5 mg/kg/day (or 3 mg/kg/day for nortriptyline) may be prescribed in selected individuals. Because children metabolize drugs more efficiently than do adults, tricyclics are usually given in divided doses.

Side effects with both SSRIs and the cyclic antidepressants are similar to those seen with adults (see chapter 9). With the SSRIs, common adverse effects are agitation, insomnia, irritability, nausea, and diarrhea. Common tricyclic side effects include dry mouth, constipation, sedation, fast heartbeat, and dizziness caused by low blood pressure. All antidepressants confer the risk of precipitating a switch from depression into hypomania/mania.

A handful of cases of sudden death of children taking desipramine have been reported. Although a causal relationship between the desipramine ingestion and the deaths has still not been well established (e.g., all the children were taking appropriate doses and had nontoxic blood levels), more aggressive monitoring of the electrocardiogram (EKG) in children taking tricyclics has become the norm (Kye and Ryan, 1995). EKGs are typically taken before treatment, after major dosage changes, and if higher than usual doses are prescribed.

Matt, age 12, was the younger of two children in a stable, upper middle-class family. He had always done relatively well in school and had friends. One year prior to being evaluated, Matt had become interested in darker, more morbid subjects and showed a new bleak view of his life and the world. He talked increasingly about the meaninglessness of all sorts of activities that had previously been interesting to him. Always an avid reader, his choice of reading material now tended to be horror stories and mysteries filled with violence and tragedies. He saw his friends less and less. In school, he was less active in class participation and his grades diminished from A-minus to C-plus. On weekends, Matt spent increasing amounts of time in his room, napping some but mostly just being isolated. To his parents, Matt freely admitted the change in his attitude and behavior but could give no explanation for it. He denied true sadness but expressed apathy and an emotional distance from everything. When directly questioned, Matt admitted that he thought about death a lot but did not have active feelings of killing himself. No drug use or alcohol abuse was evident. In Matt's family history, a maternal grandmother had been treated successfully with ECT while a maternal uncle had clear recurrent depressions, most recently treated by sertraline (Zoloft). Matt agreed to be evaluated and treated.

After two months of individual psychotherapy, Matt's depression was unchanged. After extensive discussion with him and his parents, Matt began taking sertraline 25 mg daily, increasing to 50 mg within a few days. Within three weeks, he felt significantly better with resolution of most (but not all) his depressive symptoms. Four months after beginning sertraline, he felt as if he was back to his usual self. Matt stayed on the antidepressant for six months after which the medication was tapered over one month without incident. Two years later, a similar depressive episode emerged that was again treated successfully with sertraline and psychotherapy. Now 15 years old, Matt remains on sertraline. Another trial off antidepressant is being considered.

For treating mania in children and adolescents, lithium is generally considered the treatment of choice (Botteron and Geller, 1995). At the same time, in contrast to the adult literature, not one controlled study has ever even examined lithium's efficacy in youngsters (although two are currently in progress), thereby making the statement more of a testament than a well-validated finding. Noncontrolled clinical experience is, however, consistently positive (Kafantaris, 1995). Similarly, no maintenance studies using lithium in children or adolescents exist, but here too, open experience suggests response rates similar to those for adults. Lithium discontinuation in adolescent bipolar patients is associated with high relapse rates (Strober, Morrell, Lampert and Burroughs, 1990). The technique of lithium administration with children is identical to that with adults (see chapter 10), with blood levels guiding doses. Side effects with lithium are the same as seen with adults: polyuria (increased urination), thirst, tremor, weight gain, and possible cognitive effects. It is especially important to look for the possible cognitive effects since they may affect schoolwork and may be lessened by lowering the medication dose. Long-term consequences of lithium begun in childhood and adolescence are unknown.

Experience with child and adolescent bipolar patients using the two other mood stabilizers prescribed for adult bipolar disorder—valproate (Depakote) and carbamazepine (Tegretol)—is sparse. These medications, however, are relatively commonly prescribed for childhood seizure disorders. Side effect profiles for these two medications are the same as those seen in adults, except for increased liver toxicity for valproate with children (see chapter 10).

Childhood Schizophrenia

Diagnosis

Although rare in children, the incidence of schizophrenia gradually increases during adolescence. Diagnostic criteria for schizophrenia in children/adolescents are the same as those for adults: a combination of positive/psychotic symptoms such as delusions and hallucinations, and negative symptoms such as social withdrawal, flat affect, and so on (see chapter 5). Diagnosing schizophrenia in youngsters, however, may be more difficult because of the prominence of psychotic symptoms in a number of other disorders and the ease of confusing it with some of the pervasive developmental disorders such as autism (McKenna et al., 1994). In adolescents, a history of substance abuse during the onset of psychotic symptoms may additionally confuse the diagnostic picture, especially since first psychotic breaks are often triggered (but not necessarily caused) by drug use. Nonetheless, when clear diagnostic criteria are applied, childhood/adolescent schizophrenia can be reliably distinguished from other psychotic disorders.

Pharmacotherapy

Treatment of child/adolescent schizophrenia is similar to that used with adults: a combination of antipsychotics with a variety of psychosocial treatments (McClellan and Werry, 1994). All neuroleptics are likely to be effective, although solid documentation of the efficacy of any single agent is notably lacking. Clinical experience suggests that children with schizophrenia respond less well to antipsychotics compared to adults, but this is far from proven. Akathisia or mild akinesia (see chapter 12 for descriptions) should be aggressively looked for, since youngsters may have particular difficulty expressing subjective feelings associated with these side effects. Picking one antipsychotic over another is based more on side effects than on differing efficacies. Except in very agitated patients, the high-potency, nonsedating antipsychotics are typically prescribed first because, with their lesser sedating capacities, they are likely to be associated with fewer difficulties in learning in a population that attends school. Youngsters treated with antipsychotics for extended periods of time are also at risk for tardive dyskinesia. Thus, when used in children, antipsychotics should be constantly reevaluated to ensure that the lowest effective doses are used. As with adults, for those psychotic youngsters who have shown inadequate responses to conventional neuroleptics, clozapine should be considered a viable alternative (Frazier et al., 1994).

Pervasive Developmental Disorders: Autistic Disorder, Asperger's Syndrome, and Related Entities

Diagnosis

Pervasive developmental disorders (PDD), of which the most common and well known is autistic disorder, are characterized by severe and pervasive impairment in the domains of social interactions and communication skills and the presence of restricted or peculiar behaviors. Autistic disorder has a very early onset, before age three. Core symp-

toms of the disorder include impairment in nonverbal interpersonal behaviors such as eye contact, facial expressions, poor relationships with
peers, lack of emotional reciprocity; impaired communication manifested by delay or lack of spoken language skills, stereotyped or idiosyncratic language, poor ability to initiate or sustain conversation; and
odd behaviors and activities, such as preoccupation with restricted patterns of interest, rigid adherence to rituals, and stereotyped behaviors
such as flapping. Asperger's syndrome can be distinguished from autistic disorder by its lack of language development abnormality. In
contrast to childhood schizophrenia, PDDs are not characterized by
prominent or persistent hallucinations and delusions.

Pharmacotherapy

Autistic disorder and the other PDDs are not inherently treatable by
medications. However, some of the manifestations of the disorder can
be ameliorated somewhat by empirical treatment of target symptoms
(Cook and Leventhal, 1995). Antipsychotics diminish fidgeting, hyperactivity, interpersonal withdrawal, and stereotypies in some children.
Unfortunately, patients with autistic disorder seem unusually susceptible to developing tardive dyskinesia. Because of evidence of serotonergic abnormalities in autistic disorders and the efficacy of serotonergic
antidepressants in obsessive compulsive disorder (which resembles the
ritualized behaviors of PDD), serotonergic medications have been used
to treat autistic disorder. Fenfluramine (Pondimin), a serotonin antagonist usually prescribed as an appetite suppressant and weight loss aid,
initially showed promise in reducing hyperactivity and impulsivity.
More recent studies, however, have been disappointing. Serotonergic
antidepressants—SSRIs and clomipramine (Anafranil)—that form
the mainstay of pharmacotherapy for obsessive compulsive disorder
are most likely to help autistic children with prominent ritualized behaviors. Those autistic children with prominent attentional difficulties
and/or hyperactivity might benefit from stimulants or clonidine, analogous to treatments for classic attention deficit/hyperactivity disorder.

Anxiety Disorders

Diagnosis

Systematic inquiry into the nature and treatment of many anxiety syndromes in children does not exist. As with many other childhood disorders, much of what is known about diagnosis and treatment has been
drawn from adult studies. Overall, anxiety disorders in children and

adolescents are far from rare (Popper, 1993). Most of these disorders are easily recognizable as early onset of otherwise typical adult disorders such as phobias, obsessive compulsive disorder, and post-traumatic stress disorder. From DSM-III-R to DSM-IV, considerable changes in the classification of childhood anxiety disorders were made. Overanxious disorder has been subsumed under generalized anxiety disorder while avoidant disorder has been eliminated as a diagnosis because of its similarity to social phobia, generalized subtype. Only separation anxiety disorder survives from previous DSMs to DSM-IV as a specific childhood onset anxiety disorder. In separation anxiety, children are frightened to be away from parents or from home, often complaining of physical symptoms when separation (e.g., school) is anticipated. School phobia (or school absenteeism) may be a specific manifestation of separation anxiety. School absenteeism, however, may also be caused by a variety of other disorders such as other anxiety disorders, depression, or conduct disorder.

Pharmacotherapy
With the exception of treating obsessive compulsive disorder, the use of medications for child and adolescent anxiety disorders is based primarily on anecdotal clinical experience and open studies. Studies comparing medications to other therapeutic approaches are virtually nonexistent. Pharmacotherapeutic approaches should ideally always be part of a more comprehensive multimodal treatment plan.

The only childhood anxiety disorder for which medications are well documented as effective is obsessive compulsive disorder with effective agents the same as those prescribed for adults: SSRIs and clomipramine (see chapter 4). Evidence is strongest for clomipramine and fluoxetine, although anecdotally fluvoxamine, sertaline, and paroxetine are also likely to be effective (March, Leonard, and Swedo, 1995). As with adults, obsessive compulsive disorder in children is likely to be a relatively chronic disorder, suggesting the possible if not probable need for long-term treatment (Leonard et al., 1993).

Twenty-five years ago, imipramine was shown to decrease school phobia (Gittelman-Klein and Klein, 1971). More recent studies evaluating the efficacy of tricyclic antidepressants for separation anxiety disorder (in which the vast majority of patients also met criteria for school absenteeism) have been more negative (Popper, 1993). Therefore, the exact role of tricyclic antidepressants in treating children with separation anxiety disorder manifesting in school refusal is still unclear. Experience with other antidepressant classes—especially SSRIs—for childhood anxiety disorders is just beginning. Similar to treating adult disorders, the preliminary evidence seems positive (Birmaher et al., 1994).

Benzodiazepines have been prescribed successfully for a variety of childhood anxiety syndromes such as panic disorder and separation anxiety disorder (Bernstein and Perwien, 1995). As with other pharmacotherapies, evidence for benzodiazepine efficacy in children is largely anecdotal. Side effects with benzodiazepines are similar to those seen with adults except that disinhibition, a paradoxical reaction in which the patient becomes aggressive and irritable, may occur more commonly in children. Many child psychiatrists are therefore reluctant to prescribe these medications to children with problems of impulse control. As with adults, if benzodiazepines are used for any significant period of time, tapering the dose as opposed to sudden withdrawal is appropriate.

In contrast to adult treatment, antihistamines such as diphenhydramine (Benadryl) are often used as first-line treatments for childhood anxiety disorders, especially with young children. However, since antihistamines are significantly sedating and cause cognitive effects during the day even when used the night before, their use for daytime anxiety should be limited. Tolerance to the sedating, antianxiety effects of antihistamines is also common.

Attention Deficit/Hyperactivity Disorder

Diagnosis

Previously referred to as hyperactive child syndrome, attention deficit/ hyperactivity disorder (ADHD) is the most extensively studied disorder in child psychiatry as well as the disorder for which medication is the best validated treatment. ADHD is currently defined by the criteria listed in Table 8–2. In contrast to previous manuals, DSM-IV highlights the separate dimension of inattention in addition to the long-recognized hyperactivity/impulsivity symptoms. To meet the DSM-IV criteria for ADHD, a child can show only attentional problems without hyperactivity or impulsivity. The consequence of this change has been to include more girls in the ADHD category, since they are less likely to show the disruptive behaviors characteristic of ADHD boys (Lahey et al., 1994). Most children, however, will meet criteria for the combined subtype of ADHD in which both attentional and hyperactivity/impulsivity are both prominent. Not all children show all symptoms nor are the symptoms apparent in all settings. DSM-IV requires the symptoms

Table 8–2
Diagnostic Criteria for Attention-Deficit/Hyperactivity Disorder

A. Either (1) or (2):

    (1) six (or more) of the following symptoms of **inattention** have persisted for at least 6 months to a degree that is maladaptive and inconsistent with developmental level:

Inattention

    (a) often fails to give close attention to details or makes careless mistakes in schoolwork, work, or other activities

    (b) often has difficulty sustaining attention in tasks or play activities

    (c) often does not seem to listen when spoken to directly

    (d) often does not follow through on instructions and fails to finish schoolwork, chores, or duties in the workplace (not due to oppositional behavior or failure to understand instructions)

    (e) often has difficulty organizing tasks and activities

    (f) often avoids, dislikes, or is reluctant to engage in tasks that require sustained mental effort (such as schoolwork or homework)

    (g) often loses things necessary for tasks or activities (e.g., toys, school assignments, pencils, books, or tools)

    (h) is often easily districted by extraneous stimuli

    (i) is often forgetful in daily activities

    (2) six (or more) of the following symptoms of **hyperactivity-impulsivity** have persisted for at least 6 months to a degree that is maladaptive and inconsistent with developmental level:

Hyperactivity

    (a) often fidgets with hands or feet or squirms in seat

    (b) often leaves seat in classroom or in other situations in which remaining seated is expected

    (c) often runs about or climbs excessively in situations in which it is inappropriate (in adolescents or adults, may be limited to subjective feelings of restlessness)

    (d) often has difficulty playing or engaging in leisure activities quietly

    (e) is often "on the go" or often acts as if "driven by a motor"

    (f) often talks excessively

Impulsivity

    (g) often blurts out answers before questions have been completed

    (h) often has difficulty awaiting turn

    (i) often interrupts or intrudes on others (e.g., butts into conversations or games)   *(continued)*

B. Some hyperactive-impulsive or inattentive symptoms that caused impairment were present before age 7 years.

C. Some impairment from the symptoms is present in two or more settings (e.g., at school [or work] and at home)

D. There must be clear evidence of clinically significant impairment in social, academic, or occupational functioning.

E. The symptoms do not occur exclusively during the course of a Pervasive Developmental Disorder, Schizophrenia, or other Psychotic Disorder and are not better accounted for by another mental disorder (e.g., Mood Disorder, Anxiety Disorder, Dissociative Disorder, or a Personality Disorder).

Code based on type:
314.01   Attention-Deficit/Hyperactivity Disorder, Combined Type: if both Criteria A1 and A2 are met for the past 6 months
314.00   Attention-Deficit/Hyperactivity Disorder, Predominantly Inattentive Type: if Criterion A1 is met but Criterion A2 is not met for the past 6 months
314.01   Attention-Deficit/Hyperactivity Disorder, Predominantly Hyperactive-Impulsive Type: if Criterion A2 is met but Criterion A1 is not met for the past 6 months

Coding note: For individuals (especially adolescents and adults) who currently have symptoms that no longer meet full criteria, "In Partial Remission" should be specified.

---

to be present in at least two settings for the diagnosis to be made. The disorder may be most obvious in an environment that requires behavioral stability while simultaneously providing many potential distractions, such as a schoolroom with many other children. In a different situation, such as focusing on a video game or engaging with one person, the child may not show any abnormalities. Because of this, ADHD is typically diagnosed after the child has begun school. Another situation in which ADHD symptoms are very likely to be apparent would be one that demands sustained attention, is boring and difficult—such as doing math homework. Although the diagnosis may be made at any time, the symptoms of ADHD never appear for the first time in late childhood or adolescence. A syndrome characterized by distractibility, inattentiveness, and behavioral change that first occurs in fourth grade following three years of normal school behavior may be adjustment disorder, depression, or another disorder but is not ADHD.

Because the expression of ADHD may vary across settings, an appropriate diagnostic evaluation requires the involvement of the child, the parents, and the teacher. A number of rating scales may be used to help identify and quantify the core symptoms of the disorder. No consensus exists, however, on which rating scales are best. For many children, taking a careful history of attentional, impulsive, and hyperactive symptoms in a variety of settings using the DSM-IV criteria as a guide will suffice for an accurate diagnostic evaluation.

ADHD is commonly seen in association with other disorders, especially conduct and oppositional disorders, depression, anxiety disorders, and learning disorders (Biederman, Newcoran, and Sprich, 1991). Additionally, 10 percent of ADHD patients exhibit a comorbid tic disorder including Tourette's disorder. ADHD children typically show significant psychosocial sequelae of their disorder, such as poor self-esteem, disturbed peer relations, and poor school and work performance. As ADHD children grow up, the symptoms disappear in many of them but are present in over half during adolescence and in a significant minority during early adulthood (Mannuzza et al., 1991). Chapter 6 reviews adult ADHD.

Pharmacotherapy

A number of medications, listed in Table 8–3, have been demonstrated as effective in treating child/adolescent ADHD. Without question, stimulants are the treatment of choice for children with ADHD. They have been amply documented as effective with 75% of children showing a positive response (Greenhill, 1995). The exact mechanism by which stimulants effectively treat the symptoms of ADHD is still unknown. Although stimulants' ability to slow down hyperactive children is often considered paradoxical, their effects are mediated in part by diminishing the attentional symptoms, allowing greater focus with a secondary decrease in the hyperactivity. As mentioned in the discussion of adult ADHD, the quieting effect of stimulants may also be observed in normal children. The magnitude and quality of the response to stimulants is variable. Improvements may be seen in attention, distractibility, hyperactivity, and increased mood stability. Secondary effects may be seen in improved school performance, family relations, and peer relationships. If the child has developed some of the complications of the disorder with disturbances in self-esteem and demoralization, these are

Table 8–3
Pharmacotherapies for Child/Adolescent ADHD

Medication Class/Agent	Efficacy Rating
First-line agents	
Stimulants:	
Methylphenidate (Ritalin)	+++
d-Amphetamine (Dexedrine)	+++
Pemoline (Cylert)	+++
Second-line agents	
Antidepressants:	
Tricyclics—desipramine, nortriptyline, imipramine, and others	++
Bupropion (Wellbutrin)	++
Alpha-adrenergic agonists:	
Clonidine (Catapres)	++
Guanfacine (Tenex)	++
Third-line agents	
MAO inhibitors	+
Antipsychotics	+

+++ = Definite efficacy
++ = Probable efficacy
+ = Possible efficacy

not likely to improve quickly because of an increased attention span. In these cases and with those children with concomitant conduct disorder, additional psychotherapeutic and behavioral interventions are mandatory.

The same three stimulants used in adult ADHD are prescribed for children: methylphenidate (Ritalin), d-amphetamine (Dexedrine), and pemoline (Cylert). By far, methylphenidate has been utilized the most, both in research studies and in general clinical use, although d-amphetamine is as effective. Some response is seen very quickly, typically within the first few days, at any dose. Some children respond better to one stimulant or the other. Therefore, if the first stimulant tried is ineffective, the other is generally prescribed. Optimum dosing requires careful balancing to maximize the desired effects of diminished hyperactivity and improved functioning and avoid excessive side effects. As with adults, both methylphenidate and d-amphetamine are short-acting drugs, necessitating two or three doses daily. Many clinicians feel that the sustained release forms of both medications are not as consistently effective as the standard forms. Some children, however, will do better on the sustained release form because they allow less frequent dosing and obviate the need for obtaining a medication dose from a school nurse during the school day. Fortunately, there is little evidence that tolerance develops to the positive effects of stimulants when used for ADHD, although some children will need a small dosage increase soon after the initial dose stabilization.

Pemoline may be somewhat less effective than either of the other two stimulants and takes longer to work, often up to many weeks. Its major advantage is that it needs to be taken only once daily because of its longer duration of action. Since there is a small risk of liver inflammation when pemoline is used in ongoing treatment, intermittent blood tests arc necessary.

An important issue in treating ADHD children with stimulants is whether the medications should be discontinued on weekends or summers (called drug holidays). An advantage of this approach would be to diminish some side effects and to continually reassess the need for ongoing treatment since, as mentioned, ADHD diminishes in many patients over time. Drug holidays over weekends may, however, have adverse effects on the child's relationships with family and friends. To test for the need for ongoing medication, it makes more sense to occasionally discontinue the stimulant such as during the school summer holidays. However, a significant number of ADHD patients will need to continue the medication into adolescence and beyond.

For the 25 percent of patients who do not respond adequately to stimulants, tricyclic antidepressants, bupropion, and alpha adrenergic agonists have all shown some positive effect in treating child/adolescent ADHD (Green, 1995). Among the tricyclics, desipramine has been the most commonly prescribed although imipramine, nortriptyline, and others may also be effective. Tricyclics tend to be less effective in improving concentration compared to their effects on mood and hyperactivity. For those children with comorbid tics, tricyclics may be less likely than stimulants to exacerbate the tics (Spencer, Biederman, and Wilens, 1994).

Other than antidepressants, the other important second-line medications for ADHD are clonidine (Catapres) and guanfacine (Tenex), both of which are classified as alpha adrenergic agonists. They are probably better at improving hyperactivity, impulsivity, and aggressiveness than inattention. Clonidine may be particularly helpful for children with ADHD and tics since it successfully treats both disorders. Although limited somewhat by its sedating qualities, clonidine is also effective in improving the sleep disturbances of ADHD (Wilens,

Biederman, and Spencer, 1994). Guanfacine is less sedating and is a more easily tolerated drug overall (Hunt, Arnsten, and Asbell, 1995).

Third-line agents for ADHD include the MAO inhibitor antidepressants and antipsychotics. The dietary restrictions necessary with the latter group of medications, though, probably preclude their use in most children and adolescents. Antipsychotics may be helpful for the hyperactivity symptoms, but do not improve and may exacerbate the attentional problems. Finally, despite a great deal of press and individual testimonials, dietary approaches in treating ADHD, including the Feingold Kaiser-Permanente diets, show no consistent evidence of efficacy in controlled studies (Kavale and Forness, 1983; Wolraich, et al., 1994).

Sleep Disorders

Diagnosis

Two of the major sleep disorders seen primarily in childhood are night terrors (called sleep terror disorder in DSM-IV) and sleepwalking disorder, also called somnambulism. Night terrors are characterized by episodes of sudden arousal from sleep in which the child typically sits up in bed, screams in terror, sometimes gasps for air, breathes quickly, has a rapid heartbeat, sweats, and appears completely terrified. The child is typically unresponsive during the terror and confused if awakened during an episode. Amnesia for these episodes, which usually occur during the first third of the night, is common. Night terrors occur intermittently, generally at intervals of days or weeks, and are more likely when the child is stressed or fatigued. Night terrors are unrelated to the more common occurrence of nightmares.

Sleepwalking also tends to occur during the first third of the night and is characterized by sitting or standing from a sleeping position, walking in a clumsy way, occasionally bumping into obstacles, and mumbling or talking incomprehensibly. These episodes can lead to serious injury if the child trips or falls down stairs. As with night terrors, the child is difficult to awaken during sleepwalking. Amnesia for the episodes is virtually universal, and when informed of his behavior, the child is usually ashamed and perplexed. Sleepwalking is more likely to occur when the child's bladder is distended and can be precipitated by calling the child's name. Medications such as antipsychotics and lithium may trigger these episodes. Sleepwalking tends to start around age five and typically disappears by early adolescence. It is not associated with significant psychopathology except in those patients whose disorders extend into adulthood (Kales et al., 1980).

Pharmacotherapy

Both night terrors and somnambulism begin during deeper levels of sleep and are most likely to occur during the transition to lighter levels of sleep (Dahl, 1995). They are not associated with REM (rapid eye movement) periods when most dreaming occurs. If nonpharmacological approaches—which typically focus on having the child obtain adequate amounts of sleep, regularity of bedtimes, and having the child empty his bladder before sleep—are ineffective, the medications prescribed are those that decrease delta sleep and diminish arousal between sleep stages. Benzodiazepines and tricyclic antidepressants such as imipramine are most often used with generally very good results. Medications tend to be prescribed intermittently at times of highest risk, such as when the child is physically ill or under stress, or to break a cycle of night terrors or sleepwalking.

For children with insomnia secondary to acute stress or anxiety, the most common medication approaches are the intermittent use of low-dose tricyclics such as imipramine 25 mg, benzodiazepines, or antihistamines such as diphenhydramine (Benadryl) 25 to 50 mg or promethazine (Phenergan) 12.5 to 50 mg.

Behavioral Conditions

Enuresis

Repeated episodes of urinating in the bed or clothes is a common problem of childhood, affecting 15 percent of 5-year-olds and gradually declining in prevalence for the next decade. Although primary treatments for enuresis are nonpharmacological, the antidepressant imipramine is occasionally used with some success. The mechanism by which imipramine diminishes enuresis is not well understood but is unlikely to be related to its antidepressant effect, since the antienuretic effect is seen within days of starting the medication, in contrast to the weeks needed for depression to remit. Doses used are relatively low—1 to 2 mg/kg. Tolerance to imipramine's antienuretic effects is often seen. Even when it continues to be effective, symptoms often recur after the medication is stopped. Therefore, it is usually reserved for those children who have not responded to a variety of behavioral approaches.

Conduct Disorder

As with antisocial personality in adults, which it resembles to a great degree, the defining characteristics of conduct disorder are behavioral. They describe an unruly child who consistently violates the usual norms of social behavior and commits a pattern of aggressive and deceitful acts toward others over at least a six-month period. Isolated acts of aggressive behavior are therefore not considered conduct disorder. Typical conduct disorder behaviors include stealing, lying, fire-setting, cruelty to animals, physical fights, and forcing another person to engage in sex. Early onset (at less than 10 years old) of conduct disorder predicts a worse prognosis. A significant proportion, but probably less than half, of conduct-disordered children grow up to be antisocial adults. Their long-term prognosis is generally poor.

There are no established treatments, either behavioral, psychological, or biological, for conduct disorder. Medications, when used to treat conduct disorder, should be considered to treat specific behaviors and concomitant disorders and *not* the primary condition. Therefore, in the following discussion treatment of aggressive behaviors regardless of diagnosis will be included. For those children with conduct disorder, pharmacotherapy should never be considered except as part of a more comprehensive treatment plan.

Medications that are sometimes effective in diminishing aggressive behavior in children and adolescents regardless of diagnosis include neuroleptics, lithium, carbamazepine, clonidine, beta-blockers, and antidepressants (Stoewe, Kruesi, and Lelio, 1995). Neuroleptics and lithium have the most documentation to their credit but are also associated with prominent side effects and compliance problems (especially with lithium, since its prescription requires blood tests for dose adjustments.) Carbamazepine (and possibly valproate), clonidine, and beta-blockers have shown promising results in preliminary studies but further documentation of their efficacy is needed. Finally, given the link between aggressive impulsive behavior and serotonin abnormalities, serotonergic antidepressants have recently been prescribed for aggressive children and adolescents. Trazodone is the most well-documented antidepressant for decreasing aggressive behavior, but SSRIs are likely to be explored more consistently in the future. The capacity of fluoxetine (Prozac) to cause stimulation may be problematic for some youngsters with aggressive behaviors.

Two comorbid conditions commonly seen with conduct disorders which may be amenable to psychopharmacological treatment are attention deficit/hyperactivity disorder and major depressive disorder.

Stimulants are therefore prescribed for those children with ADHD and conduct disorder. When effective, the child is likely to show diminished aggressive behavior. Intentional aggressive activities are unlikely to improve. If prescribed to treat conduct disorder in the absence of ADHD, stimulants are ineffective. When children with both depression and conduct disorder are given antidepressants, the medication may diminish conduct disorder symptoms as well as depression.

Aggressive, Destructive Behavior in Mentally Retarded Children

As currently used, the nonspecific term *mental retardation* comprises many different syndromes caused by a variety of etiologies, including genetic, viral, toxic, and traumatic. The essential features of mental retardation are subaverage intellectual functioning and deficits in adaptive functioning. Medications have no place in the treatment of the core deficits. However, since concomitant psychiatric disorders are more common in mentally retarded individuals, prescribing medications for these associated conditions should be considered as they would be for those of normal intelligence (Szymanski, Rubin, and Tarjan, 1989). Unfortunately, the most commonly used medications, antipsychotics, have often been prescribed in an abusive manner, in which the goals of the treatment have been to induce docility and enhance compliance. There is, however, a place for medications in treating the subset of mentally retarded individuals who exhibit repeated self-injurious behavior (SIB). Most well documented and most commonly used are the high-potency, relatively nonsedating antipsychotics such as haloperidol. Constant attention must be paid to possible side effects, particularly those such as the motor restlessness of akathisia (discussed in detail in chapter 12) which can easily be mistaken as anxiety, especially in individuals with lesser verbal skills who may have difficulties describing physical feelings. Reflecting the theoretical notion that the opioid system and serotonin are implicated in the biology of SIB, both opiate antagonists such as naltrexone (now marketed as ReVia) and SSRIs such as fluoxetine have recently been prescribed with occasional success in diminishing these behaviors (Bregman, 1995). Beta-blockers and buspirone (Buspar) effectively diminish aggressive behavior in some mentally retarded youngsters.

Tourette's Disorder

Diagnosis

Among the group of childhood tic disorders, Tourette's is the most severe, characterized by a chronic array of motor and vocal tics. Vocally, the tics can be grunts, coughs, clicks, or sniffs while motor symptoms can be eye blinking, tongue protrusions, hopping, or twitches in the face or body. Tics can also be complex, involving activities such as squatting, deep-knee bends, posturing, and retracing steps. A rather well-known but less common tic occurring in less than a third of Tourette's patients is coprolalia, characterized by sudden verbal outbursts of obscenities. Patients may also describe mental coprolalia which is the sudden intrusive thought of obscene words or phrases experienced as ego-dystonic. Tourette's patients are at high risk also to have a number of other psychiatric disorders, especially attention deficit/hyperactivity disorder and obsessive compulsive disorder (Coffey, Miguel, Savage, and Rauch, 1994). ADHD is present in up to half and OCD occurs in over half of Tourette's patients. Aggressive behavior is also commonly seen in Tourette's patients. In many cases, the behavioral and psychological impairment and distress associated with the symptoms of these other disorders exceed that from the tics themselves. The exact relationship between these associated syndromes and the tic disorder is still unclear but much evidence suggests a common genetic predisposition.

Tics can be voluntarily suppressed for brief periods of time. Anxiety and stress may make the tics worse, although a waxing, waning quality of the disorder is typical. Despite these observations, Tourette's is unquestionably a neuropsychiatric disorder with manifestations in both neurological and psychiatric realms (Hyde and Weinberger, 1995). It does both a patient and his family an extreme disservice to consider the tics, coprolalia, or other symptoms of Tourette's as manifestations of conflicts about hostile impulses. This does not imply that psychological intervention with the child and/or with the family is not useful for these patients. Family interactions or psychological difficulties can certainly alter the course of Tourette's—but they are not the cause.

Pharmacotherapy

With the increasing awareness that it is a neuropsychiatric disorder with varied presentations, characterized not just by tics but by obsessive compulsive, attentional, and aggressive symptoms, the pharmacotherapeutic options for treating Tourette's disorder have become increasingly complex. Although the general rule of using one medication if possible is still a reasonable conceptual approach, many

Tourette's patients require multiple agents to treat the varied manifestations of their disorder. In general, medications are used to treat symptoms that are psychologically or socially disabling. Additionally, since the tics wax and wane in severity, medication may be warranted at some times but not at others. Thus, a youngster with mild tics does not inherently need to be treated for the movements but if they worsen, pharmacotherapy would be warranted. Similarly, complete eradication of symptoms may require medication doses that cause unacceptable levels of side effects. Frequently, a 50 percent decrease in symptoms with a low dose of medication represents optimal treatment. Flexibility and an individualized approach are required elements of pharmacotherapy in Tourette's disorder.

For treating tics, high-potency neuroleptics such as haloperidol (Haldol) are well documented as effective. Typical doses used for Tourette's disorder of 0.5 to 5 mg daily are far lower than those used to treat psychotic disorders. Pimozide, an antipsychotic prescribed almost exclusively for Tourette's disorder, also diminishes tics. Clonidine is less consistently effective than the neuroleptics in treating the tics but may have a particular role in reducing aggressive behavior and hyperactivity when present along with tics. Similar preliminary findings have been demonstrated for the related medication guanfacine (Tenex) (Chappell, Leckman, and Riddle, 1995).

Unfortunately, all three medications have significant side effects that limit their usefulness. Haloperidol can cause sedation, cognitive blunting, and weight gain as well as putting these patients at risk for tardive dyskinesia (see chapter 12). Pimozide shares these side effects but may also be associated with changes in cardiac conduction, therefore requiring periodic electrocardiogram (EKG) monitoring. Clonidine does not produce weight gain or tardive dyskinesia but is very sedating. If stopped after any significant period of time, it must be tapered in order to avoid rebound hypertension, agitation, and worsening tics.

Pharmacological options for treating the syndromes associated with Tourette's disorder such as ADHD and OCD are similar to approaches generally used for these disorders. The only exception to this would be the wariness about prescribing stimulants such as methylphenidate (Ritalin) for the attentional symptoms since these medications often cause a worsening of the tics. Therefore, other medications for ADHD such as clonidine and desipramine are often prescribed first. Some children with tics and ADHD may, however, be safely treated with stimulants (Gadow, Sverd, Sprafkin, Nolan, and Ezor, 1995).

GERIATRIC DISORDERS

With the exception of the dementias, psychiatric disorders in the elderly are the same as those affecting younger patients. Unique age-specific considerations, however, affect both diagnosis and treatment plans in the elderly, especially those involving medications. Table 8–4 lists these considerations. For therapists, the meaning of these differences is that a medical evaluation is a more urgent issue when older patients present for treatment because of the greater likelihood that an undiagnosed medical disorder or a medication side effect is causing or exacerbating psychological symptoms. A second implication is that if a referral for psychopharmacological consultation is appropriate, it should be made, if possible, to a practitioner who is knowledgeable about prescribing medications for the elderly.

Compared to younger patients, the elderly are far more likely to be taking ongoing medications. Thirty percent of all prescriptions are written for those age 65 and older even though they make up only 11 percent of the population (Thompson, Moran, and Nies, 1983). The average older person takes 4.5 medications daily with those who are medically ill likely to take more—up to ten or more daily medications (Beers and Ouslander, 1989). This makes for potential additive effects or negative interactions if a psychotropic medication is prescribed. The

Table 8–4
Special Considerations in the Diagnosis and
Psychopharmacological Treatment of the Elderly

Diagnostic considerations:
  Presence of concomitant medical disorders, both diagnosed and undiagnosed, causing psychiatric symptoms
  Ongoing use of medications causing psychiatric symptoms
Therapeutic considerations:
  Possible decreased metabolism and excretion of medication leading to higher blood levels
  Greater sensitivity to having side effects
  More negative medical consequences to side effects
  Interaction of psychiatric medication side effects with ongoing medical disorders and ongoing medications
  Possible compliance difficulties, including forgetting pills, confusing pills of one type with another

most important of these interactions, since it is often unrecognized, is the additive effect of medications in causing sedation and/or confusion. Not only do many medications prescribed for psychiatric disorders cause sedation, but so do some antihypertensives (blood pressure pills), all narcotic analgesics (pain killers), and, of course, sleeping pills and alcohol. The problem is often further compounded by the use of over-the-counter remedies, many of which can also cause sedation.

Another common problem in using psychotropic medications is the elderly patient's increased susceptibility to becoming grossly confused from medications with anticholinergic properties (see chapter 12). Those medications that block the effect of acetylcholine can cause decreased memory, confusion, and, occasionally, delirium. Many antidepressants, most antipsychotics, over-the-counter sleeping pills, and medications used to block antipsychotic side effects, as well as many medications used for diarrhea, have anticholinergic effects. Taking any one of these medications would be unlikely to cause significant problems, but in combination, additive toxicity becomes more probable.

Because the elderly tolerate high doses of medications less well and are subject to greater side effects at any dose, the most important guideline used by psychopharmacologists is to start at approximately half the usual adult dose of any medication and increase doses far more slowly than usual. Side effects should be elicited more aggressively since the consequences are potentially more serious. As an example, a 30-year-old with postural hypotension (low blood pressure upon change in position) from an antidepressant, who experiences dizziness when he stands up, will usually hold onto a rail or other support and typically does not fall—or if he does, he falls gracefully, avoiding harm. A 70-year-old with the same drop in blood pressure, even without other causes for postural unsteadiness, such as arthritic hips, is more likely to miss the rail, fall, and risk breaking a hip or ribs.

Although the issues in Table 8–4 are always relevant for a psychopharmacologist to consider, they do not apply to all patients. For instance, even though those over 65 are less likely to metabolize drugs well and therefore need smaller doses of medications, some elderly patients not only tolerate high doses, but need them for a clinical response. More than any other recommendation, the most important is that the doses of medications in the elderly should be prescribed using an individualized approach.

Additionally, using a single cutoff age to define the elderly—typically age 60 or 65—ignores the potential differences between patients 60 to 75 and the quickly growing population often described as the old-

old, age 80 or above. With almost no studies examining pharmacotherapy in the old-old, good guidelines for these patients do not exist. Compliance problems form another potential obstacle to optimal treatment of geriatric patients. With more medications to take and greater likelihood of cognitive disturbances, remembering which pills to take at what time becomes increasingly difficult. Compliance problems with geriatric patients should be anticipated, asked about, and an effective plan constructed in order to avoid either a poor treatment response or toxicity.

Pharmacotherapy for Common Disorders

Mood Disorders

The key issue in evaluating and treating depression in the elderly is recognizing it. A number of factors make the diagnosis of depression more difficult in geriatric patients than in younger individuals. The most important of these reflects the bias of our society and is mirrored in the attitude of health professionals—that depression is "understandable" given the patient's difficult life circumstances. Therefore, active treatment is not considered. Other impediments to accurate diagnosis of geriatric depression include the tendency of older patients to focus on somatic symptoms as opposed to mood symptoms, the complications of ongoing medical problems which often distract patient and professional alike from recognizing the depression, and the lower functional expectations for the elderly, which allow both patient and therapist to miss the greater functional decline from the depression (NIH Consensus Development Conference, 1993).

Antidepressants are effective in geriatric depression with a 60 percent response rate. Even with treatment, however, many patients continue to exhibit residual depressive symptomatology. Elderly depressed patients may require more time—6 to 12 weeks—for antidepressant responses than do younger patients. The role of continuation and maintenance treatment for geriatric depressed patients who have had recurrent episodes, however, is identical to that for younger individuals.

The range of antidepressant treatment options is the same for elderly and younger depressed patients. Cyclic antidepressants, SSRIs, monoamine oxidase inhibitors, and electroconvulsive therapy (ECT) are all appropriate treatments. Because of the enhanced concern about potentially medically dangerous side effects such as sedation, confusion, and blood pressure effects, many clinicians prefer the newer antidepressants as first options for geriatric patients. It is not yet clear whether a specific subgroup of geriatric patients (e.g., the severely depressed) are more likely to respond to tricyclics than to SSRIs.

MAO inhibitors may be of benefit in elderly patients who have not responded to other more commonly prescribed antidepressants (Sunderland et al., 1994). For those patients for whom antidepressants are deemed medically inadvisable or have been ineffective or who need to have their mood lift quickly, stimulants may be effective (Wallace, Kofoed, and West, 1995). Stimulants may also be useful for anergic, apathetic elderly patients.

Even in the context of the many medical problems that afflict the elderly, such as Parkinson's disease, strokes, and cancer, antidepressants may be effective, albeit less consistently than in medically healthier individuals (Katz, 1993).

For older bipolar patients, the range of options is the same as with younger patients. Since the two more recently introduced mood stabilizers—valproate (Depakote) and carbamazepine (Tegretol)—are virtually untested in geriatric bipolar patients, lithium is generally considered the treatment of choice. Because kidney function is always diminished in the elderly, doses are lower. Additionally, more elderly patients seem to respond to lithium blood levels—such as 0.4 mEq/l—that would typically be subtherapeutic for younger patients. Elderly patients may also become lithium toxic more easily and at lower blood levels, suggesting that more frequent lithium levels be obtained during dose adjustments.

Psychotic Disorders

All the common side effects with antipsychotics are also seen when these medications are taken by the elderly. The sedating and hypotensive effects (lowering blood pressure) must be watched especially closely. Because the risk of tardive dyskinesia increases as patients age, maintenance treatment must be considered even more carefully than usual.

Anxiety Disorders and Insomnia

The major danger in treating anxiety or insomnia is the potential accumulation of benzodiazepines because of the slower metabolism of medications in older patients. Especially with tranquilizers with long durations of action (see Table 11–3), the amount of medication in the blood may build up, causing morning hangovers or even around-the-clock cognitive changes. In general, therefore, short-acting benzodiazepines are the preferred drugs to treat anxiety and insomnia in the elderly. If cognitive impairment from benzodiazepines occurs, it is reversible upon discontinuation of the medication. Especially when the cognitive disturbance is mild, patients may have a different evaluation of the risk/benefit ratio compared to clinicians (Salzman, 1995). As an example, is it worth an enhanced capacity to repeat serial sevens or remember the composition of last night's dinner if the price is more restless sleep or pervasive daytime anxiety? Compared to symptom and side effect ratings, quality of life is rarely measured or directly addressed in these circumstances.

Medications Used in Treating Dementias

As more people survive into old age, the group of disorders that present with dementia is an increasing problem for psychiatrists specifically, and society in general. Dementia is characterized by impairment of memory, abstract thinking and judgment, personality changes, and—ultimately—deficits in functioning. A number of different causes for dementia can be identified, the most common of which is Alzheimer's disease (called dementia of the Alzheimer's type in DSM-IV). The second most common cause is multi-infarct dementia, now called vascular dementia in DSM-IV, which is characterized by a series of small strokes in the brain. The most important treatment for dementia is diagnosing other less common but more reversible causes, such as hypothyroidism (low thyroid), vitamin deficiencies, or associated depressions that will exacerbate the dementia.

Of all the agents that have been suggested as effective in retarding or reversing the cognitive decline of Alzheimer's disease, only tacrine (Cognex), released in 1993, has shown any consistent efficacy (Knapp et al., 1994). One of the biological changes associated with Alzheimer's disease is a loss of cholinergic function (i.e., decreased acetylcholine, a neurotransmitter that seems central to memory and other cognitive functions). Tacrine enhances cholinergic function by inhibiting acetylcholinesterase, the enzyme that breaks down acetylcholine. Higher doses—160 mg daily—are more effective than lower doses. When effective, tacrine reverses the cognitive decline of Alzheimer's disease by approximately six months, but does not otherwise prevent the progression of the disorder (Winker, 1994).

Tacrine's usefulness is limited by its side effect profile, especially at the higher, more effective doses. Common side effects include nausea, abdominal distress, dizziness, and agitation. Of more concern, at higher doses tacrine causes liver inflammation, often necessitating medication discontinuation, although physical signs of liver damage are unusual. Tacrine is also very expensive.

A number of other medications are also prescribed to treat Alzheimer's disease. Most common among these are low-dose selegiline (Eldepryl) and a group of drugs called ergoloid mesylates, the most common of which is marketed as Hydergine. Selegiline is an MAO inhibitor which at higher doses is an antidepressant (see chapter 9). At low doses—5 to 10 mg daily—selegiline selectively inhibits MAO-B and has been used to retard the deterioration of Parkinson's disease. At these same low doses, selegiline may enhance cognitive functioning in Alzheimer's patients (Schneider, Olin, and Pawluczyk, 1993). Hydergine is, at best, weakly effective in treating patients with Alzheimer's disease and does not change the clinical picture substantially (Hollister and Yesavage, 1984).

Another group of medications are commonly prescribed for Alzheimer's patients to manage the behavioral disturbances: agitation, wandering, aggressiveness, insomnia, and psychosis including paranoia. In these circumstances, the goal of treatment is simple behavioral control, not altering the progression or core features of the disorders. Most commonly prescribed are the antipsychotics. As with the treatment of agitation in the mentally retarded, antipsychotics are sometimes prescribed for Alzheimer's patients abusively, in excessive doses, for unclear reasons, and for too long. When used at low doses, however, with care taken to recognize and minimize side effects, they have clear but modest effects in decreasing agitation and psychosis (Raskind, 1995).

With the increasing concern about antipsychotics, a number of other agents have been more recently prescribed with some success in decreasing the behavioral disturbances associated with Alzheimer's disease. These have included low-dose trazodone (Desyrel), buspirone (Buspar), beta-blockers, and the mood stabilizers—lithium, carbamazepine, and valproate (Sky and Grossberg, 1994). Short-acting benzodiazepine tranquilizers may also be effective but must be used cautiously in order to avoid sedation and confusion.

FEMALE-SPECIFIC ISSUES AND DISORDERS

Over the last decade, the proper use of medications in clinical situations and disorders that are unique to women has become an increasingly prominent topic. Premenstrual syndrome has been the most commonly investigated of these disorders because of its prevalence and frequent association with significant distress and impairment. The other major areas of concern are the potential use of medication during pregnancy and the postpartum period, and the relationship between menopause and depression.

Premenstrual Syndrome

Although its name frequently changes, a cyclical syndrome exists that starts some time after ovulation and disappears within the first day or two of menses. This syndrome is characterized by a variety of psychiatric symptoms such as depression, irritability, affective lability, rejection sensitivity, and changes in appetite, sleep, and energy, along with physical symptoms such as edema, breast tenderness, and headaches. Colloquially known as PMS, it was given the awful name of late luteal phase dysphoric disorder in DSM-III-R, and is now called premenstrual dysphoric disorder (PMDD) in DSM-IV, where it is listed in the Appendix and as a depressive disorder not otherwise specified (NOS). The time course of PMS shows remarkable variability—it may begin soon after ovulation, disappear, and then return before menses or may occur only for a few difficult days before the period. Although many women have mild symptoms, 5 to 10 percent have symptoms severe enough to interfere with normal functioning. A substantial proportion of women presenting with self-reported PMS will, upon prospective evaluation, exhibit a depressive disorder that is not consistently linked to their menstrual cycle (Gitlin and Pasnau, 1989). Because of this, if possible, the diagnosis of PMS should be made only after two months of mood charting that shows a consistent relationship between mood changes and the menstrual cycle. Patients with relatively severe PMS are at high risk to have a lifetime history of major depression, while women with major depression show increased premenstrual depressive symptoms.

An extraordinary variety of treatments, listed in Table 8–5, have been proposed to treat PMS (Altschuler, Hendrick, and Parry, 1995). Many of the earlier studies were hampered by a lack of consistent methods of diagnosing the disorder, thereby casting some doubt on their conclusions. A further difficulty in the area has been the high placebo response rate which often exceeds 40 percent. Nonetheless, in the last decade, better studies have allowed some reasonable generalizations on the treatment of PMS.

Given the definitional link between the menstrual cycle and PMS, the most frequently touted treatments have been hormonal. The most common of these has been progesterone supplementation during the

Table 8–5
Pharmacotherapies for Premenstrual Syndrome

Treatments	Efficacy Rating
Hormonal therapies	
Progesterone (synthetic or natural)	?
Estrogen	+
Oral contraceptives	?
GnRH agonists	+++
Danazol	+++
Nonprescription agents	
Pyridoxine	+
Vitamins A, E	+
Calcium, magnesium	+
Evening primrose oil	++
Targeted symptom interventions	
Diuretics (for bloating and edema only)	+++
Antiinflammatory agents (for cramps only)	+++
Psychotropic medications	
Fluoxetine (Prozac)	+++
Other antidepressants	++
Alprazolam (Xanax)	+++
Buspirone (Buspar)	++

+++ = Definite efficacy
 ++ = Probable efficacy
  + = Possible efficacy

second half of the menstrual cycle, predicated on a postulated relative progesterone deficit. Initial uncontrolled studies showed very positive results. Double-blind studies, however, have for the most part shown no differences between progesterone and placebo. Whether estrogen supplementation or oral contraceptives effectively diminish PMS is still unclear. Oral contraceptives, however, have also been reported to exacerbate depressive symptoms.

Two other hormonal treatments have shown more efficacy but are associated with greater medical complications. Gonadotropin-releasing-hormone (GnRH) agonists, such as leuprolide (Lupron), decrease the pituitary hormones that promote estrogen and progesterone production. GnRH agonists consistently improve PMS symptoms. Biologically, however, their effects produce a chemical ovariectomy, thereby simulating menopause. Therefore, over months or years, GnRH agonists are likely to be associated with the negative long-term consequences of menopause such as greater risk of osteoporosis and heart disease. Long-term use of these medications cannot be recommended. Danazol, a synthetic androgenic steroid, also suppresses estrogen and progesterone production and reduces PMS symptoms. However, it is associated with a number of side effects and, like GnRH agonists, its long-term safety is in question.

A variety of nonprescription treatments have been proposed to treat PMS. The most commonly used agent is pyridoxine (vitamin B_6) which is required for the synthesis of dopamine and serotonin. Evidence for its efficacy is weak. Although safe at moderate doses (50 mg daily), pyridoxine can cause neurological symptoms when taken over time at doses exceeding 100 mg daily. The efficacy of other vitamin and mineral treatments—vitamin A, vitamin E, supplemental calcium and magnesium—is still unclear. Evening primrose oil, which contains gamma-linoleic acid, a precursor of prostaglandin E_1, decreases the effects of the hormone prolactin and has been reported to reduce PMS symptoms.

Another group of PMS treatments target specific symptoms. Diuretics reduce bloating and weight gain for those women in whom these symptoms predominate. Nonsteroidal antiinflammatory agents such as naproxen (Naprosyn) may relieve menstrual cramps. These agents, however, are unlikely to improve the mood and irritability symptoms of PMS.

Most of the recent interest in treating PMS has centered around psychotropic agents, specifically antidepressants and antianxiety agents. The best studied medication is fluoxetine (Prozac) which, at a daily dose of 20 mg, consistently improves premenstrual mood and irritability (Steiner et al., 1995). Whether the other SSRIs would be just as effective is likely but not demonstrated. Similarly, other antidepressants may also be effective but few have been evaluated. The antidepressants are typically prescribed throughout the menstrual cycle. Whether antidepressants might be effective when given only during the second half of the menstrual cycle is unknown. The antianxiety agent alprazolam (Xanax) has been shown to reduce anxiety, depression, irritability, and fatigue when taken during the second half of the menstrual cycle. Buspirone (Buspar) may also be effective.

Given the wide variety of potential treatments for PMS, a reasonable treatment strategy would be: (1) Establish that the symptoms are clearly linked to the menstrual cycle. (2) If symptoms are mild, education, exercise, and reduction of exacerbating factors (e.g., salt, alcohol, and caffeine) may suffice. (3) Those patients who want to avoid prescribed medications can start with pyridoxine or evening primrose oil. (4) If more aggressive treatment is warranted, fluoxetine or alprazolam are appropriate medications. (5) For those women with specific physical symptoms (e.g., bloating or cramps), targeted interventions noted above might suffice. (6) Hormonal treatments (e.g., GnRH agonists, estradiol, and danazol) should be used as last resorts given their side effect profiles. The exact place of progesterone or oral contraceptives for treating PMS, if any, is controversial since, despite anecdotal evidence of their efficacy, the majority of studies indicate little benefit from their use (Altshuler, Hendrick, and Parry, 1995).

Medications During Pregnancy

Any sensible clinician would recommend that, if possible, women who are pregnant or planning a pregnancy avoid medications, especially in the first trimester when most fetal organ development occurs. All other therapeutic modalities are preferable to medications in these circumstances. This statement is easy to make and pure in its conclusion. In real clinical situations, however, the risks of any potential treatment must be weighed against other variables, such as the risk of not treating, or the possible benefits of treating. For mild depressions or minimal anxiety, it makes sense to avoid medications. But how does one proceed with a psychotically depressed woman who is significantly suicidal? Or a manic woman who sleeps only two hours a night, is hyperactive, drives dangerously, and takes drugs and alcohol? Or a schizophrenic woman who is delusional about her unborn child and is not eating because of her psychosis? Even with less destructive episodes, the risks of not treating may be considerable given the impairment and distress associated with, for example, untreated panic disorder and moderate depression. If nonbiological treatments are ineffective or if the disorder is severe enough to demand relatively emergent treatment, the question of prescribing medication inevitably arises. Certainly, to appropriately assess the risk/benefit ratio for pharmacotherapy in these situations, knowledge about the potential negative effects of the medications is required. Yet even with the most current information, knowledge can only take us so far. Considering the use of medications during pregnancy involves the most difficult judgments of risks vs. benefits in psychopharmacology. The final decision is a best judgment, made by the woman, possibly her family, her therapist, and the psychopharmacologist.

Potential risks to the fetus from maternal medication taken during pregnancy can be divided into three types: (1) Overt malformations of the fetus/infant, described as teratogenic effects. For teratogenic effects to occur, the fetus must be exposed to the medication during the time organs are formed. (2) Toxic effects on the fetus or newborn evident at the time of birth, caused by medications taken during the third trimester toward the time of birth. These effects would also include medication withdrawal symptoms in the newborn. (3) Behavioral teratogenicity—potential long-term effects that are not apparent until months to years after birth that result from the exposure of the developing nervous system to medication. A common concern is that the child exposed to medication in utero might have a lower IQ or slower development. Also of concern, however, might be whether maternal use of an antidepressant during pregnancy could alter the fetus/child's neurotransmitter receptor system development such that, for instance, the risk of becoming depressed during adult life would be increased. Currently, there is no solid evidence for behavioral effects in humans, although these would be the hardest to document.

Antidepressants

After over thirty-five years of clinical experience with their use, there is no consistent evidence that tricyclic antidepressants are teratogenic (Altshuler et al., in press). Some mild withdrawal syndromes without long-term sequelae have been described for those children exposed to tricyclics just before birth. SSRIs have been available for less than ten years so less long-term experience on their potential teratogenic effects is available. However, the one systematic study of fluoxetine in pregnancy did not indicate any teratogenic risk. Insufficient information has been reported for any of the other newer antidepressants to form any conclusion as to their safety during pregnancy. Very little information exists for MAO inhibitors as a possible teratogen in humans. In animals, however, these medications are associated with clear increases in fetal growth retardation and other anomalies. Most experts in the field therefore consider MAO inhibitors potentially teratogenic drugs.

Antianxiety Drugs

Benzodiazepines are the most widely used medications in this class. Although no overall increase in teratogenic effects are seen when benzodiazepines are prescribed to a pregnant mother during the first trimester, there is an increased risk for the specific development of cleft palate in exposed fetuses/infants (Altshuler et al., in press). The overall magnitude of this risk, however, remains small. Whether all benzodiazepines confer this risk is unclear. Some evidence suggests (but certainly does not prove) a lower risk in those mothers and fetuses treated with clonazepam compared to other benzodiazepines. Neonates exposed to benzodiazepines while in utero are at higher risk to show poor muscle tone and failure to feed at birth. The long-term ramifications of these findings are unclear. Behavioral teratogenic effects from prolonged in utero exposure to benzodiazepines have been described in some but not all studies. Here too, the clinical significance of these findings is not understood.

Mood Stabilizers

Until recently, lithium was considered to be among the most teratogenic of all psychopharmacological agents, conferring a marked increased risk for a cardiac abnormality called Ebstein's anomaly. More recent studies, however, indicate that even though an increased risk exists, it is far smaller than previously assumed (Cohen, Friedman, Jefferson, Johnson, and Weiner, 1994). The current estimate is that lithium exposure during the first trimester is associated with the development of Ebstein's anomaly in less than 1 percent of exposed fetuses. Infants exposed to lithium during the third trimester are occasionally reported to show transient neuromuscular abnormalities. No evidence of lithium-induced behavioral teratogenicity has been reported.

Both anticonvulsant mood stabilizers—carbamazepine and valproate—are clearly teratogenic. The use of valproate during the first trimester confers a 1 to 2 percent risk in exposed fetuses of spina bifida, an abnormality in the development of the spinal cord associated with marked neurological defects (Lammer, Sever, and Oakley, 1987). Carbamazepine may confer similar although slightly smaller risks but is also associated with other neurological abnormalities (Jones, Lacro, Johnson, and Adams, 1989). Thus far, there is no evidence of behavioral teratogenicity from either valproate or carbamazepine.

Antipsychotics

Fetal exposure to neuroleptics during the first trimester probably slightly increases the risk for fetal malformations. However, the risk is probably smaller than that resulting from simply having a psychotic disorder such as schizophrenia which is itself associated with higher rates of fetal malformations. The risk associated with the more recently released neuroleptics clozapine and risperidone is unknown. Infants exposed to neuroleptics during or just prior to birth show some neurological symptoms which seem to resolve slowly but completely. As with other medication groups, no clear evidence of behavioral teratogenicity from antipsychotics is evident.

Electroconvulsive Treatment (ECT)

ECT is among the safest of treatments for the developing fetus, partly reflecting the very brief exposure (seconds to minutes) to the treatment and the current emphasis on ensuring adequate oxygenation during the procedure itself (Miller, 1994).

Given this information, decisions for an individual woman can more easily be made. As an example, for depression, fluoxetine or the tricyclics have been the agents most well documented as safe. Therefore, they might be first choices for those women who become severely depressed during the first trimester or for those women who become pregnant but must continue on antidepressants to prevent severe relapses. For bipolar women, the need for ongoing, preventive medication during pregnancy is considerable. In contrast to conclusions drawn only a few years ago, lithium may be the safest mood stabilizer available. Furthermore, Ebstein's anomaly can be diagnosed using ultrasonography at 16 to 18 weeks, thereby allowing the possible termination of the pregnancy. An acute mania during the first trimester might be treated by a brief course of antipsychotics, followed by lithium after the first trimester. For patients with panic disorder, benzodiazepines may be slowly tapered before pregnancy. If panic recurs during pregnancy, consideration should be given to the use of tricyclics or even fluoxetine, both of which are effective. If panic attacks continue, benzodiazepines can be added as needed at low doses. Finally, although infrequently prescribed, ECT should also be considered for severely depressed or manic pregnant women since it may pose fewer risks for the fetus than medication (Sitland-Marken, Rickman, Wells, and Mabie, 1989). For each situation, however, the risks and benefits of all possible options must be thoughtfully reviewed.

Postpartum Period and Breastfeeding

A somewhat different but related set of concerns must be addressed in considering the use of medications during the postpartum period. At this point, the infant may be treated separately from the mother, thereby diminishing some concerns. However, the postpartum period is one of very high risk of relapse for depressed and bipolar patients, with new onset disorders also commonly seen during this time. Therefore, for those women with a prior history of depression, mania, or specifically postpartum mood episodes, consideration should be given to preventive treatment. Although there are few studies in this area, it appears that for those women at high risk, initiating antidepressants and/or mood stabilizers helps prevent postpartum mood episodes (Wisner and Wheeler, 1994; Stewart, Klompenhouwer, Kendall, and Van Hulst, 1991). Whether prophylactic treatment should be instituted before giving birth or right after is still unclear.

The other important pharmacological consideration during the postpartum period concerns the potential risk to the infant of breastfeeding if the mother is taking a psychotropic agent. All psychotropic medications that have been evaluated are secreted in breast milk in variable amounts. Yet when measured, plasma levels of antidepressants in breastfeeding infants are low or nondetectable (Wisner, Perel, and Foglia, 1995; Altshuler, Burt, McMullen, and Hendrick, 1995). Moreover, adverse effects to the infant have rarely been reported. In contrast, ingestion of lithium in breast milk is associated with measurable amounts of the drug in the infant (American Academy of Pediatrics, 1994).

How best to utilize this sparse information is still in some dispute. Many feel that the trivial risk to the infant who breastfeeds on milk containing medication is outweighed by the psychological and biological benefits of breastfeeding. Others are more cautious, especially when lithium is involved. As always, in these situations the woman needs to know whatever information is available for that medication and make a best informed decision.

Menopause

Finally, menopause has often been considered to be associated with a specific increase in depression. Theoretically, menopause and mood could be linked either biologically, psychologically, or both. Biological considerations point to the relative increase in estrogen/progesterone ratio at the beginning of menopause, followed by a marked but gradual decrease in both hormones by the end of menopause. Psychologically, changes in physical body characteristics in a society that strongly links youth and sexuality, loss of childbearing capacity leading to an alteration in self-image, adolescent children leaving home leading to a change in the role within the family are all postulated as links to depression. Most studies, however, show no increase in either recurrences of major depression or new episodes of major depression during the menopausal years (Gitlin and Pasnau, 1989). These findings do not exclude the possibility of milder mood symptoms and syndromes that may arise during menopause (Schmidt and Rubinow, 1991). However, as a generalization, menopause should not be considered a time of particular risk for serious depressive disorders in women (Matthews et al., 1990).

SECTION

FOUR

9

Antidepressants

I T IS NOW THIRTY-FIVE YEARS since the initial reports on the effects of the first tricyclic and monoamine oxidase (MAO) inhibitor antidepressants were published almost simultaneously. During this time, the number of antidepressants with documented efficacy has expanded dramatically; there are now twenty-one antidepressants available, and more are likely to be released over the next few years. In addition, the use of the antidepressants has continued to expand for both psychiatric and nonpsychiatric disorders. Within psychiatry, antidepressants are prescribed for panic disorder, obsessive compulsive disorder, bulimia nervosa, attention deficit/hyperactivity disorder and more; in general medicine, they are used to treat migraine headaches, chronic fatigue syndrome, irritable bowel syndrome, and chronic pain. Additionally, as noted in chapter 3, the accepted use of antidepressants for depressive disorders has dramatically expanded to include their prescription for milder depressive spectrum disorders that were previously considered not amenable to pharmacotherapy. With their broad spectrum of efficacy, antidepressants should be considered a woefully misnamed class of medications. More properly, they should be called anti-broad-spectrum-psychiatric-syndromes drugs—but antidepressants is much easier to say. Whatever we call them, antidepressants have increasingly become the mainstay of modern psychopharmacology.

HISTORY

Prior to the late 1950s, the somatic treatment of depression consisted of three options. The first was stimulants resembling amphetamine which had the effect of increasing energy and activity. Their capacity in treating severe depression, however, was limited. Electroconvulsive therapy (ECT), the second option, had been first used in the late 1930s. Although ECT was unquestionably effective as a treatment for depression, it was a frightening and dangerous treatment at that time. (See chapter 13 for modern and safe use of ECT). The third option was time. One of the most important "treatments" for depression prior to the modern era was waiting. Since the majority of depressions were, and are, time limited in nature (albeit lasting many months), simply keeping the patient from committing suicide during that time would allow spontaneous recovery to take place.

As with so many other discoveries in medicine, imipramine, the first tricyclic antidepressant, was discovered serendipitously through the careful observations of a researcher/clinician. In the early 1950s, soon after the discovery of the antipsychotic properties of chlorpromazine, a European investigator, R. Kuhn, was testing a similar compound, hoping to find another effective antipsychotic. The drug he tested, imipramine, was ineffective as an antipsychotic but improved the mood of some of the depressed schizophrenics. Further testing showed imipramine to be effective with depressed patients. The tricyclic antidepressant era had begun.

At the same time, iproniazid, an antitubercular drug known to inhibit monoamine oxidase (MAO), an important intraneuronal enzyme (see chapter 2), was noted to elevate the mood of tuberculosis patients, even causing euphoria and overactivity in some. By 1958, the same year that Kuhn's research on imipramine was published, two independent studies reported that iproniazid was effective in treating depressed patients. Thus, within one year, the two most important discoveries in the pharmacological treatment of depression were reported (Ayd and Blackwell, 1970).

In the twenty years following those first discoveries, the clinical and research gains consisted of elucidating some of the biological abnormalities in depression, finding uses for antidepressants in treating other disorders, and developing other but very similar tricyclic and MAO inhibitor drugs. Clinically, however, these new medications did not translate as major breakthroughs since the antidepressants released were so similar to imipramine and the first MAO inhibitors. In the early 1980s, a small group of antidepressants were released that had different chemical structures from the tricyclics—that is, they did not have three rings. For clinical purposes, however, these agents were very similar to the older tricyclics in overall efficacy and general side effect profiles. The new era of antidepressants began in late 1987 with the release of fluoxetine (Prozac), the first selective serotonin reuptake inhibitor (SSRI). The SSRIs and the other new antidepressants released since then are much easier to use, have far fewer (and different) side effects, seem to be qualitatively more effective than the tricyclics in treating a number of disorders, and are far more acceptable, even desirable, to many patients. Within an amazingly short period of time, these newer agents—both the SSRIs and other newer medications released in the 1990s—have come to dominate the prescription of antidepressants.

What has often been forgotten in the publicity surrounding these new antidepressants, however, is that they are no more effective than the older tricyclics in treating classic major depression. In antidepressant trials, imipramine, the first tricyclic, is still the "reference drug"; new antidepressants are tested to see if they are *as* effective as imipramine, not more effective. Thus, after thirty-five years of research, we still do not have an antidepressant that treats major depression more successfully than imipramine.

The evolution of the MAO inhibitor class of antidepressants has followed a somewhat different path. The early MAO inhibitors were toxic to the liver and were ultimately withdrawn from clinical use. The currently available MAO inhibitors are not significantly toxic but all share the same side effects (although in slightly different proportions) and the same problem with dietary restrictions because of the attendant risks of hypertensive (high blood pressure) reactions if the wrong foods are eaten (see below). In these ways, as with the cyclic antidepressants until the advent of the SSRIs, the MAO inhibitors have not progressed much as a class of medications in thirty-five years. With the emergence of the SSRIs, the MAO inhibitors have gone into somewhat of a decline, becoming the third-line antidepressants (with the newer antidepressants and the tricyclics first and second). One MAO inhibitor, isocarboxazid (Marplan), has been withdrawn from the market because of poor sales. The long awaited breakthrough for the MAO inhibitors has been the release of a medication of this class without dietary restrictions. Unfortunately, the domination of the SSRIs has made the expense of releasing a new medication in the United States increasingly risky. Thus, a clearly effective MAO inhibitor without dietary restrictions widely available elsewhere in the world (moclobcmide—see below) was recently withdrawn from further testing in this country because of the shrinking niche for this class of antidepressants. Although some agents will continue to be available and are very effective antidepressants for many patients, the long-term future of the MAO inhibitors is now in some doubt.

CLASSIFICATION

There is no universally accepted method of classifying antidepressants. The two most common classification schemes are based on chemical structure—tricyclics (three rings) vs. nontricyclics—and presumed mechanism of action—selective serotonin reuptake blockade (SSRI) vs. mixed reuptake blockade vs. MAO inhibition. The newer antidepressants released in the 1990s further complicate the situation since, for instance, venlafaxine (Effexor) bears some similarity to the tricyclics in its effects on multiple neurotransmitters but resembles the SSRIs in its side effect profile and powerful effect on serotonin. Bupropion (Wellbutrin), on the other hand, shares no similarity either structurally or biologically with any other antidepressant. For the purposes of this chapter, then, the antidepressants will be divided (albeit somewhat arbitrarily) into four subtypes acknowledging that medications within one class may be more alike than those in another. These four classes are the SSRIs, novel antidepressants, tricyclic and related compounds, and the MAO inhibitors. Additionally, since clinical decisions are often made by choosing among the SSRIs, novel antidepressants, or tricyclics (avoiding the MAO inhibitors as a first choice), these three classes will sometimes be lumped together and called the cyclic antidepressants.

CYCLIC ANTIDEPRESSANTS

Clinical Uses

The cyclic antidepressants (ADs) are used to treat a variety of disorders, both psychiatric and medical, listed in Table 9–1. Not all cyclic ADs have been tested in all the disorders listed.

Certainly, all the cyclic ADs are effective in treating depression, both unipolar and bipolar. For the majority of patients, no one cyclic AD is more effective than any other in treating either of these depressive subtypes. The only clear exception to this is in treating atypical depression, which responds to the SSRIs and probably some of the novel antidepressants, but is less effectively treated by the tricyclics. Among the other depressive subtypes, only psychotic depression has been demonstrated to be poorly responsive to the cyclic ADs. (The use of antidepressants for depression is discussed extensively in chapter 3.)

Cyclic ADs are well documented as effective treatments for panic disorder with or without significant agoraphobic symptoms (Ballenger, 1993). The primary therapeutic effect of the medications is thought to be the blocking of spontaneous panic attacks. The medications are probably not as effective in treating the phobic or behavioral symptoms in panic disorder. Rather, the blocking of the panic attacks allows pa-

Table 9–1
Disorders for Which Cyclic Antidepressants Are Useful

Disorder	Efficacy Rating
Depression, both unipolar and bipolar	+++
Panic disorder	+++
Obsessive compulsive disorder	+++
Bulimia nervosa	+++
Social phobia	++
Milder depressive disorders	++
Premenstrual dysphoric disorder	+++
Personality disorders	++
Chronic pain syndromes	++
Attention deficit/hyperactivity disorder	++
Paraphilias	+
Chronic fatigue syndrome	+
Generalized anxiety disorder	+
Post-traumatic stress disorder	+
Anorexia nervosa	+
Cocaine abuse	+

+++ = Definite efficacy
 ++ = Probable efficacy
  + = Possible efficacy

tients to decrease and eliminate phobic behavior, either by themselves or with the help of a behavioral program.

The tricyclics, especially imipramine, are the most well-documented antidepressants for treating panic disorder. Despite a relative paucity of research evidence, SSRIs are also very effective for panic disorder. Among the cyclic ADs, only bupropion and possibly trazodone and amoxapine are likely to be ineffective.

There is some controversy as to the appropriate doses of cyclic ADs in treating panic disorder. Most controlled studies indicate that the doses should be comparable to those used in treating depression. Numbers of clinicians, however, myself included, have seen excellent results with low doses of antidepressants in treating panic disorder, far lower than is generally effective for depression. It may be, of course, that since panic patients are unusually sensitive to certain side effects, we tend to increase the doses more slowly than when treating depressed patients, thereby allowing more patients to respond in this low-dose range.

The antidepressants that effectively treat obsessive compulsive disorder (OCD) are those with powerful serotonergic effects. The well-documented agents in this regard are all four SSRIs and clomipramine (Anafranil). Serotonergic antidepressants are effective in reducing both obsessions and compulsions regardless of whether depression is present. Appropriate doses of SSRIs when prescribed for obsessive compulsive disorder are usually thought to be higher than those required to treat depression, although recent studies have demonstrated the efficacy of fluoxetine and sertraline for OCD at typical antidepressant doses (Tollefson et al., 1994b; Greist et al., 1995a). Clomipramine doses for OCD are the same as those used for treating depression. Maximal clinical effects may take up to twelve weeks to be fully evident in treating OCD, far longer than needed for other disorders such as panic disorder or depression. So called OCD spectrum disorders, such as trichotillomania (compulsive hair pulling), onchyphagia (compulsive nail biting), and the like may also be effectively treated with SSRIs, although the evidence is far less consistent for these disorders (Christenson, Mackenzie, Mitchell, and Callies, 1991).

Without question, cyclic ADs are effective in decreasing binges and purges in patients with bulimia nervosa (American Psychiatric Association, 1993a). The effect of cyclic ADs on binging is independent of the presence of depression. (See chapter 6 for further discussion.) It is likely, although not proven, that all cyclic ADs are effective in bulimia nervosa, with imipramine, desipramine, and fluoxetine being the most well-documented medications. Bupropion, however, should not be prescribed for bulimic patients because of a significant risk of grand mal seizures (Davidson, 1989). For most cyclic ADs, doses used for treating bulimia nervosa approximate those for depression, although fluoxetine (and possibly other SSRIs) seems to possess stronger antibulimic efficacy at higher than antidepressant doses (Fluoxetine Bulimia Nervosa Collaborative Study Group, 1992).

Although large-scale studies are still lacking, social phobia has recently been demonstrated to be effectively treated by SSRIs (Jefferson, 1995). Even though fluoxetine has been the medication most consistently evaluated, three of the four SSRIs have shown efficacy, indicating that all agents of this class are likely to be effective.

Milder depressive disorders, described more in chapters 3 and 7, are anecdotally very effectively treated with SSRIs and possibly some of the other new antidepressants. These disorders include dysthymic disorder, rejection sensitivity syndromes, mild mood reactive depressions, and possibly depressive personality.

Premenstrual dysphoric disorder (a.k.a. premenstrual syndrome) is effectively treated by a variety of antidepressants. Fluoxetine is the most well-documented of these (Altshuler, Hendrick, and Parry, 1995). As in the treatment of other disorders, it is likely that the other SSRIs are also effective although systematic evidence is lacking. Some tricyclic antidepressants are also effective in treating PMS, although most women and psychopharmacologists would probably prescribe fluoxetine first because of side effect considerations.

Patients with Cluster B personality disorders, such as borderline personality, often show a decrease in symptoms such as mood lability, impulsiveness, and irritability when treated with SSRIs (Gitlin, 1995a). As with many other recently described effects of the newer antidepressants, the research studies in this area lag far behind the clinical practice in the community. In contrast to the serotonergic antidepressants, tricyclics are unlikely to be effective for treating borderline personality disorder or traits.

Chronic pain syndromes from a variety of causes including diabetes, back pain, and facial pain have been effectively treated with antidepressants for over thirty years (Philipp and Fickinger, 1993; Watson, 1994). Most studies have used the more serotonergic tricyclic antidepressants, such as amitriptyline (Elavil), doxepin (Sinequan), and clomipramine (Anafranil). This reflects both the long-standing clinical tradition in which sedating antidepressants were preferentially used (the tricyclic serotonergic ADs tend to be more sedating than noradrenergic ADs) as well as the evidence that serotonin is centrally involved in the neurotransmission of pain sensation and relief. However, the notion that antidepressants diminish pain purely by serotonergic activity seems highly unlikely. As an example, in one double-blind study, desipramine (a noradrenergic tricyclic AD) was more effective than fluoxetine (Prozac, a serotonergic AD) in treating diabetic neuropathy pain (Max et al., 1992). As with other nonaffective syndromes, the presence of depression does not consistently correlate with clinical response to antidepressants in chronic pain patients. Most studies have used smaller doses of antidepressants to treat pain than are used to treat depression. Whether this reflects the more conservative use of antidepressants by nonpsychiatric physicians or true responses at lower doses is not known.

Some cyclic antidepressants—most commonly bupropion and desipramine—are prescribed for adult patients with attention deficit/ hyperactivity disorder (ADHD) (March, Erhardt, Johnston, and Conners, 1995). A few case reports suggest that fluoxetine may be effective in treating ADHD in children, but there are no studies evaluating its efficacy in adults.

Paraphilias and related disorders, characterized by intensely arousing sexual urges and behaviors that are either considered socially deviant or interfere with normal sexual functioning, have been increasingly successfully treated with SSRIs, specifically fluoxetine and sertraline (Kafka, 1994). These effects are independent of comorbid depression and, in many reports, allow for the continuation or even enhancement of normal sexual relations. Nonserotonergic antidepressants have not been evaluated for treating paraphilias.

Chronic fatigue syndrome is frequently treated with antidepressants. Both serotonergic and noradrenergic agents seem to show beneficial effects (Goodnick and Sandoval, 1993). Antidepressant doses typically prescribed for chronic fatigue syndrome are lower than those used for depression.

Cyclic ADs have been infrequently studied or prescribed for treating generalized anxiety despite evidence for their efficacy. Numerous studies from pre-DSM-III days used cyclic ADs for patients with mixed anxiety-depression syndromes. Unfortunately, the change in classification schemes since then precludes knowing the nature of the patients treated in these earlier studies. Two controlled studies over the last decade have demonstrated the efficacy of imipramine in treating generalized anxiety disorder with trazodone additionally shown as effective in one of these (Kahn et al., 1986; Rickels, Downing, Schweizer, and Hassman, 1993).

Cyclic antidepressants are somewhat effective in treating symptoms of post-traumatic stress disorder. Three different tricyclic antidepressants and fluoxetine have shown some efficacy, although not all symptoms seem to improve with pharmacotherapy (Sutherland and Davidson, 1994).

In contrast to bulimia nervosa, anorexia nervosa is only minimally responsive to antidepressants (American Psychiatric Association, 1993a). Greater difficulties with side effects often preclude adequate medication trials with anorexic patients. Uncontrolled studies indicate that fluoxetine may be somewhat beneficial in treating anorexia nervosa when used as part of an overall treatment program (Kaye, Weltzin, Hsu, and Bulik, 1991).

In contrast to earlier reports, desipramine, a tricyclic antidepressant, is now thought to be only minimally effective in decreasing self-reported craving and abstinence in cocaine abusers (Meyer, 1992). The subgroup of desipramine responders may be those patients who have less severe cocaine abuse (Carroll et al., 1994). Fluoxetine seems to decrease cocaine craving in some studies, but its efficacy in clinical settings is less impressive (Grabowski et al., 1995).

Biologic Effects

The effectiveness of cyclic ADs in treating as wide a variety of disorders as those listed in Table 9–1 is both exciting and confusing. How can we understand all these actions in concert? Are chronic pain syndromes "masked" depressions, or masked obsessive compulsive disorders? In what way is bulimia related to panic disorder?

One possible answer is predicated on the existence of "affective spectrum disorders" defined by the diverse group of disorders that respond to a variety of antidepressant classes (Hudson and Pope, 1990). This model suggests that there may be core physiological abnormalities (as yet undiscovered) shared by all of these disorders. If this were so, one would expect higher rates of classic depressive disorders in the families of patients with affective spectrum disorders. At present, there are insufficient data to either confirm or exclude this hypothesis.

Another possible explanation for the multiple clinical effects of the antidepressants is their diverse biological properties. This model is based on the assumption that considering all disorders that respond to the same treatment as the same disorder is inconsistent with clinical experience. Both medicine and psychiatry/psychology are filled with examples of different disorders responding to one treatment. (As just two of many possible examples, calcium channel blockers are used to treat migraine headaches and angina; hypnosis can be effective both in treating chronic pain syndromes and in enhancing sleep.) As noted in chapter 2, all medications used in psychiatry (and probably all medications used in any field) are impure; that is, they do not have a single biological effect—that being the one we want—and no others. Side effects, as an example (as opposed to symptoms from a toxic overdose), are due to the unwanted diverse biological effects of the drug. Thus, many antidepressants cause dry mouth by blocking cholinergic receptors (anticholinergic effect). Yet there is no evidence that blocking that particular receptor is in any way related to the capacity of the medication to alleviate depression. The perfect antidepressant, therefore, would be devoid of cholinergic blocking properties, and of dry mouth. The perfect medication—one that affected only the parts of the brain that we wanted, and had only the specific clinical effect that we wanted—would have no side effects.

At present, it is not possible to decide which of the two proposed models—that antidepressant-responsive disorders all share some core abnormalities or that these different disorders are treated by the diverse properties of the antidepressants—better explains the medications' effects. Certainly, one might imagine one core abnormality for the depressive disorders listed in Table 9–1, and another core abnormality for the anxiety disorders. But to assume that the depressive disorders, anxiety disorders, personality disorders, bulimia nervosa, and others all share some core neurotransmitter dysfunction, especially when we do not have a coherent biological explanation for any one of these disorders, seems a leap far beyond our current knowledge. Conversely, assuming that the positive effects of the antidepressants are simply the skillful use of side effects or diverse biological properties seems rather

Table 9–2
Effects of Cyclic Antidepressants on Neurotransmitter Systems

Antidepressant Name	Norepinephrine Reuptake Blocking	Serotonin Reuptake Blocking
Amitriptyline	+	+++
Amoxapine	++	+
Bupropion	0	0
Clomipramine	++	+++
Desipramine	+++	0
Doxepin	+	++
Fluoxetine	0	+++
Fluvoxamine	0	+++
Imipramine	++	+
Maprotiline	+++	0
Nefazodone	+	+++
Nortriptyline	++	+
Paroxetine	0	+++
Protriptyline	++	+
Sertraline	0	+++
Trazodone	0	++
Trimipramine	+	++
Venlafaxine	++	+++

0 = None
+ = Minimal
++ = Moderate
+++ = Strong

coincidental given the comorbidity of so many of the disorders listed in Table 9–1. What is clear is that the cyclic antidepressants have a variety of biological effects. But which of these effects are important in treating depression, which in treating panic? Until more is known of the biological abnormalities of the disorders for which cyclic ADs are helpful, these questions cannot be answered. (Chapter 2 reviews the current hypotheses of depression, panic disorder, and obsessive compulsive disorder.)

With the exception of bupropion, all the cyclic ADs currently available block the reuptake of norepinephrine, serotonin, or both into the presynaptic neuron (see chapter 2 for background). Figure 9–1 shows this schematically; Table 9–2 shows the effect of each cyclic AD on both of these neurotransmitters. This blockade has the initial biologic result of increasing the amount of neurotransmitter available to the postsynaptic neuron. As discussed in more detail in chapter 2, according to the original monoamine hypothesis of depression, increasing the amount of norepinephrine (NE), serotonin (5-HT), or both would correct the presumed deficit in these chemicals and cause a clinical remission. This hypothesis ignored the fact that reuptake blocking is immediate (within hours of the first dose of an antidepressant) yet clinical response is delayed for weeks. Therefore, an additional biologic effect beyond reuptake blocking was needed to explain the antidepressant capacity of the medications. Ultimately, what became apparent was that cyclic antidepressants shared the capacity not only to block the reuptake of neuro-

Figure 9–1   Cyclic Antidepressants as Reuptake Blockers

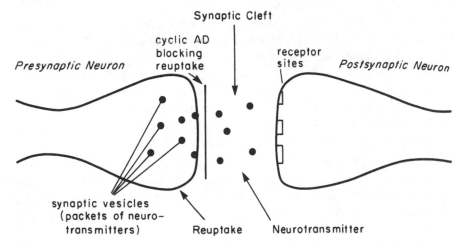

transmitters but, with chronic use (a few weeks), to alter a number of other cellular functions. As reviewed in chapter 2, these functions include neurotransmitter synthesis, aspects of receptor function, and the responsivity within the cells to receptor activation. Because the time course of these changes parallels the time course of antidepressant efficacy, it has been hypothesized that these chronic changes are likely to be important in explaining the medications' clinical effects. What is still unclear is which of these chronic changes are most central to the clinical properties of the cyclic ADs.

Moreover, there may be more than one mechanism to alter the overall function of the neurotransmitter/receptor/intracellular system. As an example, bupropion, which has no reuptake blocking properties at all, changes the sensitivity of adrenergic receptors, a capacity that may in part explain its antidepressant efficacy (Ferris and Cooper, 1993). Probably the best way to summarize our understanding of antidepressants' mechanism of action in treating depression is that they each alter NE or 5-HT via one of a variety of mechanisms. These alterations then cause a series of changes that results in a more normally functioning system and, ultimately, a clinical response. Of course, understanding the mechanism by which antidepressants work implies nothing about the "cause" of depression, nor does it preclude the effectiveness of other treatments for depression, such as psychotherapy.

Research on the mechanism of action of cyclic ADs in treating panic disorder has focused on the medications' effect in decreasing the excitability of the brainstem areas regulated by norepinephrine (locus ceruleus) and/or serotonin (dorsal raphe) (Gorman, Liebowitz, Fyer, and Stein, 1989). (See chapter 2.) As with the research in depression, current hypotheses suggest that cyclic ADs work by reregulating adrenergic and/or serotonergic neurotransmission, altering the receptor sensitivities and ultimately decreasing the system's responsivity (Charney, Bremer, and Redmond, 1995).

Since all cyclic ADs that are effective in treating obsessive compulsive disorder have powerful serotonin reuptake blocking properties, and those cyclic ADs without strong serotonergic effects are relatively ineffective, the mechanism of therapeutic effect is assumed to be related to alterations in serotonergic function. Unfortunately, little direct evidence suggests that obsessive compulsive disorder is caused by or even characterized by serotonergic dysfunction (Price, Goddard, Barr, and Goodman, 1995). Additionally, the observation that the vast majority of obsessive compulsive patients responding to serotonergic antidepressants have only partial responses further highlights the distinction between efficacy and cause. (See chapters 2 and 4 for more details.)

Since there is little research that suggests a coherent biologic explanation for bulimia nervosa, the mechanism of action of cyclic ADs in treating this disorder is equally obscure. Common hypotheses discussed in more detail in chapter 6 are that (1) bulimia is a "depressive equivalent"; therefore, the mechanism of action of the medications is the same as for depression; (2) antidepressants decrease bulimic symptoms by diminishing the anxiety that builds before a binge; (3) since food intake is controlled in the brain by a complex system that includes norepinephrine and serotonin, cyclic ADs may reduce bulimic symptoms by altering the activity of these two neurotransmitters.

Altering serotonergic function is the current dominant hypothesis explaining the efficacy of antidepressants in treating personality disorders. This hypothesis, reviewed in greater detail in chapter 7, is based on two findings: (1) serotonergic abnormalities are associated with certain personality traits commonly seen in Cluster B personality disorders; and (2) the antidepressants most likely to be helpful with these patients are those with powerful serotonergic effects.

The two major hypotheses for the efficacy of antidepressants in chronic pain syndromes are that (1) antidepressants work via their mood-enhancing effect, and (2) since both norepinephrine and serotonin play an important part in the neurological pathways that mediate pain and its inhibition, the effect of cyclic ADs is due to direct action on pain mechanisms. The fact that antidepressants decrease pain even in the absence of depression is supportive of the second hypothesis.

Multiple explanations have been presented to explain the efficacy of the SSRIs in treating paraphilias. These include considering the disorder a variant of obsessive compulsive disorder, linking the paraphilia to depression, and using the common SSRI side effect of decreased sexuality in a therapeutic manner.

The two antidepressants with the most well-documented efficacy in treating attention deficit/hyperactivity disorder—bupropion and desipramine—both increase catecholamine (dopamine and norepinephrine) activity. This observation is consistent with the effects of the stimulants as first-line agents in treating ADHD, since they too increase dopamine and norepinephrine.

Most research into the biological abnormalities of post-traumatic stress disorder has focused on arousal and anxiety mechanisms, similar to those related to panic. Since these clinical phenomena are thought to be mediated by norepinephrine and dopamine, antidepressants affecting these neurotransmitters might be effective in PTSD by decreasing their activity (Charney, Deutch, Krystal, Southwick, and Davis, 1993). The efficacy of fluoxetine, a serotonergic antidepressant, is less easily explained but may reflect the inhibitory role of serotonin on emergency responses (van der Kolk, 1994).

Choosing a Cyclic Antidepressant

Table 9–3 shows the currently available cyclic ADs, their classification (SSRI, novel, or tricyclic), trade names, usual beginning doses, and usual dosage range. The choice of a specific antidepressant depends on the disorder being treated and the individual medication's efficacy for

Table 9–3
Cyclic Antidepressants

Name (Trade Name)	Beginning Dose (mg daily)	Usual Dosage Range (mg daily)
Selective Serotonin Reuptake Inhibitors (SSRIs)		
Fluoxetine (Prozac)	10–20	10–80
Fluvoxamine (Luvox)	50	100–300
Paroxetine (Paxil)	10–20	20–50
Sertraline (Zoloft)	25–50	50–200
Novel Antidepressants		
Bupropion (Wellbutrin)	100–150	300–450
Nefazodone (Serzone)	100–200	300–600
Trazodone (Desyrel)	50	150–400
Venlafaxine (Effexor)	50–75	150–300

Tricyclics and Related Compounds

Amitriptyline (Elavil, Endep)	25–50	100–300
Amoxapine (Asendin)	50–100	150–400
Clomipramine (Anafranil)	25–50	100–250
Desipramine (Norpramin, Pertofrane)	25–50	100–300
Doxepin (Sinequan, Adapin)	25–50	100–300
Imipramine (Tofranil)	25–50	100–300
Maprotiline (Ludiomil)	25–50	100–225
Nortriptyline (Aventyl, Pamelor)	10–25	50–150
Protriptyline (Vivactil)	10	15–60
Trimipramine (Surmontil)	25–50	100–300

Note: These doses are for general guidelines only.

that disorder, as well as side effect considerations. These topics are covered in the chapters on individual disorders and earlier in this chapter.

As shown in Table 9–3, cyclic antidepressants are classified by chemical structure (tricyclic) or by biological effect (selective serotonin reuptake inhibitor). Tricyclics are all distinguished by their chemical structure—they all have three rings, hence the term (see Figure 9–2). The newer medications—those released over the last decade or more—have nontricyclic structures (see Figure 9–3). However, the number of rings in a compound's chemical structure is clinically irrelevant except that it may predict some common side effects (at least for the tricyclics). Chemical structure does not predict a specific effect on the various neurotransmitters (e.g., norepinephrine, serotonin, or both) nor efficacy in specific disorders.

Figure 9–2   Typical Tricyclic Structure

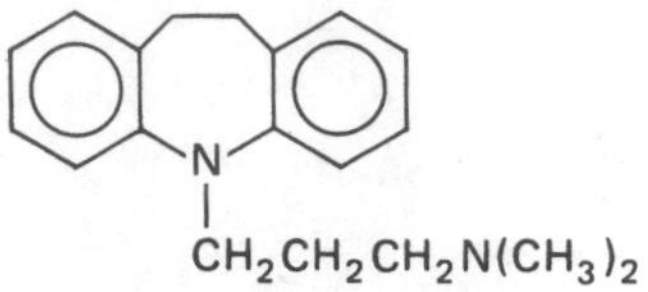

$$CH_2CH_2CH_2N(CH_3)_2$$

IMIPRAMINE

Antidepressant Classes: Prescribing Techniques and Side Effects

General Principles

With the release of the newer antidepressants that differ in a variety of ways from the older tricyclics, it has become more difficult to generalize on the practical aspects of treatment. How to start and raise doses, likely side effects, and toxic effects differ between cyclic AD classes and even between medications within a class. A few principles, however, still apply to all agents in all classes.

The most important of these principles is that antidepressants may take up to six weeks for full effect. Some patients begin to show some positive effect within the first week or two while others may show no response until the fourth week or later. It has been estimated that up to one quarter of antidepressant responses only become evident between weeks four and six (Quitkin, Rabkin, Ross, and McGrath, 1984). There is no consistent evidence that any one antidepressant works more quickly

Figure 9–3   New Cyclic Antidepressant Structure

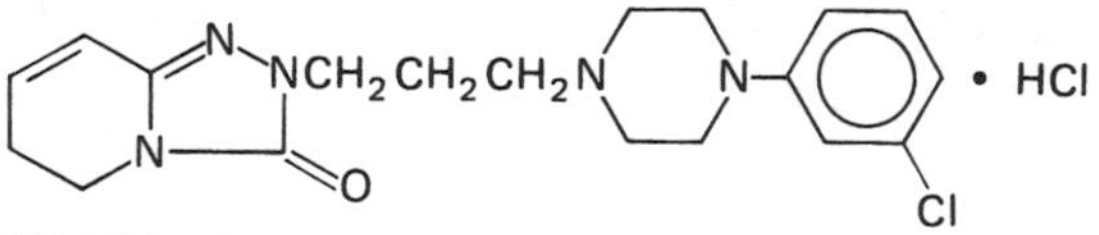

$$NCH_2CH_2CH_2N \qquad N \qquad \bullet \ HCl$$

TRAZODONE

$$F_3C \qquad O—CHCH_2CH_2NHCH_3$$

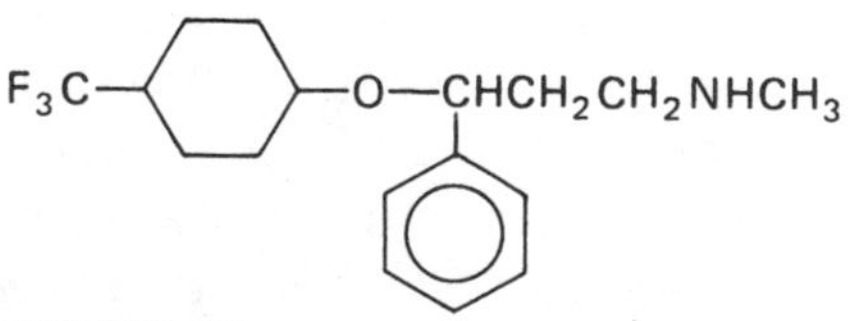

FLUOXETINE

than the others. Despite this generalization derived from controlled studies, all psychopharmacologists have observed a subgroup of patients who seem to improve markedly within days of starting an SSRI, and whose response maintains for months or years. It is possible that some of these early responses are either placebo effects or a therapeutic response to side effects. For example, a patient with psychomotor retardation taking fluoxetine may feel more energetic within days; the major effect of the medication on the depression will not emerge for four to six weeks. Yet the frequency and sustaining nature of the early positive responses seen with the SSRIs differs from what is seen with other agents. For now, this phenomenon should be considered a clinical observation without research validation.

Another important general principle of prescribing techniques concerns strategies for managing side effects. Antidepressants cause at least some side effects in the majority of patients who take them. It is important, though, not to think of side effects as a unitary phenomenon that are either present or absent. Some side effects may be common and only minimally bothersome. Others may be common early in treatment and then disappear over time. As with so many other treatment decisions, the possible use of an antidepressant must be evaluated using a risk/benefit ratio, with side effects being one of the risks. Thus, simply rattling off a list of side effects that are occasionally seen in association with an antidepressant to a patient who is considering taking that medication is unwise and unfair. (Unfortunately, this is the approach taken by the *Physicians' Desk Reference* [PDR], which, as discussed in chapter 1, should be considered more of a marketing and medicolegal document than a clinical guide.)

Depressed patients also commonly attribute depressive symptoms to side effects from the antidepressant. Therefore, it is sometimes helpful for the psychopharmacologist to ask about various complaints (such as constipation, anxiety, or sexual difficulties) that are frequently seen as either symptoms or side effects before beginning medication treatment. In an interesting study that examined the emergence of side effects during treatment with the tricyclic desipramine, subjective complaints were associated with *pre*treatment symptoms and depression scores, and not desipramine blood levels, implying that much of what distresses the patient who is taking an antidepressant may be due to or subjectively magnified more by the disorder than by the medication (Nelson, Jatlow, and Quinlan, 1984).

When the topic of side effects is discussed with the patient before the antidepressant is prescribed, four points should be emphasized: (1)

the difference between likely and unlikely side effects; (2) the need to distinguish between uncomfortable and dangerous side effects; (3) the accommodation to side effects that commonly occurs, and (4) ways to diminish side effects such that the patient's anxiety is contained rather than heightened. Different patients want and need different levels of detail. For some patients, anticipating the unwanted effects confers mastery; for others, it promotes anxiety. The exact presentation must therefore be tailored to the individual patient.

The therapeutic use of time in increasing the likelihood of a response and in diminishing side effects cannot be overemphasized. In a most interesting study examining this point, patients who had not responded to fluoxetine 20 mg daily for three weeks were randomly assigned in a double-blind fashion either to continue with 20 mg daily for five more weeks or to switch to 60 mg daily (Schweizer et al., 1990). At the end of the five additional weeks (eight weeks total treatment time), the response rate in the two groups was the same, although the group that was switched to the higher dose had more side effects.

Increasing the dose too quickly—either in the first week of treatment or after two to three weeks—ignores the body's ability to accommodate to side effects. A dose of medication that causes significant sedation (in the case of a tricyclic) or agitation (from an SSRI) may, after a few weeks, be neither sedating nor activating, but the body needs those days and weeks to accommodate. If the dose is raised too quickly, the unpleasant side effect that may result will scare the patient away from taking the medication again. It is generally not worth saving a few days at the cost of such a negative physical and psychological reaction to the medication.

When first seen in consultation, Patty had been depressed for three months. Her internist had already tried her on two of the newer antidepressants, neither of which she tolerated. Fluoxetine (Prozac), prescribed initially at a dose of 20 mg daily had made her so agitated that she stopped the medication after two days. The unpleasant side effects took three additional days to subside. Following that, she was given paroxetine (Paxil) 20 mg with the thought that since it was less activating than fluoxetine, it might be better tolerated. Similar activating side effects ensued and Patty stopped the medication again within two days. Understandably, Patty felt pessimistic about finding an antidepressant she could tolerate, especially since she had been given two of the newer medications that supposedly caused fewer side effects than the older agents. Although the doses given were those recommended in the PDR, for Patty, they were excessive. She was then referred to a psychiatrist who heard about the patient's experience and restarted her on paroxetine at one quarter tablet (5 mg) daily along with a mild tranquilizer to be taken as needed for agitation. During the first week of treatment, Patty was wary about the medication and noted no benefit, but was at least able to take it. Over the next two weeks, she was able slowly to raise the paroxetine dose to one full tablet (20 mg). Four weeks after the initiation of the low dose of paroxetine, Patty began to improve and by six weeks, she was clearly better with only minor side effects.

It is often very difficult for patient, therapist, and psychiatrist to wait four to six weeks for an antidepressant response to occur. Time is slowed down during depression; the patient may be suffering greatly and asking for relief daily, and suicidal ideation may be present, worrying everyone. There is a great temptation to switch medications if no response is evident after three weeks. I have often prescribed an adjunctive medication (see chapter 3 for options) during the fourth or fifth week simply to do *something* to alleviate the seemingly interminable wait. Still, a significant number of patients will respond during the fifth and sixth weeks of treatment. Be patient; try to help your patient be patient.

Selective Serotonin Reuptake Inhibitors (SSRIs)

The SSRIs share not only a relatively specific effect on serotonin, but a common prescribing technique and side effect profile. One of the most important advantages of the SSRIs for patients and prescribers alike is that the antidepressant does not require a gradual dosage increase to a full therapeutic dose. For many patients, the starting dose of each of the four SSRIs may be the final optimal dose. However, many psychopharmacologists, myself included, often start with a somewhat lower dose than recommended by the manufacturers. As examples, fluoxetine 10 mg, sertraline 25 mg, or paroxetine 10 mg (both of the latter two doses are one half the smallest single-pill dose available) are often prescribed as the initial dose, following which the dose can be raised after a few days to 20 mg, 50 mg, or 20 mg respectively if the patient tolerates the initial dose without difficulties. (Fluvoxamine is likely to be similar to the other SSRIs. Since it was only released in 1995, experience with the nuances of its dosing are limited at this time.) Patients who are likely to have particular difficulties with SSRI side effects—those with a history of medication sensitivities, patients with panic disorder or prominent anxiety, or the elderly—can be started at even lower doses. Alone among the SSRIs, fluoxetine is available as a liquid, allowing the prescription of very low doses for very sensitive patients by use of a dropper. Technical considerations—the difficulty in cutting pills into smaller than half or quarter tablets—preclude similar very low-dose strategies with the other SSRIs. Assuming the patient can tolerate the SSRI, most psychopharmacologists continue the typical dose of fluoxetine 20 mg, sertraline 50 to 75 mg, or paroxetine 20 mg for at least a few weeks before considering raising the dose.

Although the half-life (a measure of how long the medication stays in the body and brain before being metabolized and/or excreted) of the SSRIs markedly differ, fluoxetine, sertraline, and paroxetine are all effective when taken once daily at any dose. It is recommended that fluvoxamine be taken in a split dose. The time of day when the patient takes the medication depends purely on side effects. For most patients, fluoxetine and sertraline are mildly stimulating and are therefore taken in the morning. Paroxetine, associated with both sedation and activation, is taken at either time, depending on the individual patient, while the largest part of a fluvoxamine daily dose is typically taken at night because of its mildly sedating properties.

Common side effects for all the SSRIs are nausea, insomnia, anxiety, diarrhea, anorexia (poor appetite), headache, somnolence, and sexual side effects. (See Table 9–4.) In contrast to the tricyclics, SSRIs are not generally associated with weight gain or blood pressure changes. For the minority of patients who gain weight on SSRIs it is unclear whether this is due to enhanced appetite (or decreased dietary vigi-

Table 9–4
Common Side Effects Seen with Cyclic Antidepressants

Name (Trade Name)	Anticholinergic Effects	Stimulation	Sedation	Postural Hypotension
Selective Serotonin Reuptake Inhibitors (SSRIs)				
Fluoxetine (Prozac)	0	+++	0	0
Fluvoxamine (Luvox)	+	+	+	0
Paroxetine (Paxil)	+	+	+	0
Sertraline (Zoloft)	0	++	0	0

Novel Antidepressants

Bupropion (Wellbutrin)	+	++	0	0
Nefazodone (Serzone)	+	0	++	+
Trazodone (Desyrel)	+	0	+++	+++
Venlafaxine (Effexor)	+	+	0	0

Tricyclics and Related Compounds

Amitriptyline (Elavil, Endep)	+++	0	+++	+++
Amoxapine (Asendin)	+	0	+	++
Clomipramine (Anafranil)	+++	0	+++	+++
Desipramine (Norpramin, Pertofrane)	+	+	+	++
Doxepin (Sinequan, Adapin)	++	0	+++	++
Imipramine (Tofranil)	++	+	++	+++
Maprotiline (Ludiomil)	+	+	++	+
Nortriptyline (Aventyl, Pamelor)	+	0	++	+
Protriptyline (Vivactil)	+++	+	+	++
Trimipramine (Surmontil)	+++	0	+++	++

0 = None
+ = Minimal
++ = Moderate
+++ = Strong

lance) secondary to diminished anxiety or to another more primary weight-gaining mechanism. SSRIs occasionally cause anticholinergic side effects, such as dry mouth, constipation, and urinary hesitation, but more infrequently and in far milder form than do the tricyclics. (See the subsection on tricyclics below for more details on anticholinergic side effects.) The stimulation effects seen with SSRIs are dose related, often diminish over time, and can be effectively treated with either low doses of tranquilizers or the adjunctive use of trazodone (Desyrel), a sedating antidepressant which, at low doses, is an effective sleeping aid.

In many ways, the sexual side effects, seen in 20 to 40 percent of patients, are the most difficult to manage. All SSRIs are equally likely to cause sexual side effects although some patients might have fewer problems with one medication than another. A variety of specific side effects can occur, such as decreased libido or arousal, erectile dysfunction, and delayed time to orgasm (or anorgasmia). Other than erectile dysfunction of course, men and women are equally likely to have sexual side effects. Since a number of these same symptoms may be seen in association with either depression itself or other psychiatric disorders, a careful history is imperative in order to correctly ascertain the cause of the sexual dysfunction. General strategies to treat sexual side effects are time (waiting for accommodation to occur), decreasing the medication dose, or switching to a different medication, such as another SSRI, bupropion, or nefazodone. A number of antidotes to treat sexual side effects are available such as cyproheptadine (Periactin, a serotonin antagonist), yohimbine (Yocon), buspirone (Buspar), or even bupropion itself, but none is consistently effective (Gitlin, 1995b).

A controversial fear surrounding the SSRIs was that fluoxetine might be associated with an increase in suicidal ideation and/or violent behavior (Teicher, Glod, and Cole, 1990). However, multiple studies reviewing the treatment course of thousands of patients have consistently and conclusively demonstrated that, compared to those treated with other antidepressants, patients treated with fluoxetine are *not* at increased risk for suicidal ideation or violence (Tollefson, Rampey, Beasley, Enas, and Potvin, 1994a). Overall, rates of suicidal ideation substantially decrease with fluoxetine use because of the improvement in overall depressive symptoms. These findings do not preclude the possibility of a small subset of patients becoming suicidal from fluoxetine secondary to either agitation/restlessness or to a paradoxical response to a serotonergic medication (Hamilton and Opler, 1992; Mann and Kapur, 1991). However, such reactions are unusual and, overall, the SSRIs should be neither considered dangerous nor withheld from depressed patients with suicidal ideation. SSRIs are relatively safe when taken in overdose.

SSRIs block the hepatic (liver) metabolism of some, but not all medications, resulting in increased blood levels of these drugs. The most important interaction of this type occurs when tricyclic antidepressants and SSRIs are prescribed in combination, potentially increasing tricyclic levels to high and possibly toxic levels (deVane, 1994). Sertraline may have fewer effects in this regard than the other SSRIs (Preskorn et al., 1994). Fluvoxamine specifically may affect the metabolism of some antihistamines such as terfenadine (Seldane) and astemizole (Hismanal). For all SSRIs, however, the prescribing physician must always be aware of other medications a patient might be taking, measure blood levels of the drug if possible, and adjust the dose if needed.

In order to avoid a serotonin syndrome, a potentially fatal reaction characterized by fever, muscular rigidity, hypotension (low blood pressure), convulsions, and coma, SSRIs should never be combined with an MAO inhibitor (Sternbach 1991; Beasley, Masica, Heiligenstein, Wheadon, and Zerbe, 1993). SSRIs should not be prescribed until fourteen days after the discontinuation of an MAO inhibitor. The appropriate washout period following an SSRI before the safe prescription of an MAO inhibitor varies according to the half-life of the drug. Five weeks are required for fluoxetine to wash out while two weeks will suffice for sertraline, paroxetine, and fluvoxamine.

When SSRIs are discontinued, a transient withdrawal syndrome may be seen. This is far more likely with those antidepressants with shorter half-lives which therefore are excreted far more quickly. Thus, withdrawal symptoms are seen rarely with fluoxetine, unusually with sertraline, and commonly with paroxetine. Based on its half-life, fluvoxamine is also likely to be associated with withdrawal syndromes. The withdrawal syndrome is characterized by intense dizziness, lightheadedness, irritability, nausea, and generalized malaise. Although uncomfortable and distressing, these symptoms are not dangerous and disappear in two to ten days. To avoid these symptoms, paroxetine and probably fluvoxamine should be tapered over days to a few weeks when possible.

Novel Antidepressants

In contrast to the SSRIs, the atypical antidepressants comprise a heterogenous group of medications that share few similarities with each other except that they differ from the other available antidepressants.

Trazodone (Desyrel) has selective but weak serotonergic reuptake blocking effects with virtually no effect on norepinephrine reuptake. Despite clear evidence of its efficacy in research studies, many clinicians (myself included) find trazodone less effective than other antidepressants except in treating mild depressions with prominent anxiety. With its short half-life, theoretically, trazodone may be more effective if prescribed in divided doses. Clinically, though, this does not seem to be true. Since it is one of the most sedating medications, it is sometimes difficult for patients to take it during the day. Because it is so sedating, trazodone is effective in quickly diminishing both insomnia and anxiety. It has very few anticholinergic side effects but can produce marked dizziness. Trazodone is relatively safe if taken in overdose.

Trazodone is the most likely of the antidepressants to cause priapism—a prolonged painful erection not associated with sexual stimulation. Priapism can cause permanent impotence by decreasing blood flow to the penis. If a patient reports this, have him stop taking the medication and go to the emergency room immediately.

Bupropion (Wellbutrin), released in 1989, does not block the reuptake of either norepinephrine or serotonin, in contrast to all other cyclic antidepressants. However, it does increase noradrenergic function through other mechanisms, which may explain its antidepressant efficacy (Ascher et al., 1995). Bupropion must be taken on a divided dose regimen with no more than 150 mg ingested at any one time because of the risk of grand mal seizures if the entire daily dose is taken at once. Since bupropion is also stimulating, the doses are generally given in the earlier part of the day. Bupropion's major side effects are related to its stimulating properties; it can cause insomnia, anxiety, tremor, and headaches. It causes few blood pressure effects, no sedation, is only minimally anticholinergic, and probably causes fewer sexual side effects than other antidepressants. Much concern has been raised about whether bupropion is more likely than other antidepressants to cause seizures. However, at the recommended doses (not more than 450 mg daily given in divided dose), the seizure risk of 0.4 percent is probably the same as or only minimally increased compared to most other antidepressants (Rosenstein, Nelson, and Jacobs, 1993). Bupropion should not be prescribed for patients with a history of seizures or active eating disorders (who are at higher risk to have some metabolic abnormality such as low potassium which may increase the seizure risk). Like all of the newer cyclic ADs, bupropion is relatively safe in overdose.

Venlafaxine (Effexor), released in 1994, strongly blocks the reuptake of both serotonin and norepinephrine (Montgomery, 1993). In this way, it bears some resemblance to many of the tricyclic antidepressants. Also similar to the tricyclics, venlafaxine is typically started at a low dose which is gradually increased over a few weeks. Because of its short half-life, venlafaxine should probably not be given once daily. Dosage regimens of twice to three times daily are typical.

In many other ways, however, venlafaxine resembles the SSRIs. As an example, its side effect profile is virtually identical to all the SSRIs. Common side effects are nausea, headache, somnolence, insomnia, anxiety, anorexia, sexual dysfunction, and dry mouth (Wyeth-Ayerst, 1994). Also similar to the SSRIs, venlafaxine should not be combined with a MAO inhibitor. At least seven days must elapse between the last dose of venlafaxine and the first dose of a MAO inhibitor. Venlafaxine infrequently causes hypertension, especially when prescribed in higher doses. Therefore, patients on venlafaxine need to have their blood pressure occasionally monitored. It is relatively safe in overdose. Because of its short half-life, venlafaxine should be discontinued gradually, since its sudden discontinuation is associated with the type of withdrawal symptoms described above for short half-life SSRIs.

Nefazodone (Serzone), released in 1995, is a serotonergic drug that has activity in blocking reuptake (like an SSRI), as well as possessing other more complex serotonergic effects. It has mild noradrenergic activity. Because it was so recently released, its place among the antidepressants is still unclear. With its short half-life, nefazodone is given in divided doses. Common side effects are somnolence, dizziness, fatigue, nausea, dry mouth, and constipation. Nefazodone reportedly causes fewer sexual side effects than other serotonergic drugs, but this is far from confirmed.

Tricyclic Antidepressants (and Related Compounds)

Within this class are the classic tricyclic agents, including clomipramine (Anafranil) which, although best known for its efficacy in obsessive compulsive disorder has a tricyclic structure, along with two compounds (amoxapine [Asendin] and maprotiline [Ludiomil]) that share sufficient similarities with the tricyclics to be generally considered with them.

The technique of starting a tricyclic is similar for all agents. The initial starting dose is low and is gradually increased over seven to fourteen days to the lower end of the therapeutic range. Using imipramine as a prototype for those antidepressants with the same dosage range, this would translate to starting at 25 or 50 mg daily for one to three days, then increasing by 25 mg every day or two or by 50 mg every three days up to 150 mg daily. The analogous starting dose for nortriptyline is 10 to 20 mg, increasing to 75 mg over the first one to two weeks. Amoxapine's doses are higher than imipramine's, maprotiline's slightly lower.

Since the tricyclics as a group are somewhat sedating (although some are more sedating than others), most psychopharmacologists tend to prescribe them all at bedtime, no matter what the daily dose. The advantage to taking the entire dose at night is that whatever sedation exists is maximum during sleep (a fine time to be sedated). There is no evidence that dividing the daily dose increases efficacy. Finally, since compliance is a major problem with all medications, the more times during the day patients have to remember to take their pills, the more likely they are to forget at least one dose.

A subgroup of patients will become stimulated by one of the less sedating ADs, such as desipramine, imipramine, nortriptyline, protriptyline, or amoxapine. If a patient experiences insomnia, jitteriness or a feeling of being "wired," taking the medication earlier in the day and possibly in divided doses can alleviate the problem.

Typically, if no response is seen after two or three weeks and side effects are minimal, the tricyclic is gradually raised to the maximum dose shown in Table 9–3. If no response is seen despite the increased dose, it is appropriate to ensure that the patient is taking an optimal amount of the tricyclic by obtaining a plasma level of the antidepressant. (Plasma is the liquid portion of blood, as opposed to the cells. All chemicals in the blood are actually in the portion of blood that is plasma. Most psychopharmacologists use the terms plasma and blood levels interchangeably.) Technically, this involves drawing a small amount of blood (only one tube is needed) and measuring the amount of the antidepressant in the circulation. Blood levels allow for a more accurate dose adjustment: the body "sees" the blood level, not the dose. True toxicity occurs when the blood level is too high, no matter what the dose.

For some—but not all—tricyclics, a blood level within a certain range will correlate with maximum improvement of depression. Table 9–5 shows the four tricyclics for which blood levels correlate best with therapeutic response when treating depression (Perry, Zeilmann, and Arndt, 1994). For the three tricyclics with upper limits shown in Table 9–4, too high a blood level is just as likely to be associated with a poor response as too low a level. When the level is too high, the dose of the tricyclic should be decreased. For desipramine, no obvious upper level has been established, although levels above 500 ng/ml should generally be avoided. With careful monitoring of the blood level, tricyclic doses can be increased until the level is in the therapeutic range. As an exam-

Table 9–5
Antidepressants for Which Therapeutic Blood Levels
Are Established

Drug	Therapeutic Blood Level in ng/ml (approximate)	Comment
Nortriptyline	50–150	Most well established
Desipramine	> 125	No obvious upper limit
Imipramine	200–350	Blood level = combination of imipramine and desipramine (its major metabolite) levels
Amitriptyline	95–140	Least well established. Blood level = combination of amitriptyline and nortriptyline levels.

ple, if a patient is taking imipramine 300 mg daily (generally considered a maximum dose) and has a combined blood level (imipramine plus its metabolite desipramine) of 105 ng/ml, raising the dose would be an appropriate therapeutic maneuver. If the blood level is 325 ng/ml, raising the dose would be unlikely to be helpful.

These therapeutic blood level ranges may not apply when a tricyclic is prescribed for other disorders. For example, when imipramine is prescribed for panic disorder, optimal blood levels (of combined imipramine plus desipramine) are in the 110–140 ng/ml range (Mavissakalian and Perel, 1995).

For all the other cyclic ADs, one can measure the blood level, but the "correct amount" needed for maximum effect is unknown. (Unfortunately, there are no correlations between blood levels of the SSRIs or the other newer agents and clinical response.)

Table 9–4 presents the most common types of side effects seen with the tricyclics and the likelihood of seeing them with any individual medication. Table 9–6 lists other side effects sometimes seen with these medications.

The most common side effects seen with the tricyclics are the anticholinergic side effects, so called because they are due to the blockade of cholinergic receptors. The anticholinergic effects are dry mouth (the most common), constipation, urinary hesitation, and blurry vision.

Table 9–6
Other Side Effects of Cyclic Antidepressants

Sexual dysfunction: anorgasmia, erectile dysfunction

Stimulation: nervousness, irritability, palpitations, tachycardia (fast heartbeat), tremor, sweating

Weight gain

Indigestion

Edema (swelling)

Extrapyramidal symptoms: stiffness, slowness, restlessness (rare except with amoxapine)

Rash

Speech blockade (rare)

Seizures (rare but more common with high doses of maprotiline, clomipramine, and bupropion)

Additionally, some patients, especially the elderly, have decreased memory and poor concentration because of anticholinergic effects. (Of course, since depression itself is characterized by these two cognitive symptoms, caution must be used in interpreting these symptoms as side effects.) Occasionally, a patient who is on multiple medications with anticholinergic effects can exhibit an anticholinergic delirium. This unusual and serious condition is a toxic psychosis characterized by confusion, visual hallucinations, and disorientation. Anticholinergic delirium must be distinguished from an exacerbation of the primary psychiatric problem since the treatments are, not surprisingly, very different.

Anticholinergic side effects that are extremely bothersome can be treated by reversing the cholinergic blockade at the various affected organs or by taking bethanechol, a cholinergic medication. Thus, dry mouth can be treated by cholinergic mouth wash (along with cheaper and easier maneuvers, such as chewing sugarless gum) or bethanechol. Constipation can be a significant problem, especially with the elderly. It is best treated by the use of bulk, either in food such as bran, or bethanechol. If these remedies are ineffective, laxatives can be used cautiously. Urinary hesitation can be especially troublesome for elderly males who have enlarged prostates (which also obstruct urine flow). In general, the use of "antidotes" for side effects such as dry mouth is recommended only when the symptoms are extremely bothersome. Otherwise, the patient might end up taking five medications—one for the primary disorder and the others to treat various side effects!

Sedation is an extremely common side effect, seen with most of the tricyclic antidepressants. Luckily, it is also a side effect to which patients often experience significant accommodation, such that at the end of a few weeks of treatment, a profoundly sedating medication may be only minimally sedating. Unfortunately, this is not always the case. If a patient has significant anxiety or insomnia, a possible strategy (other than prescribing a sedating antidepressant) is to prescribe a relatively nonsedating antidepressant plus a tranquilizer; the tranquilizer can then be withdrawn when the depression lifts. If sedating antidepressants are used, patients will still be taking a sedating medication even after they are no longer agitated. The best ways to manage medication-induced sedation are to give all of the antidepressant at night, or to wait for sedation to diminish, as it will over time. Caffeine in the morning can help, but it can also cause anxiety.

Postural hypotension is a relatively common side effect that is manifested by a drop in blood pressure upon change of position, especially when standing up. The subjective complaint associated with this blood pressure drop is a feeling of dizziness or lightheadedness when getting up or starting to walk. When severe, it can cause loss of balance or even fainting, potentially resulting in serious injury. This is a significant problem when treating elderly patients, who may have poor balance to begin with. As noted in Table 9–4, the cyclic ADs differ markedly in their capacity to produce postural hypotension. Among the tricyclics, nortriptyline is the least likely to cause postural hypotension but the SSRIs and atypical antidepressants cause blood pressure changes far less frequently than any of the tricyclics. Potential treatments for postural hypotension include increasing salt intake or adding one of a number of medications.

Some patients will experience a variety of stimulation side effects from tricyclic ADs, especially those with marked noradrenergic effects (see Table 9–2). Stimulation effects are manifested by a fast heartbeat (tachycardia), insomnia, anxiety, and/or a tremor. The tachycardia may be frightening or uncomfortable but is not dangerous, except for some patients with preexisting heart disease. The insomnia can frequently be controlled by taking the antidepressant early in the day. The tremor (and the tachycardia) can be treated by low-dose propranolol.

Sweet craving and weight gain are important tricyclic side effects. With some patients, this can be a problem of monstrous proportion, causing great anguish and precipitating noncompliance. The statement, "I would rather be depressed than get fat" is often heard during the discussions of medication-induced weight gain. In one study using imipramine, 15 percent of patients gained more than ten pounds within four months (Fernstrom, Krowinski, and Kupfer, 1986). The weight gain is real and does not just reflect regaining the weight frequently lost as a symptom of depression. There are no predictors of weight gain (Garland, Remick, and Zis, 1988). Desipramine may cause less weight gain than the other tricyclics. The mechanism of the weight gain is unknown. Hypoglycemia is clearly *not* the cause. Proposed mechanisms include histaminic blocking properties of the antidepressants and changes in serotonin and norepinephrine function in the hypothalamus, the area of the brain that regulates appetite, feelings of satiety, and carbohydrate hunger.

The best treatment for the antidepressant-induced sweet craving and weight gain is prevention. Warning the patient *before* treatment can be very helpful. Drinking high-calorie drinks when thirsty from antidepressant-induced dry mouth is also preventable. Once the weight has been gained, dieting and exercising are always helpful, just as they are for losing weight from any cause. Patients frequently get discouraged, however, because they find that a vigorous program that would ordinarily allow them to lose two pounds weekly when not on an antidepressant causes only a half pound weight loss while on medications. Anorectic (decreasing appetite) medications are sometimes used but their ultimate effectiveness is unknown.

Alone among the tricyclics, amoxapine (Asendin) can cause the types of side effects typically associated with antipsychotics, including tardive dyskinesia (see chapter 12 for more details on side effects of antipsychotics). These antipsychotic side effects are caused by one of the major metabolites of amoxapine that possesses clear antipsychotic activity.

Clomipramine (Anafranil) is a tricyclic antidepressant with powerful (but not selective) serotonergic effects, which explains its efficacy in treating obsessive compulsive disorder. Its side effect profile includes those common to the tricyclics and others that are typical of the SSRIs. It possesses strong anticholinergic, sedating, and orthostatic effects, while at high doses it is more likely than other antidepressants to cause epileptic seizures. Like the SSRIs, it causes high rates of sexual side effects. Clomipramine should never be combined with an MAO inhibitor. Two weeks should elapse between the prescription of clomipramine and an SSRI, regardless of which medication is used first.

Finally, a significant drawback of the tricyclic antidepressants concerns their lethality if taken in overdose. Paradoxically, the patients at highest risk for suicide are sometimes prescribed the most dangerous medications—ingestion of as little as one week's dose of antidepressants is potentially lethal. Patients who take more than one extra day's dose should be taken to the emergency room immediately.

MONOAMINE OXIDASE (MAO) INHIBITORS

Even though MAO inhibitors were first shown to have antidepressant efficacy at the same time as the tricyclics, they have been used only a fraction as much since then. This stems from two separate but important early observations, one of which suggested a lack of efficacy in severe depressions, while the other focused on life-threatening side effects. In the last fifteen years, both of these clinical observations have been shown to be gross overstatements. With the luxury of our current vantage point, MAO inhibitors should be considered equivalently effective to cyclic ADs for treating major depression, and more effective than the tricyclics in treating atypical depression. Additionally, the dangerousness of the MAO inhibitors, due to the effect of ingesting tyramine-containing foods or stimulant-containing medications, can be minimized greatly with proper patient education and cooperation. Two reviews have estimated the risk of serious hypertensive reactions as 1 to 3 percent (Robinson and Kurtz, 1987; Rabkin, Quitkin, McGrath, Harrison, and Tricamo, 1985).

Unfortunately, even as psychiatrists became more aware of the efficacy of the MAO inhibitors and their unique advantage in treating atypical depression, and also became more comfortable with the MAO dietary restrictions, the SSRIs were released and quickly dominated the antidepressant market. Despite a lack of controlled trials, the SSRIs became the antidepressants of first choice among clinicians for atypical depression because of their perceived efficacy, far greater ease of administration, lower side effect profile, and general patient acceptability. The MAO inhibitors have therefore become the third choice of antidepressant classes, behind the SSRIs and other new agents, and the tricyclics. With a decreasing share of the antidepressant market resulting in less financial gain for the medications' manufacturers, one of the MAO inhibitors was recently withdrawn from manufacture and release, while clinical research in the United States with another MAO inhibitor already available in other countries was suspended. Thus, the future of the MAO inhibitors as a class of antidepressants is in some doubt unless there is a change in the rules regulating the financing of medications with small market shares.

Clinical Uses

Just as with the cyclic ADs, the MAO inhibitors show efficacy in a variety of different disorders. These disorders, listed in Table 9–7 overlap substantially with the cyclic AD list. The comparative efficacy of the antidepressant classes for each disorder, and the pros and cons of using each, are discussed in the chapters on each disorder.

As noted above, it was initially thought that the MAO inhibitors had their only significant effect in atypical depressions (defined in a variety of ways) and were relatively ineffective in the classical and more severe depressions. In retrospect, this was in large part due to the small, probably inadequate doses used in those early studies. Over the last fifteen years, a number of studies have demonstrated that, when prescribed in higher doses, MAO inhibitors are clearly effective in melancholic and nonmelancholic depressions (Davis, Wang, and Janicak, 1993). Because they are simpler to use (due to the dietary restrictions needed with all available MAO inhibitors) and the evidence for their efficacy is far greater, the cyclic ADs should still be considered the appropriate first treatment for most cases of major depression. Although there is a paucity of studies on the topic, bipolar and unipolar depressions are probably equally likely to respond to MAO inhibitors. Bipolar depressions with anergic features (psychomotor retardation, fatigue, and hypersomnia) may show a preferential response to MAO inhibitors (Himmelhoch, Thase, Mallinger, and Houck, 1991).

Table 9–7
Disorders for Which MAO Inhibitors Are Useful

Disorder	Efficacy Rating
Depression, unipolar, bipolar, and atypical	+++
Panic disorder	+++
Social phobia	+++
Bulimia nervosa	++
Borderline personality disorder	++
Post-traumatic stress disorder	+
Obsessive compulsive disorder	+
Chronic pain syndromes	+
Attention deficit/hyperactivity disorder	+

+++ = Definite efficacy
 ++ = Probable efficacy
  + = Possible efficacy

Atypical depression responds preferentially to MAO inhibitors compared to tricyclics (Liebowitz, Quitkin et al., 1988). Atypical depressions are those characterized by mood reactivity and two of four of: hyperphagia, hypersomnia, heavy feelings in arms and legs (leaden paralysis), and interpersonal rejection sensitivity. (See chapter 3 for more details.)

No study has systematically compared the antidepressant efficacy among the three MAO inhibitors. At this point, then, it seems warranted to consider them equal, with the choice of a specific medication decided by other criteria, such as side effect profile.

MAO inhibitors are very effective in the treatment of panic disorder, with therapeutic effects seen irrespective of any depressive component (Pohl, Berchou, and Rainey, 1982). The MAO inhibitors may also be effective in diminishing the anticipatory anxiety and phobic avoidance seen in panic disorder (as opposed to the seemingly more pure effect of the tricyclics in blocking the panic attacks without changing other symptoms) (Sheehan, Ballenger, and Jacobsen, 1980). Among the MAO inhibitors, phenelzine is the most well studied in panic disorder, although it is likely that all are effective. Tranylcypromine, with its greater stimulant properties, will cause more unwanted stimulation/anxiety. Doses used for treating panic disorder and the time to response are the same as in depression.

Generalized social phobia is very effectively treated by MAO inhibitors (Liebowitz et al., 1992). Phenelzine has been the most well studied in this regard but all agents, including those available in Europe, are likely to be effective. Positive effects seen are global with patients showing less anxiety, less avoidance of social and work activities resulting in better overall functioning, and fewer avoidant personality traits.

MAO inhibitors are occasionally prescribed to treat normal weight bulimia nervosa. Clinically, using these medications for bulimia is appealing for two reasons (Walsh, 1987): first, bulimic patients often present with a mixed anxiety/depression picture along with their eating symptoms in a manner reminiscent of the atypical depressions thought to be responsive to MAO inhibitors. Second, the anxiety/tension that seems to be a precipitant to many binges suggests the possible use of medications with powerful antianxiety effects, such as the MAO inhibitors. Two controlled studies (Walsh et al., 1988; Kennedy et al., 1988) and many anecdotes using all the MAO inhibitors have demonstrated the success of these medications in diminishing both binges and purges. However, the strict requirement for dietary controls when using these medications makes their use with bulimic patients tricky at best. Interestingly, one study using phenelzine with bulimic patients noted no problems with hypertensive reactions (presumably because of careful patient selection), but found that the usual MAO inhibitor side effects such as postural hypotension and sedation severely limited their utility. Eighty-nine percent of the patients who *improved* in that study discontinued treatment during the follow-up phase, the majority due to side effects (Walsh, et al., 1988).

MAO inhibitors have been used to treat impulsive borderline personality disorder patients. In one double-blind study comparing many different psychopharmacological treatments in a group of borderlines with depressed mood, rejection sensitivity, and extensive destructive behavioral outbursts (such as wrist cutting or physical violence), but without a current major depression, tranylcypromine was effective in improving mood, rejection sensitivity, and suicidality with some effects on decreasing behavioral outbursts (Cowdry and Gardner, 1988). Consistent with this, patients with atypical depression with prominent borderline features showed excellent responses to an MAO inhibitor (Parsons et al., 1989). Further studies are needed to confirm the generalizability of these results. Similar to treating those with bulimia or ADHD, prescribing MAO inhibitors with their dietary restrictions for impulse-driven borderline patients can be dangerous. Patients must therefore be selected carefully.

Post-traumatic stress disorder (PTSD) has been successfully treated with MAO inhibitors in a few open trials and in one recent double-blind study (Frank et al., 1988). Theoretically, MAO inhibitors are attractive for treating PTSD because of their mixed antipanic/antidepressant properties. Phenelzine has been used the most in these reports, although all medications in this class are likely to be effective. However, the dietary restrictions, side effects, and contraindication to the use of MAO inhibitors in the context of drug abuse preclude their use in many traumatized patients.

MAO inhibitors are effective for some patients with obsessive compulsive disorder. Obsessive compulsive patients who are most likely to respond to MAO inhibitors may be those with comorbid anxiety or depressive disorders, although one controlled study demonstrated efficacy in an unselected group of OCD patients (Vallejo, Olivares, Marcos, Bulbena, and Menchon, 1992).

The use of MAO inhibitors with chronic pain syndromes has been infrequent despite the preliminary evidence that they may be helpful. This is due to the general decreased use of the MAO inhibitors, the dietary restrictions required for their use, and because pain clinics tend to be directed by anesthesiologists who are wary of, and inexperienced with these medications. Chronic pain patients frequently exhibit atypical depression syndromes with anxiety, somatic preoccupation, and reversed vegetative symptoms, suggesting the use of MAO inhibitors on this basis alone (Dworkin and Caligor, 1988). In one older study, phenelzine was superior to the tricyclic amitriptyline in patients with chronic pain and depression (Raft, Davidson, Mattox, Mueller, and Wasik, 1979).

Attention deficit/hyperactivity disorder (ADHD) in adults is another disorder for which MAO inhibitors, especially tranylcypromine, have been occasionally prescribed. A major problem with the MAO inhibitors is that tolerance may develop during treatment, a phenomenon rarely seen with other agents used to treat ADHD (Wender, 1988). Additionally, prescribing medications with dietary restrictions for patients with problems of impulse control is a real concern. If tranylcypromine's effects in adult ADHD are similar to those seen when it is used to treat childhood ADHD, results may be seen within the first few days of treatment, far sooner than is seen when MAO inhibitors are used in depression.

Biologic Effects

As shown in Figure 2–4, MAO is an intraneuronal enzyme that metabolizes a variety of neurotransmitters. These neurotransmitters include norepinephrine, serotonin, dopamine, phenylethylamine, tyramine, and others. Given the number of different neurotransmitter systems affected by MAO, it is not surprising that, like the cyclic ADs, MAO inhibitors have such a broad range of effects. Because MAO inhibitors decrease an enzyme that metabolizes neurotransmitters, their initial effect, like those of the cyclic ADs, is to increase the amount of norepinephrine, serotonin, and other neurotransmitters. However, as with cyclic ADs, it cannot be assumed that the increased availability of neurotransmitters soon after the MAO inhibitors are taken is the mechanism by which these medications cause a clinical effect.

It is also clear that MAO exists in two forms, MAO-A and MAO-B. MAO-A primarily metabolizes norepinephrine and serotonin while MAO-B metabolizes dopamine and phenylethylamine. The currently available MAO inhibitors are nonselective; that is, they affect the A and B forms equally. Investigations with selective MAO inhibitors suggest that it is inhibition of the A form that is more important for antidepressant activity. This contrasts with the observation that in human brains (as compared with kidney, liver, and other organs in which MAO is found), 75 percent of the MAO is in the B form (Robinson and Kurtz, 1987). However, a statement about the brain as a whole tells us nothing of what is occurring in the specific parts of the brain that are relevant to antidepressant mechanisms. It is possible that MAO-A is preferentially utilized in the parts of the brain regulating mood, affect, and cognition, despite MAO-B being the more common form in the brain overall.

Choice of Agents and Techniques for Prescribing

Table 9–8 lists the currently available MAO inhibitors. Two of the medications listed, phenelzine (Nardil) and tranylcypromine (Parnate), have been the most commonly prescribed MAO inhibitors for years. Isocarboxazid (Marplan), another MAO inhibitor, had also been available for decades until the end of 1993 when the manufacturers withdrew it from the market, seemingly because of financial considerations. (There were no reports or evidence of any medical problems associated with its use.) It is possible that isocarboxazid will become available again if another pharmaceutical firm buys its patent, but for now, it is a piece of MAO inhibitor history.

Selegiline (Eldepryl), the other available MAO inhibitor, is marketed and FDA indicated as an adjunctive treatment for treating Parkinson's disease. Therefore, many physicians are unaware that, at higher doses than used for Parkinson's disease, selegiline is a classic MAO inhibitor with well-documented antidepressant efficacy (Mann et al., 1989). At the low doses (5 to 10 mg daily) that are prescribed for treating Parkinson's disease, selegiline is a selective MAO-B inhibitor. As noted above, it is MAO-A inhibition that seems to mediate antidepres-

Table 9–8
Monoamine Oxidase Inhibitors Currently Available

Name (Trade Name)	Dosage Range (mg daily)	Comments
Phenelzine (Nardil)	45–90	Most well studied
Tranylcypromine (Parnate)	30–60	Most stimulating
Selegiline (Eldepryl)	20–60	Least used, fewer side effects, very expensive

sant effects. Therefore, at low doses, selegiline is neither an antidepressant nor does it require dietary restrictions (see below). When the dose of selegiline is increased beyond 10 mg daily, it begins to inhibit MAO-A, antidepressant efficacy is seen, and the dietary restrictions are required.

No agents of its kind are currently available in the United States (although at least one medication—moclobemide, marketed as Aurorix or Manorix—is widely used in Europe), but reversible MAO inhibitors represent the next wave of medications in this class. The three MAO inhibitors listed in Table 9–8 are all irreversible; that is, they bind to the MAO enzyme permanently, requiring the synthesis of new enzyme to reverse their effect. The reversible MAO inhibitors, also known as RIMAs (reversible inhibitors of MAO-A) can be displaced from the MAO enzyme. The end result of this reversibility is that virtually no dietary restrictions are required. Similar to irreversible agents, reversible MAO inhibitors seem to be effective in melancholic depression, social phobia, and atypical depression (Rudorfer, 1992). Along with their lack of dietary restrictions, reversible MAO inhibitors also have fewer side effects than the classic agents. Unfortunately, the makers of moclobemide recently stopped the progress of clinical trials within the United States, thereby retarding or precluding its release here. Since moclobemide is available in Europe, Canada, and Mexico and has not been associated with medical problems, the only explanation for the cessation of the research in the United States is, as noted with the withdrawal of isocarboxazid, financial.

The same guidelines presented above for prescribing the tricyclic antidepressants are also used with the MAO inhibitors: They are initially prescribed at low doses and then gradually raised. Because the MAO inhibitors are less sedating than the tricyclics, the doses may be raised slightly faster. An additional consequence of lesser sedation with the MAO inhibitors is that they are usually not taken at bedtime. Morning administration of MAO inhibitors is also helpful for decreasing the insomnia frequently seen with these medications.

MAO inhibitors are taken either in one daily dose or in divided doses. Although the half-lives of all three medications are short (measured in a few hours), their effects on MAO inhibition last far longer. Thus, taking the entire daily dose once daily should—and does—work just as well as divided doses. The major reason to divide the dose is to prevent intense side effects one to two hours after taking the entire daily dose. The most common symptom from ingesting a large amount of an MAO inhibitor is postural hypotension, manifested as dizziness or even fainting, especially upon changing position from lying or sitting to standing.

A reasonable beginning dose for each MAO inhibitor is two pills daily (20 mg for tranylcypromine, 30 mg for phenelzine, and 10 mg for selegiline). For a patient who may be particularly frightened by the medication, starting with one pill daily for a few days before increasing to two pills daily is often helpful. This can then be increased to three pills after three to seven days. Doses of tranylcypromine and phenelzine can then be increased by one pill every week to ten days depending on side effects and therapeutic response; selegiline doses may be raised somewhat faster.

The MAO inhibitors are similar to the cyclic ADs in that from three to six weeks may be needed for a therapeutic response to occur. Certainly, earlier responses are sometimes seen. Tranylcypromine frequently causes an early, usually helpful, stimulant response, with patients noting increased energy and mood. This is generally not the same as the later more global antidepressant response.

If a patient is taking a reasonably high dose of an MAO inhibitor, has few side effects, and shows insufficient clinical response, the dose may be cautiously increased until a positive response or significant side effects ensue. Accurately measuring the blood or plasma levels of an MAO inhibitor is, unfortunately, not possible, and, although some research and university laboratories can measure percent MAO inhibition as a marker of dose adequacy, this test is neither consistently available nor sufficiently reliable to justify its routine use.

Among the three MAO inhibitors, the choice of a specific medication should be made by either history of past response, side effect profile, or cost. Tranylcypromine is the most stimulating of the three MAO inhibitors. Sometimes, this is a useful side effect—for example, in treating a depressed patient with psychomotor retardation—while for others, it is a significant problem, requiring a switch to a different medication if the stimulation doesn't resolve over time. Phenelzine, conversely, is the most sedating, while selegiline is in the middle. In general, selegiline causes the same side effects as the other two MAO inhibitors, but of lesser severity (Mann, 1991). Compared to the other two agents, selegiline's major drawback is price; it is staggeringly expensive, costing from $9 to $30 daily, depending on the dose.

Until the 1995 edition when the warning was deleted, the *Physicians' Desk Reference* stated that Parnate (tranylcypromine) should not be prescribed for patients over 60 years of age. However, elderly depressed patients are clearly responsive to MAO inhibitors (Georgotas et al., 1986). In fact, theoretically, they may be more likely to respond, since monoamine oxidase increases as a normal concomitant of aging (Plotkin, Gerson, and Jarvik, 1987; Sunderland et al., 1994). Increased MAO would decrease the amounts of neurotransmitters, which might then make certain elderly individuals more vulnerable to clinical depression. As with the cyclic ADs, side effects may be more of a problem in the elderly, especially the postural hypotensive effects. Selegiline may have somewhat of an advantage over the other two MAO inhibitors in treating the elderly, given its more benign side effect profile.

Food and Drug Interactions

The most salient aspects of treatment with MAO inhibitors are the dietary and medication restrictions (especially the former). Patients always remember if they have ever been treated with an MAO inhibitor if you simply ask "Did the doctor say you couldn't eat cheese while taking the medication?" Furthermore, the warnings about what might happen if dietary restrictions are ignored—a sudden increase in blood pressure (hypertensive reaction), stroke, or even death—are certainly enough to scare anyone, especially if the person is depressed, somatically preoccupied, or anxious. A great deal of the lore about MAO inhibitors is a residue of twenty-five years ago, when neither patients nor doctors knew the cause of the hypertensive reactions. At that time, these medications *were* dangerous in unpredictable ways and their reputation was justified. Unfortunately, reputations are difficult to change. A quick perusal of the way the *Physicians' Desk Reference* describes the risks and side effects of these medications should be enough to convince anyone that terrifying warnings, albeit unjustified, still abound. It must be remembered that the MAO inhibitors can be dramatically effective with a great number of patients. The risks mentioned above are all real—but preventable in the vast majority of cases given our current knowledge. We must also remember that the potential morbidity and even mortality of depression or severe anxiety disorders is far from trivial itself. As always, potential risks and potential benefits must be weighed and compared in order to truly assess a treatment's dangerousness.

A review of tyramine, the most common amino acid in food that raises blood pressure, will help clarify the MAO inhibitor/food list. Tyramine is found in a variety of foods, the majority of which are aged foods. Anyone—on MAO inhibitors or not—will experience a rise in blood pressure if enough tyramine is absorbed into the bloodstream. Therefore, one important variable is how much tyramine gets absorbed.

Ordinarily, when a person not on MAO inhibitors ingests a tyramine-containing food (such as aged cheese), the enzyme monoamine oxidase (MAO) which exists in the lining of the intestinal tract and in the liver (through which all absorbed foods pass first) metabolizes the tyramine so that very little gets into the bloodstream. Thus, anyone on an MAO inhibitor will absorb an increased amount of tyramine. Once tyramine is absorbed, it is taken up into the cells where it releases norepinephrine, and this in turn raises the blood pressure. Since MAO metabolizes norepinephrine within the cells, patients on an MAO inhibitor have greater stores of norepinephrine to be released, thereby raising the blood pressure even more. These two mechanisms—the increased absorption of tyramine and the increased release of norepinephrine—explain why patients on MAO inhibitors can have hypertensive reactions when they ingest tyramine-containing foods. Some foods capable of causing a hypertensive reaction do not contain tyramine but contain other amines with similar properties. With these other foods, the explanation is identical to that for tyramine.

There are many different lists that enumerate all the foods that have ever been reported to cause a hypertensive reaction in patients on MAO inhibitors. Most of these lists are absurdly long and do not distinguish between foods that may have caused a reaction in one individual on one occasion and those likely to cause reactions frequently. Unless the patient on MAO inhibitors also has an obsessional personality disorder, these long, overly inclusive lists are likely to result in random noncompliance. It is far better to have a shorter list with which a reasonably cooperative patient will be able to comply.

This seemingly simple task—that of giving an appropriate list of proscribed foods with MAO inhibitors—can demonstrate the difference between working with a knowledgeable psychopharmacologist and dealing with a competent psychiatrist who is inexperienced in psychopharmacology. Moreover, as with explaining side effects in general, how the information is presented is as important as what is presented. The MAO/food list can induce fear and dread, or a sense of realistic dangers that is mastered with minimal effort, depending on the person presenting it. Psychotherapists are not expected to know the nuances of these lists. It is extremely helpful, however, if you are knowledgeable enough to help your patient deal with the appropriate concerns, as well as allay inappropriate fears that surround the MAO inhibitors.

Table 9–9 lists the foods that are likely to provoke hypertensive reactions in patients on MAO inhibitors. As is clear, some foods must never be eaten, while others can be consumed in limited quantities.

Table 9–9
Food Restrictions for Patients on MAO Inhibitors

Foods and Beverages to Avoid Completely

Cheese—all kinds except cottage cheese, ricotta, and cream cheese

Smoked or pickled fish (canned tuna is OK)

Fermented meats—such as summer sausage, salami, mortadella

Sauerkraut

Yeast/protein extracts—such as Marmite and Bovril spreads

Red wines, especially chianti; imported or tap beers; sherry, vermouth (white wine and champagne are OK)

Fava or broad bean pods (Italian green beans). The beans themselves are OK; string beans are OK

Beef liver or chicken liver (unless absolutely fresh)

Overripe figs or overripe bananas (young bananas with white pulp are OK)

Foods and Beverages to Be Used in Moderation

Canned or packeted soups

Soy sauce

Other alcoholic beverages

Yogurt

Sour cream

Avocados

Raspberries

Note: These instructions must be followed for two weeks after stopping the MAO inhibitors.

Even among lists that distinguish appropriately between likely and unlikely risks, there may be some differences. This stems from the lack of extensive chemical analysis for a great number of the foods listed. The major offenders, however, are almost always the same. With only rare exceptions (e.g., broad bean pods, which contain dopamine), these forbidden foods are aged. As food ages or ferments, tyramine is formed. Thus, even a food that has little tyramine when absolutely fresh, such as liver, can contain a significant amount of tyramine when it is left out, even for a few hours.

There are two important reminders regarding this list. One, a food that causes no reaction the first ten times it is eaten can provoke a reaction the eleventh time. In the case of cheese, for example, this happens because each wheel of cheese contains a different amount of tyramine. Also, the amount of tyramine varies greatly depending on whether the particular slice comes from the rind or the center of the wheel. Thus, there is simply no way of knowing that any cheese (other than cottage cheese or cream cheese) is safe, no matter how many times the patient has eaten it without problems. If your patient describes a cavalier attitude towards an MAO diet, you should not only refer the patient back to the psychiatrist for clarification and education about the diet, but also consider exploring any possible psychodynamic roots of the dietary indiscretions. Is it a rebellion against parental authority as represented by the physician? Is there a flirtation with self-destructive behavior? Is limit testing in other situations part of the patient's character style? If the patient confides in the therapist that he is "cheating" on the MAO diet, encouraging the patient to deal with the psychiatrist directly would be best. If the patient refuses and continues to risk a major medical catastrophe through dietary indiscretions, informing the psychopharmacologist yourself is appropriate if a working relationship has previously been established with the patient's knowledge and consent.

The second reminder is that it is the amount of tyramine ingested (and absorbed) that is important in understanding the risk of hypertensive episodes. The foods listed under "consume in moderation" generally contain a small amount of tyramine; if a great deal of any of them is eaten, however (such as four ripe avocados in one sitting), a hypertensive reaction is possible.

Table 9–10 lists the medications that must be avoided by patients taking an MAO inhibitor. Two types of reactions may be seen, each caused by a different class of medications: hypertensive crises and serotonin (hyperpyrexic–high fever) syndromes.

Those medications causing hypertensive reactions are all stimulants and provoke hypertension by the increased release of norepinephrine, as explained above for foods. Tyramine is not involved with the medication-induced reactions. The major dangers are with the cold medications, many of which are sold over the counter. There are a few safe cold tablets that are pure antihistamines, but most of them contain decongestants which can easily provoke a hypertensive episode. A good general rule is to have the patient call the psychiatrist about any new medication.

A hypertensive headache is described by most patients as a severe, pounding headache, very unlike a typical tension headache and somewhat reminiscent of a severe migraine. It typically starts explosively, usually within minutes to an hour of ingesting the offending substance. Associated symptoms of a hypertensive reaction may be nausea, visual

Table 9–10
MAO Inhibitors—Medications to Avoid

Medications with Stimulant Properties Causing Hypertensive Reactions

Virtually all cold, cough, or sinus medications (except pure antihistamines such as
Benadryl, Chlortrimeton, or Seldane)

Weight reducing or pep pills

Asthma inhalants (except for steroid sprays or Intal)

Epinephrine in local anesthesia, such as is used in dental work (the local anesthesia itself is safe)

Cocaine

Amphetamines, speed

Other antidepressants (except in special circumstances)

Medications Causing Serotonin (Hyperpyrexic) Syndromes

Antidepressants with strong serotonergic effects—clomipramine (Anafranil), fluoxetine (Prozac), sertraline (Zoloft), paroxetine (Paxil), fluvoxamine (Luvox), venlafaxine (Effexor), nefazodone (Serzone)

Some opiates—Meperidine (Demerol), dextromethorphan (found in many cold and
cough preparations, usually labeled as DM)

Note: For the serotonergic antidepressants listed, two weeks must elapse between their discontinuation and the
prescription of an MAO inhibitor, except for venlafaxine and nefazodone where the washout is one week, and
fluoxetine which requires a five-week washout. All antibiotics are safe, as are aspirin, plain Tylenol, Advil, or
Motrin.

Patients should check with their psychiatrists before taking any other medicines. They must also tell their doctors or dentists that they are taking an MAO inhibitor.

After stopping the MAO inhibitors, two weeks must elapse before the ingestion of any of the medications
listed.

disturbances, sweating, and anxiety. Any blood pressure rise that is of
medical concern is associated with a severe headache. Small rises of
blood pressure may occur without any symptoms. These are not of concern since they are not dangerous.

Psychiatrists vary in the instructions they give patients to follow in
the event of a sudden headache while taking an MAO inhibitor. My
recommendations are to go to an emergency room where the patient's
blood pressure can be measured. If it is high, a number of medications
can be given that will lower the blood pressure promptly. Other psychopharmacologists give patients a small dose of a medication, nifedip-
ine (Procardia) that will lower blood pressure so that they can treat
their hypertension themselves. Except in situations in which patients
are likely to be far away from any help (e.g., backpacking or traveling in

exotic places), I am wary of this approach since not all headaches are hypertensive, and I would rather have patients evaluated and treated under carefully monitored conditions. Certainly, if a patient calls you in a situation in which a hypertensive headache seems likely, have him go to the nearest emergency room.

All currently available MAO inhibitors are capable of causing hypertensive episodes, although tranylcypromine may be somewhat more likely to do so than the other two. It is difficult to accurately state the risk of hypertensive episodes from MAO inhibitors. As noted above, two studies have estimated the probability of having a hypertensive episode that resulted in the patient going to the emergency room as 1 to 3 percent. Assuredly, the risk of actual harmful events, such as a stroke, is far less, and in the range of one per many thousands. Nonetheless, the food and medication list must be taken seriously or the MAO inhibitor should be stopped.

A serotonin syndrome (see p. 299) may be seen when an MAO inhibitor is combined with either of two types of medications: antidepressants with strong serotonergic effects, or either of two opiates—meperidine (Demerol) or dextromethorphan (found in many cold/cough medicines and usually labeled as DM). (See Table 9–10 for a list of the strongly serotonergic antidepressants.) MAO inhibitors and serotonergic antidepressants should *never* be combined. The washout time for a serotonergic antidepressant before an MAO inhibitor can be safely prescribed varies depending on the medication's half-life from one week for venlafaxine (Effexor) to five weeks for fluoxetine (Prozac). As noted above, if a serotonergic antidepressant and an MAO inhibitor are taken together or without sufficient washout time between them, the potential reaction—a serotonin syndrome—constitutes a medical emergency (Sternbach, 1991). Similar reactions may be seen with the combination of the MAO inhibitor and the two opiates listed in Table 9–10.

One of the most important messages about the MAO diet that is often accidentally omitted concerns methods of stopping the medication. In general, patients must stay on the diet and avoid potentially dangerous interacting medications for fourteen days after stopping an MAO inhibitor. (If a switch is made from one MAO inhibitor to another, fourteen days between the two medications is also required). It takes that long for the cells to resynthesize MAO in sufficient quantity to make a hypertensive episode unlikely after a pizza with anchovies and sausage, washed down by a Chianti.

Other Side Effects

Beyond the hypertensive risks, the MAO inhibitors can cause a host of side effects, listed in Table 9–11. The previous discussion about how to present side effects with cyclic ADs, distinguishing between minor and major side effects, applies equally to the MAO inhibitors.

Paradoxically, for a class of medications for which the major danger is a hypertensive reaction, the most common side effect is postural hypotension. Only when certain foods or medications are ingested does hypertension typically occur; otherwise, the MAO inhibitors are decidedly hypotensive. The hypotension is clinically manifested by the same complaints as described when it is caused by a tricyclic—a feeling of dizziness, especially upon standing up quickly or getting out of bed. It can occur with any of the MAO inhibitors, although tranylcypromine may cause it less frequently, presumably due to its stimulant-like effects. Clinically, the hypotensive effects with the MAO inhibitors are more troublesome than with most tricyclics. The treatments for postural hypotension are the same as when it is caused by the cyclic ADs—switching medications, increasing salt ingestion, and taking various medications that increase blood pressure.

Weight gain can be a woeful problem with phenelzine, less so with selegiline, and rarely with tranylcypromine. Presumably, the amphetamine-like properties of tranylcypromine help curb any appetite increase that might be seen. My own clinical experience is that the MAO inhibitor-induced weight gain more commonly reflects increased sweet craving and actual increases in caloric ingestion than with the tricyclics for which a variety of weight-gaining mechanisms may be operating. As

Table 9–11
Common Side Effects of MAO Inhibitors

Postural hypotension
Weight gain (less with tranylcypromine)
Sexual dysfunction—anorgasmia, erectile dysfunction, retarded ejaculation
Insomnia
Energy slumps
Stimulation (especially with tranylcypromine)—nervousness, irritability, tremor, sweating, tachycardia, palpitations
Edema (swelling)
Muscle twitching

with the cyclic ADs, the only real treatments are prevention, diet, and exercise.

Sexual side effects are relatively common with MAO inhibitors. Difficulty in sexual arousal, difficulty with erections, and/or anorgasmia have all been reported. Retarded ejaculation is also seen, a side effect that when mild is enjoyed by some. Sexual side effects are likely to be dose-related; one hopes that the threshold for the side effect is not at the same dose as the threshold for therapeutic effects. The sexual difficulties may also diminish over time. As with the SSRIs, some "antidotes" exist, although, in my experience, they are not effective often enough.

Although many systematic studies do not mention it as a significant problem, insomnia and "energy slumps" are among the most disturbing and refractory of MAO inhibitor side effects. These seem to be separable from insomnia from overstimulation. Typically, patients describe being able to initiate sleep, but awaken during the night "wide awake." They can usually distinguish this from depressive insomnia—they don't feel anxious, just very awake. Simultaneously, they will describe a period of profound exhaustion in the late afternoon that lasts up to two hours and then remits either spontaneously or after a brief nap. Varying the time of taking the medications is generally not helpful, although it should be tried. The MAO inhibitor-induced insomnia is notably resistant to treatment. Typical remedies include benzodiazepine hypnotics, or trazodone.

A variety of stimulation side effects can be seen with MAO inhibitors, especially tranylcypromine. The most obvious of these is that of feeling "buzzed," as if one had taken amphetamines or drank too much coffee. A second stimulation effect is a mild hand tremor which can be socially embarrassing. An early cue to this is a subtle change in handwriting. Switching to taking the medication in the morning can be helpful with some of these side effects (such as the overstimulation), as can lowering the dose. Changing to a different MAO inhibitor should also be considered. Beta-blockers must be used with caution, but can decrease the tremor effectively.

Edema (swelling) is sometimes seen with MAO inhibitors. Diuretics can be helpful in diminishing it. The edema is usually not severe enough to warrant discontinuing treatment.

Finally, as with the older tricyclic antidepressants, MAO inhibitors are potentially lethal when taken in overdose.

10

Lithium and Other Mood Stabilizers

SINCE BIPOLAR DISORDER is characterized by recurrent episodes of
mania and depression, there has long been an emphasis on finding
medications that would treat and/or prevent both states. These medications are generally thought of as mood stabilizers, although they have
both discrete antimanic and antidepressant qualities as well as overall
mood stabilizing properties. Lithium is the oldest, most well known and
well studied of these mood stabilizers. Following the initial glow of
lithium's success, however, psychiatry became increasingly aware of the
substantial number of patients who either did not respond or could not
tolerate lithium. Over the last fifteen years, therefore, a number of other
medications have been studied that have true lithium-like mood stabilizing qualities. At present, then, psychopharmacologists have a number of options for prescribing in order to diminish abnormal mood
swings.

HISTORY

The first report of lithium's efficacy in treating acute mania was published in 1949, years before the discovery of the antidepressants or of
the first antipsychotic. Yet lithium's widespread acceptance and use did
not occur until years after these other agents were firmly ensconced as
part of modern psychopharmacology. The primary reason for the delay
was rooted in the disastrous results that occurred when lithium was
used as a salt substitute for hypertensive patients in the 1940s and
1950s. At that time, it was hoped that by using lithium chloride instead
of sodium chloride (table salt) in flavoring food, hypertensive patients
would be able to cut down on salt intake, thereby lowering their blood
pressure. Unfortunately, virtually nothing was known at that time of
lithium toxicity or of the dangers of unrestricted lithium ingestion without monitoring. Not surprisingly, this uncontrolled use of lithium in
soups, meats, french fries, and the like resulted in serious lithium toxicity and, tragically, some deaths. After this experience, the medical com-

munity was wary of using lithium in any dose for any reason. The United States was notably behind Central Europe and Scandinavia in recognizing lithium's efficacy. Indeed, in 1961, twelve years after the initial report of lithium's efficacy and more than five years after two other studies done in Europe documented lithium's positive effect in mania, an editorial in the *Journal of the American Medical Association* declared that there were no accepted medical uses for lithium in medicine (Wingard, 1961). A second reason for lithium's delayed acceptance was that the initial study in 1949, written by John Cade, was published in the *Medical Journal of Australia,* a journal that was not well circulated in Western Europe or the United States. Furthermore, Cade's original rationale for using lithium in mania was filled with incorrect assumptions. Despite this, however, he demonstrated that lithium did control manic symptoms (Cade, 1949). Cade's ultimate discovery of lithium's effect can be best ascribed to serendipity with a large dose of careful observation. With the past negative experiences of lithium still fresh in physicians' minds, Cade's observations and those of Schou after him were viewed with great skepticism. A final reason for the delay in lithium's acceptance by the medical community was the lack of interest on the part of pharmaceutical firms to investigate and promote lithium. Since lithium is a natural product (see below), it is unpatentable. It was, therefore, not profitable for drug companies to spend money investigating a compound that any other firm could then produce without the research costs.

Despite the delay in accepting the efficacy of lithium in treating acute mania and in the prophylaxis of mania, ongoing research continued to document the extent of lithium's effect in bipolar and unipolar mood disorders. By the mid 1970s, lithium was regarded as somewhat of a wonder drug in psychiatry with acute and prophylactic effects, able to dramatically ameliorate or abolish the symptoms of a most severe disorder with only minimal side effects. Initial skepticism had evolved into the honeymoon period. The bubble burst in 1977 when the first report of lithium's potential destructive effect on the kidney was published (Hestbech, Hansen, Amdisen, and Olsen, 1977). Moreover, within the last five years, evidence derived from naturalistic studies (in which patients are treated in uncontrolled ways, mimicking usual treatment in the community) has suggested that lithium is effective as a single-agent mood stabilizer for a far smaller group of bipolar patients than was previously thought (Sachs, Lafer, Truman, Noeth, and Thibault, 1994). Now, lithium's considerable therapeutic effects, its limitations, and side effects are perceived more clearly. On balance, lithium should be considered a very effective treatment for patients with mood disorders, lifesaving for some, the benefits of which outweigh the risks in most—but not all—cases.

The other two major mood stabilizers, valproate (Depakote) and carbamazepine (Tegretol) similarly took long and circuitous routes before their establishment as viable treatments for mood disorders. Both of these medications were originally marketed in the United States as anticonvulsants with carbamazepine released in 1968 and valproate in 1978. Yet, their histories as mood stabilizers followed somewhat different paths. For instance, valproate's efficacy in treating bipolar disorder was first described in 1966. Still, it was not until the mid 1980s that there was consistent exploration of valproate's mood stabilizing effects and the best research emerged only in the 1990s and is ongoing. Carbamazepine has been prescribed most commonly for the treatment of seizures arising in the temporal lobes and limbic structures, the areas of the brain that are central in the regulation of mood, and for paroxysmal disorders such as trigeminal neuralgia, a disorder of the facial nerve characterized by excruciating episodes of facial pain. It too was first noted to have mood stabilizing properties by investigators in the 1960s who observed that the medication not only controlled seizures, but decreased the affective instability often seen in patients with temporal lobe seizures. Because of these observations, carbamazepine was then prescribed to patients with mood disorders in the late 1970s and 1980s with clear efficacy. Unfortunately, because of the expiration of the patent for Tegretol, the brand name for carbamazepine, research on its efficacy for mood disorders has diminished precipitously over the last few years.

LITHIUM

Clinical Uses

The appropriate uses for lithium, listed in Table 10–1, are predominantly in the treatment of mood disorders. Some other, less established indications do exist and will be discussed below.

Lithium is prescribed for a variety of clinical reasons in treating mood disorders. The two most common and well-documented uses are for the treatment of acute mania and in the maintenance (preventive) treatment of bipolar disorder. Its effect in treating acute mania and/or hypomania has been documented for over thirty years and is, at this point, an observation beyond question (Jefferson, Greist, Ackerman,

Table 10-1
Disorders for Which Lithium Is Useful

Disorder	Efficacy Rating
Acute mania, hypomania	+++
Bipolar disorder—maintenance	+++
Bipolar II disorder—maintenance	++
Cyclothymia—maintenance	++
Mixed states	++
Acute depression—bipolar	++
—unipolar	+
Unipolar depression—maintenance	++
Adjunct to antidepressants in treatment-resistant depression	++
Schizoaffective disorder	++
Schizophrenia	+
Aggressive outbursts	+

+++ = Definite efficacy
 ++ = Probable efficacy
  + = Possible efficacy

and Carroll, 1987). Because it takes at least seven to ten days for its an-timanic effect to be significant and because acute mania frequently re-quires a quicker behavioral effect, lithium is often combined with a neuroleptic or a benzodiazepine initially (see chapter 3). Nonetheless, if prescribed alone, lithium would show the desired effect, although slightly delayed. Most patients describe the effect of lithium as normal-izing a manic mood state as opposed to being tranquilized.

Lithium's other well-documented effect is as a maintenance treat-ment in bipolar disorder. As with acute mania, this clinical effect is firmly established (Goodwin and Jamison, 1990). Preventive treatment with lithium is equally effective against both manias and depressions. Nonetheless, many patients complain that lithium more effectively pre-vents manias than depressions. Whether this means that residual mild depressions are not prevented by lithium or that mild depressions are more remembered (and disliked) than mild hypomanias is unknown. It is also important to remember that a positive effect only *sometimes* means a complete eradication of episodes. In many patients, a positive effect means a diminution of frequency, intensity, or length of episodes that still occur. Thus, partial effects with lithium are common. Lithium may also decrease the milder mood swings commonly seen in bipolar patients (Keller et al., 1992). Although these mood swings are not severe or long enough to be described as manic, hypomanic, or depressive episodes, they are common, add substantially to the overall morbidity of bipolar disorder, and are predictive of full-blown relapses. The full preventive therapeutic effect from lithium may not occur until six to twelve months after beginning treatment (Schou, 1986).

Lithium's prophylactic effect in Bipolar II disorder (bipolar disorder NOS in DSM-III-R) is much less well studied. At present, however, it should still be considered the best treatment available (Kane et al., 1982).

Cyclothymia is the third of the bipolar subtypes for which lithium is frequently prescribed. Although no controlled studies exist, a wealth of anecdotal material suggests the positive effect of lithium in diminishing the rapid and short-lived mood swings of cyclothymia (Akiskal, Djenderedjan, Rosenthal, and Khani, 1977).

Mixed states (those with simultaneous features of both mania and depression) may also respond to lithium, although less well than classic mania (Secunda et al., 1985). The appropriate treatment of mixed states has not been studied systematically.

In treating acute depression, lithium is effective for both bipolar and unipolar depression, though the evidence is more consistent for the former (Souza and Goodwin, 1991). Because of the risks of precipitating a manic episode if an antidepressant alone (i.e., without a mood stabilizer) is prescribed for a bipolar patient, lithium is often prescribed first for bipolar depression with an antidepressant prescribed later if needed. For unipolar depressed patients, although lithium is effective for some, it is rarely prescribed as a first- or even second-line agent, since unipolar patients do not share the same risk of an antidepressant-precipitated manic episode.

In contrast to its effect in treating acute unipolar depression, lithium is clearly effective in preventing unipolar depressions (Prien and Kocsis, 1995). Since most patients are not treated with lithium during their acute depressions, compared to antidepressants lithium is not as commonly used prophylactically with these patients.

Another use of lithium in mood disorders is as an adjunctive treatment to antidepressants in treatment-resistant unipolar depression (Joffe, Singer, Levitt, and MacDonald, 1993). When used in this manner, lithium is added after the antidepressant has been prescribed without success for a number of weeks. Lithium blood levels seem to be irrelevant when it is used adjunctively, and positive responses are seen equally with levels ranging from 0.3 to 1.0 mEq/l.

Schizoaffective disorder is also treated with lithium. Given the murkiness of this diagnosis and its shifting definitions, convincing and consistent evidence characterizing lithium's efficacy for schizoaffective disorder is unavailable. Nonetheless, most clinicians and researchers assume both that lithium is effective in treating a substantial proportion of schizoaffective patients and that the presence of more prominent affective than schizophrenic features predicts a good response (Maj, 1988). In addition, there is evidence, although not convincing, that some patients with excited schizoaffective disorders will show a better response to lithium plus an antipsychotic than to an antipsychotic alone (Biederman et al., 1979).

Lithium is occasionally prescribed in the treatment of pure schizophrenia (without schizoaffective features) (Delva and Letemendia, 1982). It is unusual, however, for lithium to be effective in schizophrenia when used alone (as opposed to a combination treatment with antipsychotics). In general, lithium is reserved for use with schizophrenic patients who are refractory to treatment with neuroleptics. The presence of affective features is not required for lithium's efficacy in treating schizophrenia.

Lithium may also be used with some success in decreasing aggressive outbursts from a variety of causes in individuals, ranging from the mentally retarded to prisoners who are neither mentally retarded nor bipolar. Clinically, it is prescribed more for spontaneous outbursts in response to minor provocations, than for premeditated violence (Schou, 1986).

Given their inherent mood instability, patients with borderline personality disorder are often considered for lithium treatment. However, both anecdotally and in a few studies, evidence for lithium's efficacy in this population is slim at best (Gitlin, 1995a).

A number of other disorders have been explored as potentially lithium-responsive, including alcohol abuse and premenstrual syndrome (premenstrual dysphoric disorder in DSM-IV) with negative results. Initially, it was thought that lithium might be effective in treating alcoholics. As an example, lithium has been shown to decrease alcohol-induced confusion and the desire to drink without altering the alcohol-induced high (Judd and Huey, 1986). In contrast, the results of a number of well-designed studies over the last decade have demonstrated that in treating alcoholics with or without depression, lithium is ineffective for either the depressive symptoms or in altering the course of the alcohol abuse (Lejoyeux and Ades, 1993). Of course, those patients with bipolar disorder and alcohol abuse should be treated for both disorders (which would include lithium or another mood stabilizing agent) but without the hope that lithium by itself would treat the alcoholism.

Lithium is often mentioned as a treatment for premenstrual syndrome (PMS) despite substantial evidence that it is ineffective (Altschuler, Hendrick, and Parry, 1995). Lithium may be of some benefit to those women who show a more pervasive mood disorder throughout the menstrual cycle with premenstrual exacerbation (Steiner, Haskett, and Osmun, 1980).

Biologic Effects

Unlike all other medications used in psychiatry, lithium is a naturally occurring compound, discovered in 1817 and found in rocks, water, plants, and animals. Most of the lithium used for medicinal reasons in the United States is mined in North Carolina. (The word is derived from the Greek word *lithos,* which means stone.) Lithium is commercially available in a variety of preparations, such as lithium carbonate or lithium chloride, commonly referred to as lithium salts. (This use of the term "salt" should not be confused with table salt, which is the colloquial term for the compound sodium chloride.) The specific lithium salt prescribed is irrelevant   it is the lithium ion that is effective. Currently, virtually all lithium prescribed in the United States is lithium carbonate, but lithium citrate is just as effective.

Nowadays, the idea of a medication being "natural" is assumed to be a good thing. It simply is not so. Lithium is natural, but, as we will see, is as toxic or more toxic than most other medications in psychiatry with clear negative effects on the thyroid and kidney that are not shared by the synthesized medicines.

Lithium's mechanism of action in treating mood disorders, either acutely or preventively, is unknown. Lithium has well-documented capacities to alter the function of some neurotransmitters, especially serotonin. Yet these effects cannot easily explain lithium's effect in treating mania or its capacity to prevent both manias and depressions. Of more interest, lithium has also been shown to modulate a number of intracellular processes that translate the effects of all neurotransmitters into cellular activity (Manji, Potter, and Lenox, 1995). These include affecting two second-messenger systems (adenylate cyclase and phosphoinositol) and G proteins which link receptor effects to the second messengers (see chapter 2). By inhibiting intracellular processes, lithium alters the activities of many neurotransmitter systems, consistent with its diverse clinical effects.

Techniques for Prescribing

All preparations of lithium are equally effective for any and all uses of the medication. The only important differences among the preparations are whether they are capsule or tablet, liquid or pill, slow release or regular release, and 150 mg, 300 mg, or 450 mg pills. The standard, most commonly used preparations are the 300 mg capsules, marketed by a variety of pharmaceutical firms. There is no difference among these preparations, although patients can be frightened if the pharmacist gives them yellow and gray capsules when their last bottle contained pink capsules. The liquid form of lithium is rarely used except for those who have significant problems swallowing pills or with manic inpatients who may be surreptitiously "cheeking" their lithium pills. The slow-release forms of lithium are indeed absorbed more gradually than regular lithium carbonate; however, it is not clear whether this is at all advantageous to patients. Initial side effects such as nausea may be slightly less if slow-release tablets are prescribed, especially in the beginning of treatment. Within a few weeks, though, the nausea usually disappears, leaving increased cost as the major difference between slow-release and generic lithium carbonate. Moreover, slow-release lithium preparations may increase the incidence of diarrhea (Jefferson, Greist, Ackerman, and Carroll, 1987).

Before starting lithium (or, at the latest, within the first week of treatment), it is mandatory to obtain measures of thyroid and kidney function since these organs are sometimes adversely affected by the drug (see below). Most psychopharmacologists obtain a panel of blood tests (including a test for kidney function—called creatinine) that measure a number of bodily functions and chemistries, and a thyroid test. Sometimes, especially with older patients, an electrocardiogram is ordered, although this is not mandatory with younger patients.

More than any other medication in psychiatry, lithium is regulated by blood levels, so much so that in communicating about lithium, doses are not relevant. Lithium is measured as a concentration in the blood (or serum, which, similarly to plasma, refers to the liquid part of blood) in units of milliequivalents per liter, or mEq/l. Lithium levels have achieved this importance for three reasons. First, because there is only a small difference between therapeutic and toxic lithium levels, there is a need for careful dosage regulation. Blood levels allow more "fine tuning" for dose adjustment than does following the daily dose. Second, the appropriate blood level range within which maximum response to lithium will be seen has been well established (in contrast to our ignorance about the appropriate blood levels for most antidepressants or other mood stabilizers). Third, also in contrast to blood levels of most other medications, lithium levels are both inexpensive and easy to do. Therefore, patients can afford them and the results from most laboratories can be trusted.

The proper way to measure a lithium level is to draw the blood approximately twelve hours (between ten and fourteen hours is acceptable) after the last lithium dose. Since lithium levels are typically drawn in the morning before the first medication dose, patients often accidentally take their morning pill(s) and then get their lithium level drawn. Since a lithium level of 0.6 mEq/l taken twelve hours after the last dose will be 1.3 or more two hours after the dose, the accidental ingestion of the morning pills will dramatically change the blood test result and render it meaningless.

Food does not interfere with lithium levels; therefore, patients can eat within the twelve hours. They do need to have taken their lithium without missing doses for four days prior to the blood test for accurate results. After initiating therapy, or following a dosage change, five to seven days should elapse before testing the new level. (In the elderly, waiting seven to ten days is needed, since they take longer to achieve a "steady state"   a constant level after a dosage change.)

Optimal lithium levels vary across individuals. In general, levels needed for an acute antimanic response are higher than those needed for a prophylactic response. Additionally, geriatric patients both need lower lithium levels and tolerate higher levels less well. Lithium levels generally required to effectively treat acute mania are between 0.7 and 1.2 mEq/l, while 0.6 to 0.8 mEq/l is the usual targeted range for preventive maintenance treatment. Some patients, though, may show a response at levels of 0.4 mEq/l but exhibit intolerable side effects at 0.7. Conversely, some individuals, albeit rare, may need levels of 1.3 or above to achieve a therapeutic response and may tolerate that level easily. As always, careful observation and common sense will ensure the most appropriate treatment.

Consistent with these suggestions, the single best study examining the relationship between lithium levels and efficacy in maintenance treatment compared the effects of levels of 0.4 to 0.6 to levels of 0.8 to 1.0 mEq/l (Gelenberg et al., 1989). (Unfortunately, the usually targeted range of 0.6 to 0.8 mEq/l was not evaluated in this study.) Patients in the high lithium level group had significantly fewer relapses but more side effects, more noncompliance, and were more likely to drop out of the study. Thus, patients who are doing well at a level of 0.5 mEq/l should not have their dosage increased, just as those with profound side effects at 0.7 must have their dose decreased.

There is no right way to start lithium. In general, inpatients, acutely manic patients, or younger patients are started at higher doses than are those who are either hypomanic, depressed, older, or need prophylactic treatment. The more urgent patients can be started at doses of three to four tablets daily (300 mg each) in at least two and preferably three divided doses, with lithium levels measured every two to three days until the desired blood level and clinical effect are achieved. In less urgent situations, starting at two tablets daily and waiting five days before the first level is drawn is reasonable. In this situation, adjustment to the correct blood level may take a number of weeks. Quicker and more aggressive methods of dose adjustment may make an early response more likely but also increase the risk of side effects which are not only unpleasant but may affect future compliance. When initially prescribed, lithium is taken after meals to decrease potential nausea. This nausea almost always disappears within weeks.

After doses are adjusted to the desired level and clinical effect, most psychopharmacologists will try to simplify the medication regimen as much as possible. For virtually all patients, this means taking the entire daily dose in no more than one or two divided doses. Moreover, there is some evidence that some of lithium's negative effects on the kidney may be lessened by taking a single daily dose (Plenge and Mellerup, 1986). Therefore, the only reasons to take lithium more than twice daily are if side effects are significantly less when the dose is taken three or four times daily or if the patient is more comfortable with more frequent doses and doesn't forget to take the medication.

Once the lithium level is established and is steady—that is, two consecutive blood levels do not vary by more than 10 to 15 percent at the same dose—levels may be checked far less frequently. Checking lithium levels every three to four months in a clinically stable outpatient is sufficient. There are a number of clinical situations, listed in Table 10–2, in which levels must be checked more frequently. In virtually all of these situations, changes in lithium levels occur in conjunction with alterations in kidney function, hydration, and/or salt intake. Unlike any other medication in psychiatry, lithium is not metabolized. (Lithium is therefore not dangerous in patients with liver disease.) Rather, it is filtered by the kidneys and excreted unchanged in the urine. Any situation in which kidney function or salt and/or water balance (which alters the way the kidney handles lithium) is changed will result in an increase or decrease in lithium levels. The most interesting of these is the way the

Table 10–2
Situations in Which Lithium Levels Should Generally Be Checked

After a change in dose (5–7 days later for younger patients, 8–10 days later in the
  elderly)
During major changes in weight (e.g., diet)
During treatment with diuretics
During a change in mood (both to check compliance and because lithium levels
  decrease in mania and increase in depression)
During physical illness, including the flu. Occasionally, lithium is stopped until the
  illness remits
If lithium toxicity is suspected

kidneys excrete lithium during mood changes. It is clear that even with complete compliance, lithium excretion increases (with a decreased lithium level) in mania and decreases (causing an increased level) in depression (Kukopulos, Minnai, and Muller-Oerlinghausen, 1985). The exact mechanism for this change is not known.

Other than the occasional lithium levels, the two other blood tests taken routinely during maintenance lithium treatment are thyroid and kidney tests since these two organs are the ones that are potentially adversely affected by long-term lithium treatment (see below). These simple blood tests are drawn less frequently, typically every six to twelve months. If subtle abnormalities are found, the frequency of the blood tests is increased.

Side Effects

Lithium can cause a great number of side effects. Because patients may be on lithium for many years to a lifetime, there is an understandable concern about both the distressing and potentially dangerous aspects of these side effects. Yet at the same time, a common side effect is not necessarily distressing, and a distressing side effect is not always dangerous. As an example, Table 10–3 shows the most common and most distressing side effects seen with lithium in one study (Gitlin, Cochran, and Jamison, 1989). Whereas thirst and increased urination are the most common side effects, cognitive effects and weight gain are the most distressing. And, as always, risks must be weighed against potential benefits. If lithium decreases the number of manic episodes by 70 percent, is that worth a mild tremor and increased urination? Is it worth

Table 10–3
Lithium Side Effects

Most Common	Most Distressing
1. Thirst	1. Weight gain
2. Excessive urination	2. Cognitive effects
3. Weight gain	3. Excessive urination
4. Fatigue	4. Nausea
5. Dry mouth	5. Fatigue

Adapted from Gitlin et al., *Journal of Clinical Psychiatry, 50* (1989), 127–131. Copyright 1989 Physicians Post-graduate Press. Reproduced with permission.

a significant tremor and weight gain? The balance must be decided separately for each individual.

The most common side effects with lithium are increased urination (polyuria) and increased thirst (Vestegaard, 1983). (An associated side effect, dry mouth, is also commonly seen.) Almost always, these two side effects coexist, since the polyuria causes mild dehydration which then causes the thirst. These symptoms are due to lithium's effect on promoting the excretion of a more dilute urine in a manner similar to alcohol. The polyuria may be progressive; that is, the longer someone has been on lithium, the more likely and greater the problem. As long as the patient's thirst mechanism is intact (which it virtually always is) and the patient has access to fluids, these symptoms are not dangerous. And most importantly, the presence of polyuria is unrelated to the possibility of dangerous kidney damage (Schou, 1988). If the increased urination is profound, the careful use of certain diuretics can be helpful in decreasing the urine volume.

Tremor is another common side effect (although it was seen infrequently in the study from which Table 10–3 was taken). It is typically increased with effort of some sort, such as stretching out the arms, holding a coffee cup, or writing. Occasionally, the tremor is first noticed by a change in handwriting. It is worsened by any of the factors that worsen tremors, such as caffeine ingestion or anxiety. If the tremor is particularly distressing, propranolol, a beta-blocker, can be extremely effective in diminishing or abolishing it.

Although not as common as polyuria, weight gain is a potentially significant side effect, in large part because of how distressing it is to many patients and how difficult it can be to lose the weight. Weight gain can be substantial. One study found that 20 percent of lithium-treated patients gained more than 10 kilograms (22 lbs) (Vestergaard, Amdisen, and Schou, 1980). The cause of the weight gain is unknown, although a number of factors may all contribute. One of the most preventable and treatable causes of the weight gain is the ingestion of high-calorie drinks in response to lithium-induced thirst. Drinking noncaloric drinks would clearly help. A second possible cause is hypothyroidism, seen in a small percentage of lithium-treated patients. Accurate diagnosis is possible via a simple blood test, and appropriate treatment (with thyroid hormone) can then be instituted. Third, lithium sometimes causes edema, a retention of salt and water which can be treated with diuretics, if needed. Finally, however, it does seem that lithium has some unexplained direct effect on fat and/or carbohydrate metabolism such that patients can gain weight even in the absence of increased caloric intake. Treatment for the weight gain includes prevention, education about diet, exercise, treating associated medical side effects (such as hypothyroidism), and combating discouragement when the weight loss is slower than expected.

The most underappreciated side effects from lithium are those related to altered cognition. Patients frequently complain of a variety of thinking changes that they attribute to the medication, such as poor concentration, impaired memory, or a sense of dullness in their thinking. Among the many studies that have examined this topic, most, but not all, do not find demonstrable cognitive changes from lithium. Since these same cognitive changes can be symptoms of mild depression or may express the loss of heightened hypomanic creativity, many psychopharmacologists and researchers are skeptical that lithium causes cognitive problems. My own experience with patients, however, convinces me that these effects are real and that the tests of cognition used in these studies are, in general, too insensitive to delineate the cognitive changes.

An associated complaint about lithium is that creativity is diminished. Clearly, this is a very important issue given that a disproportionate number of artists are bipolar. The most interesting study on this topic demonstrated that the number of associations to target words as well as the number of "idiosyncratic associations" as a measure of creativity were diminished by lithium (Shaw, Mann, Stokes, and Manevitz, 1986). For most bipolar artists, though, the generally increased productivity on lithium (since the artist no longer spends significant periods of time hospitalized or psychotic or profoundly depressed) makes up for the potential loss of short-term creative bursts.

Since lithium's effects on both general cognition and creativity are probably correlated with the lithium level, a useful strategy for patients who complain of these side effects is to lower the lithium dose. If the cognitive problem continues on the lower dose, or if breakthrough episodes begin to occur, switching to another mood stabilizer may be necessary.

Subtle coordination problems may also be caused by lithium. The complaints usually relate to mild clumsiness or dropping things.

The last two commonly reported side effects from lithium are edema (swelling) and diarrhea. If severe, the edema can be treated with diuretics. It is unusual that the diarrhea is severe enough to warrant either adding an antidote or switching to another medication.

Lithium's Effects on Thyroid and Kidneys

The two organ systems that are adversely affected by lithium are the thyroid gland and kidneys. Because this statement is sometimes incorrectly translated as "lithium causes kidney failure," or "lithium is an extremely dangerous drug," the topic is worth reviewing.

Lithium decreases both the synthesis and release of thyroid hormone in the thyroid gland. Subtle evidence of these changes can be found in a substantial proportion of lithium-treated patients. In the majority of these patients, such changes do not cause any symptoms. However, between 5 and 35 percent of patients may show evidence of hypothyroidism, from abnormal blood tests to symptoms such as fatigue, apathy, sluggishness, weight gain, hypersomnia, dry skin, and coarse dry hair (Goodwin and Jamison, 1990). Since most of these symptoms are the same as those seen in depression, distinguishing between the two can be very difficult in the absence of thyroid blood tests. Women are at higher risk for lithium-induced hypothyroidism, just as they are for hypothyroidism from any cause. Luckily, a low thyroid state is among the easiest conditions in medicine to treat. A once-daily dose of thyroid hormone can easily supply the necessary thyroid hormone. Thus, although lithium does indeed cause thyroid dysfunction, a knowledgeable psychopharmacologist will be able to diagnose it if it occurs and treat it with ease. Typically, thyroid blood tests are obtained every six months to one year. This often allows the psychiatrist to discover an abnormality on the tests before the patient has any symptoms of hypothyroidism.

Lithium's effect on the kidney is more complicated. A brief digression on kidney function will help. The kidney has two major functions— filtering toxins, which takes place in the glomeruli, and regulating salt and water balance, which occurs in the tubules. When people are in renal failure, a condition that necessitates either dialysis (an artificial kidney machine) or a kidney transplant, it is because the filtering mechanism is lost. The tubular system can sustain significant damage, but as long as the brain is correctly regulating salt and water craving (thirst), and there is free access to salt and water, no significant problems should arise. Lithium has well-documented negative effects on the tubular system, as exemplified by the commonly observed increased urination in lithium-treated patients. For the vast majority of patients, though, lithium does *not* cause progressive destruction of the glomeruli with loss of filtering function. However, there may be a very small group of patients who seem to sustain substantial renal damage from lithium (Gitlin, 1993a). Because of this, psychopharmacologists measure the serum creatinine, a measure of the kidneys' filtering capacity, every six months to one year, with the frequency of the test increased if the creatinine begins to rise. If the creatinine rises to between 1.6 and 2.0 mg/dl, consultation with a renal specialist is indicated.

Lithium Toxicity

Because the difference between therapeutic and toxic doses of lithium is relatively small, it is important for anyone who treats patients on lithium to be aware of the signs of lithium toxicity. These are listed in Table 10–4. The earliest signs are usually a worsening tremor (often described as progressing from a fine to a coarse tremor), significant diarrhea, nausea, and ataxia (poor balance). If the toxicity is recognized at this stage, the lithium dose can be lowered and significant damage is rare. If the toxicity continues to the point of mental confusion or de-

Table 10–4
Signs of Lithium Toxicity

Mild	Moderate	Severe
Mild apathy, lethargy	Increased lethargy	Somnolence
Weakness	Confusion, drowsiness	Gross confusion
Unsteady balance	Gross ataxia	Profound loss of balance
Nausea	Vomiting	Urinary incontinence
Decreased concentration	Slurred speech	Random muscle twitching
Worsening hand tremor	Muscle twitching	Coma
Diarrhea		

creased consciousness (which can occur at levels of 1.8 or above), the possibility of significant neurological damage exists. Thus, early recognition is key. If a patient you are seeing shows any of these signs, tell him to not take any more lithium until he speaks to his psychiatrist, who should be called immediately.

The causes of lithium toxicity are all related to changes in hydration or salt balance, as noted in the section on lithium levels. Thus, a new diet (especially if it involves decreasing salt intake), fasting, fever, a virus that causes significant vomiting, and/or diarrhea are all potential causes. Interestingly, exercise may cause a *decrease* in lithium levels, despite the relative dehydration involved, because lithium is excreted in sweat at greater than serum levels (Jefferson et al., 1982). Certain medications, such as some antiinflammatory drugs (including ibuprofen, now sold over the counter), diuretics, and others, can cause lithium toxicity, as can a kidney infection, although this is relatively rare.

Lithium Discontinuation

Given the number of bipolar patients who do not respond adequately to lithium or cannot tolerate its side effects, the question of how best to discontinue lithium has become an important practical issue. It is now apparent that lithium discontinuation is associated with a marked increased risk of a mood episode, especially mania, within the first six months. This risk seems far greater than the simple reemergence of bipolar disorder in patients no longer on a mood stabilizer. As an example, in one recent study patients who, on average, cycled into a mood episode every 11.6 months before treatment experienced a new episode following lithium discontinuation after a mean of only 1.7 months, a dramatic difference (Suppes, Baldessarini, Faedda, and Tohen, 1991). Furthermore, patients whose lithium is discontinued rapidly (within two weeks) relapse at a far faster rate than do those who have had their lithium dose discontinued gradually (over two to four weeks) (Faedda, Tondo, Baldessarini, Suppes, and Tohen, 1993). A third troubling observation is that when lithium is discontinued because the patient has been doing well for an extended period of time (sometimes for many years), if the patient relapses and lithium is reinstituted, it is not always effective the second time (Post, Leverich, Altshuler, and Mikalauskas, 1992).

These findings indicate the need for caution when discontinuing lithium. Yet in none of these studies were patients switched directly to another mood stabilizer, which is the most common scenario when patients are taken off lithium. Because of this, it is still unclear whether the "rebound" episodes would occur or whether lithium needs to be discontinued slowly when another mood stabilizer has already been prescribed. Finally, it is unknown whether similar difficulties would arise when patients are taken off other mood stabilizers such as valproate or carbamazepine.

ANTICONVULSANT MOOD STABILIZERS

Aside from lithium, the two other medications with documented efficacy—both acutely and prophylactically—in the treatment of mood disorders are two anticonvulsants, carbamazepine (Tegretol) and valproate, also known as sodium valproate or divalproex (usually marketed as Depakote). Although these two medications are anticonvulsants, there is no evidence that mood disorders are unusual seizure disorders (such as grand mal seizures). As was noted earlier when discussing the various uses of antidepressants, it is common for different disorders to respond to the same treatment. Neither medication has been investigated in either research studies or clinical practice to the extent that lithium has, but the common occurrence of partial responses, nonresponses, and refusals of lithium treatment make the use of the anticonvulsants increasingly common in treating bipolar disorder. Furthermore, a number of particularly well-designed studies have convinced many (myself included) that either of these medications is an equivalent first choice to lithium in many clinical situations (especially the use of valproate in treating acute mania.)

Carbamazepine

Clinical Uses

Table 10–5 shows the disorders for which carbamazepine may be effective. Clinically, the evidence that is most convincing is carbamazepine's efficacy in treating acute mania and in the prophylactic treatment of bipolar disorder (Calabrese, Bowden, and Woyshville, 1995). In this way, its profile of efficacy is similar to lithium. When used for acute mania, positive effects are seen by the second week, with improvement continuing for at least the first three weeks of treatment. Carbamazepine is also clearly effective in the maintenance treatment of bipolar disorder, preventing both manias and depressions. Loss of prophylactic efficacy after a few years of successful treatment has been reported (Post, Leverich, Rosoff, and Altshuler, 1990). Whether this

Table 10–5
Disorders for Which the Anticonvulsant Mood Stabilizers Are Useful

Disorder	Carbamazepine	Valproate
Acute mania	+++	+++
Other bipolar mood disorders (e.g. Bipolar II, cyclothymia)	++	++
Alcohol withdrawal	++	?
Benzodiazepine withdrawal	+	?
Aggressive outbursts (including those associated with borderline personality)	+	?
Post-traumatic stress disorder	+	+
Panic disorder	0	+

+++ = Definite efficacy
++ = Probable efficacy
+ = Possible efficacy

differs from the other mood stabilizers is unknown. Proposed (but not well-validated) predictors of a good response to carbamazepine have been mixed states and rapid cycling.

Carbamazepine's efficacy in treating acute depression, both unipolar and bipolar, is far weaker and less well established than its effects in acute mania or as a maintenance treatment for bipolar disorder. At this point, it can be recommended as an acute antidepressant treatment for treatment-resistant patients only. Side effects of carbamazepine (discussed below) have limited its utility in depressed patients (Cullen et al., 1991). Carbamazepine's efficacy as a preventive treatment for recurrent major depression continues to be virtually unexplored except for small case series.

Carbamazepine is also used to diminish withdrawal symptoms associated with alcohol or benzodiazepine withdrawal. In treating alcohol withdrawal, although it is not commonly prescribed, carbamazepine effectively blocks withdrawal symptoms and diminishes the risk of seizure (Stuppaeck et al., 1992). A potential advantage for carbamazepine in this clinical situation is its lack of potential for dependence, in contrast to the benzodiazepines. Carbamazepine's utility in diminishing benzodiazepine withdrawal symptoms is less consistent, with side effects often precluding adequate treatment (Schweizer, Rickels, Case, and Greenblatt, 1991; Roy-Byrne, Sullivan, Cowley, and Ries, 1993). (See chapter 11.)

Carbamazepine may also be effective in the treatment of aggressive outbursts. Unfortunately, no controlled studies exist in this field, but anecdotal experiences are encouraging (Mattes, 1990). The positive effects of carbamazepine for treating aggressive outbursts do not depend on evidence of a seizure disorder or even EEG abnormalities. As with other medications used to treat behavioral outbursts, it is thought that the medication is most effective in the more "eruptive violence" that occurs impulsively as an exaggerated response to a provocation and is less effective or ineffective for violence that is premeditated.

Consistent with its effects on aggressive outbursts, carbamazepine has also been prescribed in the treatment of patients with borderline personality disorder with behavioral outbursts, such as physical violence or self-mutilation (e.g., wrist cuts, cigarette burns, or multiple overdoses) (Cowdry and Gardner, 1988). When administered in a double-blind manner, carbamazepine significantly decreased behavioral outbursts in an objective measurable way. Its effects on decreasing dysphoric mood were less consistent.

Anecdotal, uncontrolled evidence exists to support the use of carbamazepine in the treatment of post-traumatic stress disorder (PTSD) (Lipper et al., 1986). Because the symptoms of PTSD can be thought of as the reexperiencing of traumatic events and because carbamazepine may have a specific effect in decreasing responses to repeated triggered phenomena (see next section), this line of clinical investigation is likely to continue.

Biologic Effects

The most common hypothesis that has been used to explain carbamazepine's effect in treating mood disorders relates to its effects on decreasing kindling in the limbic area of the brain (Post, Uhde, Putnam, Ballenger, and Berrettini, 1982). Kindling can be thought of as the progressive increase in neural excitability with repeated stimulation. Experimentally, this would be demonstrated by needing less and less electrical stimulation to cause an overt behavioral effect (Post, Rubinow, and Ballenger, 1984). With repeated electrical stimulation, it is even possible to cause spontaneous electrical discharges in the absence of stimulation. Thus, a system that was initially barely responsive to a low-dose stimulus can ultimately spontaneously discharge.

Kindling is analogous to behavioral sensitization, a process in which repeated applications of unchanging doses of chemical substances result in increasing behavioral effects with subsequent doses. Both these processes—kindling and sensitization—can be thought of as the opposite of tolerance, in which it takes more and more of a stimulus to achieve the same response. Tolerance is common with many substances of abuse. After repeated use of barbiturates, for example, progressively higher doses are needed to achieve the same sedative effect that was initially achieved by a small dose.

Carbamazepine effectively inhibits the development of some types of kindling in the limbic area, a property that is probably linked to its anticonvulsant properties. The exact mechanism by which it blocks seizures is still unclear but may involve its effects on peripheral benzodiazepine receptors (benzodiazepines are the most common class of tranquilizers, discussed in chapter 11). The original hypothesis explaining carbamazepine's efficacy in mood disorders linked its prophylactic effect to its ability to prevent the easily provoked electrical and biological changes seen when a particular stress, be it the time of year (for those patients whose episodes occur on a seasonal basis), sleep deprivation, or the loss of a relationship, causes a biological response in a susceptible patient.

Consistent with this hypothesis is the observation in some studies that the first few manic episodes in a bipolar patient are more likely to be related to stressful life events than are later episodes (Ambelas, 1987). After a number of precipitated episodes, the system may become kindled, or more sensitive, requiring less and less of a provocation to be triggered. Ultimately, as is seen with individual neurons, the system may spontaneously discharge; that is, affective episodes may occur without a precipitating event. Instead, at this point, the patient would show the pattern of endogenously occurring episodes without relation to life events or stresses (Post and Weiss, 1995).

Although clearly speculative, the changing relationship over time between life events and affective episodes could have important treatment implications. Early intervention, both psychopharmacological or psychological (including cognitive/behavioral and psychodynamic approaches), might be helpful in altering the long-term course of the mood disorder. By instituting prophylactic pharmacotherapy earlier in the disorder (e.g., after a first episode), the mood stabilizers might be more effective when the disorder is more stress-responsive. Consistent with this notion, there is soft evidence that a greater number of prior episodes before treatment predicts a poorer prophylactic response to lithium (Post and Weiss, 1995). Similarly, psychotherapeutic intervention might diminish the magnitude of the person's responses to certain stressors either by desensitization or, in psychodynamic therapy, by diminishing the power of an event by divorcing it from the affective intensity of the earlier childhood event. This diminished response to stressful events would then make precipitation of episodes less likely. The same intervention years later, after "spontaneous episodes" have arisen, might be less useful in altering the course of the disorder.

Unfortunately, this line of reasoning, although theoretically satisfying both lacks documentation and is based on some shaky observations. First, there is no direct evidence linking the antikindling effect of carbamazepine with its efficacy in mood disorders. The antiepileptic and most of the antikindling effects of carbamazepine occur rapidly, within twenty-four to forty-eight hours, whereas the mood stabilizing effects take far longer to be established. (This is similar to the theoretical problems explaining the mechanism of action of antidepressants discussed in chapter 9.) Carbamazepine's later effects that temporally coincide with its mood stabilizing activity are still obscure. The second major problem with this hypothesis is that the oft-quoted statement describing the first few mood episodes as being more likely to be triggered by life events than later episodes is based on poor evidence and should not be considered as well established. For now, then, the kindling hypothesis should be considered an intriguing idea that may or may not lead us to a better explanation of the mechanism of action of anticonvulsants in mood disorders or provide a deeper understanding of the recurrent nature of mood disorders. Nonetheless, the indirect evidence as well as the links of the hypothesis to what is known about the course of mood disorders suggest it as a useful model for further studies.

Carbamazepine has a variety of different effects on a number of the neurotransmitter systems (Post, Weiss, and Chuang, 1992). Its effects on noradrenergic mechanisms, GABA, and on the benzodiazepine receptor sites may be especially relevant to its clinical actions. It is not currently possible, though, to correlate the clinical and biochemical effects of carbamazepine with each other.

Techniques for Prescribing

Carbamazepine is available in 100 mg and 200 mg tablets. Before starting carbamazepine, a complete blood count (CBC), a chemistry panel including electrolytes, and liver and kidney tests are required. For most patients, starting doses are either 100 or 200 mg twice daily. Average doses are generally 800 to 1000 mg daily, although therapeutic effects can be seen in daily doses as low as 400 mg or as high as 1200 to 1600 mg. As with other medications, when it is prescribed for an acute syndrome such as mania, carbamazepine is increased more rapidly than when it is being used prophylactically. For acute mania, the dose can be raised by 200 mg every few days to 800 or 1000 mg by the end of seven or eight days. For maintenance treatment, raising the dose by 200 mg every three to four days is more common. When carbamazepine is prescribed for other than bipolar disorder, patients consistently have problems tolerating its side effects, necessitating lower doses than those just noted.

Because it has a short half-life, carbamazepine needs to be prescribed in divided doses. Optimally, it would be given three or four times daily to keep the level in the blood constant as well as to diminish side effects. Because it is often difficult to remember midday or late afternoon doses, many patients take it on a twice-daily regimen. There are no studies examining whether the pharmacologic regimen (i.e., the number of daily doses) has any relationship to carbamazepine's efficacy.

Obtaining carbamazepine blood levels to help regulate the dose is very common. Most laboratories will declare that the therapeutic range for carbamazepine blood levels is 4 to 12 mg/l. Unfortunately, no relationship between blood levels and therapeutic response has been established (Post et al., 1983). This range should therefore be used as an approximate guide only.

Side Effects

Carbamazepine can cause a variety of side effects that are of potential concern. What is always remembered by patients and clinicians alike about this medication, however, is the very rare possibility of a bone marrow reaction called agranulocytosis or aplastic anemia, in which the production of white blood cells (which fight infection) and/or platelets (which promote blood clotting) is diminished or ceases. Reading the *Physicians' Desk Reference* warning about this possibility is a frightening experience. Certainly this risk needs to be taken seriously, because the reaction is potentially fatal (as, of course, penicillin allergy is). It must be remembered, though, that the incidence of this bone marrow suppression has been estimated to be between one in 40,000 and one in 125,000 patients, with some experts estimating an even lower risk. As always, the risks and benefits of any treatment must be weighed, but the risk for carbamazepine-induced life-threatening agranulocytosis seems very small.

The appropriate frequency of blood counts during carbamazepine treatment varies between treatment settings. A conservative regimen would be to obtain blood counts weekly for the first month, then monthly for the next six months, and then every six months. In contrast, some neurologists do not recommend any routine blood monitoring (Pellock and Willmore, 1991). The middle-ground approach taken by the APA Practice Guidelines suggests blood counts every two weeks for two months, followed by tests every three months (American Psychiatric Association, 1994b). The overwhelming majority of cases of bone marrow suppression have occurred within the first six months of treatment (Pisciotta, 1982). Whatever the frequency of blood count monitoring, it must be acknowledged that the frequent checking of blood counts is more reassuring psychologically and medicolegally than it is clinically helpful since the idiosyncratic bone marrow suppression can occur explosively, without warning, making random tests unlikely to diagnose it early. It is more important, therefore, that patients know to call their doctor and to obtain a blood count immediately at the first sign of infection or unusual bleeding.

This rare but disastrous bone marrow suppression is sometimes confused with the very common but benign lowering of the white blood cell count (Joffe, Post, Roy-Byrne, and Uhde, 1985). Typically, carbamazepine lowers the white count by 25 to 35 percent, an amount that still leaves the number of white cells well within the normal range.

Aside from the risk of severe bone marrow depression, other less dangerous effects can also be seen with carbamazepine. The most common of these are dizziness, ataxia (poor or unsteady balance), diplopia (double vision), sedation, lethargy, low sodium, rash, and nausea. Most of these side effects (but not nausea or rash) are typically dose related. As with many other medications, side effects can be diminished by increasing doses more slowly. Occasionally, a patient who has shown only a partial response to lithium will be prescribed a combination of lithium plus carbamazepine. At times, this combination can cause a marked increase in the neurological side effects, such as ataxia and diplopia. In these cases, lowering the dose of one or both medications can be very helpful. Similarly, interactions between carbamazepine and valproate are complex with each altering the metabolism of the other, resulting in unpredictable changes in blood levels and side effects. When these two anticonvulsants are combined, periodic checks of liver enzymes (easily accomplished through a blood test) are generally done in the hope of detecting the rare liver toxicity attendant with their simultaneous use.

Valproate

Clinical Uses

Table 10–5 shows the disorders for which valproate may be effective. Befitting a medication that has been prescribed only recently in psychopharmacology, many potential uses for valproate have simply not been evaluated.

Valproate's most well documented effects are in treating acute mania, and secondarily in the maintenance treatment of bipolar disorder. In treating acute mania, two well-controlled studies have demonstrated valproate's efficacy compared to placebo and, more importantly, its equivalent effectiveness compared to lithium (Pope, McElroy, Keck, and Hudson, 1991; Bowden et al., 1994). Because of this, many clinicians perceive valproate as a viable alternative to lithium as a first-line treatment for acute mania. Valproate's ability to prevent manias and depression seems clear from open studies, but since no controlled trials have yet been published, this effect is still not considered established. Nonetheless, considering that bipolar disorder is generally unresponsive to placebos, these open studies are persuasive. Valproate's efficacy in treating acute depression is probably weak.

Among the suggested predictors of response to valproate in treating mood disorders are rapid cycling and mixed states (Calabrese, Bowden, and Woyshville, 1995). The evidence that a mildly abnormal EEG predicts a good response to valproate is conflicted (McElroy, Keck, Pope, and Hudson, 1992; Stoll et al., 1994). However, because the patients treated in most of these studies were not randomly assigned to different treatments, the validity of all of these predictors is still in question.

Valproate is also occasionally helpful for patients with mild bipolar spectrum disorders such as cyclothymia (Jacobsen, 1993). In these ways, valproate is probably no different than lithium or other mood stabilizers.

As with carbamazepine, valproate may also be effective in treating post-traumatic stress disorder, especially in diminishing hyperarousal/hyperreactivity symptoms (Fesler, 1991). Although the evidence is still small and emerging, valproate seems to possess antipanic properties (Woodman and Noyes, 1994).

Biologic Effects

Most explanations of valproate's effects in treating both neurological and psychiatric disorders have centered on its ability to potentiate the effects of GABA (gamma-aminobutyric acid), an important inhibitory neurotransmitter found throughout the central nervous system (Post, Weiss, and Chuang, 1992). Enhancing GABA effects would have the effect of potentially decreasing electrical activity, explaining valproate's effects in diminishing seizures. It is still unclear how increasing GABA would specifically treat manias while also preventing both manias and depressions. In this way, our understanding of valproate's mechanism of action is similar to that of carbamazepine: their clinical effects *and* biological effects are well-documented but we have great difficulty specifically linking the two.

Techniques for Prescribing

Valproate is available in a generic form and in an enteric coated form, divalproex or Depakote. (Enteric coating is used to decrease stomach irritation and nausea.) Divalproex is available in 125, 250, and 500 mg forms. Before starting valproate, general chemistry screening tests (including a blood count and liver enzyme tests) are obtained. As with carbamazepine, valproate doses can be increased more quickly when used acutely than prophylactically. For inpatients, valproate can be started at 250 mg three times daily or even faster, with doses rapidly escalating to 1,500 mg daily within a few days. For outpatients, the starting dose is 250 mg twice daily with increases of 250 mg every three to five days. Daily doses of valproate may range between 500 and 3,000 mg or more. Because of its short half-life, valproate is usually started on a two to three times daily regimen. After dose stabilization, it may be taken twice or even once daily.

Valproate blood levels are available to help find the optimal dose. Unfortunately, as with carbamazepine, the correlation between valproate levels and therapeutic responses is weak. Therefore, blood levels should be used as general guides only, with side effects and therapeutic effects being more important in determining the final dose. Nonetheless, the published recommended blood level range for a therapeutic trial of valproate (derived from its use as an antiepileptic) is 50 to 100 mcg/ml.

Side Effects

Valproate probably has the fewest and mildest side effects of the three mood stabilizers. The most common side effects seen with valproate are nausea, diarrhea, hair loss, sedation, tremor, and weight gain. (Both the tremor and weight gain are less severe than are typically seen with lithium but are additive when both medications are prescribed simultaneously.) Many of these side effects are treatable: tremor by a beta-blocker, nausea by using Depakote or by certain gastrointestinal medications such as famotidine (Pepcid) or ranitidine (Zantac).

The rare bone marrow suppression seen with carbamazepine does not occur with valproate. The major concern is a rare idiosyncratic hepatotoxicity (liver toxicity) that has occurred with valproate use. However, all cases of fatal hepatotoxicity have emerged when the medication was prescribed for infants, in combination with other anticonvulsants such as phenytoin (Dilantin) or phenobarbital, or in patients with multiple neurological disorders (Dreifuss, Santilli, and Langer, 1987).When carbamazepine and valproate are prescribed together, for example, for bipolar patients who are insufficiently responsive to either agent, hepatotoxicity may occur, albeit rarely. The usual monitoring procedure in this case is to obtain liver enzyme tests every few months initially with the frequency diminishing over time.When used by itself in adolescents or adults, valproate never causes serious hepatotoxicity. Therefore, the risk for psychiatric patients is nil.

11

Antianxiety Medications and Hypnotics

H UMAN BEINGS HAVE BEEN USING chemicals to relax and to induce sleep since prerecorded history. Many individuals distinguish medications that decrease anxiety—tranquilizers, which are technically called anxiolytics (literally the loosening of anxiety)—from others used to induce sleep, called hypnotics. It is often assumed that since the two goals are different, the medications to treat them must be too. This is largely untrue. Most medications used to treat anxiety also treat insomnia, often in the same dose. The myth of two separate treatments has largely been due to patterns of individual consumption ("I take a Xanax to relax and Dalmane to sleep") and to the advertising patterns of pharmaceutical firms which want the public to think of a medication as a treatment for a specific condition and not as one of many that are broad in their effects. Thus, flurazepam (Dalmane) became a hypnotic while diazepam (Valium) became a tranquilizer, although they could easily have been reversed without sacrificing effectiveness. Of course, as we will see, all tranquilizers are not identical, even within the same medication class, but the similarities far outweigh the differences. In this chapter, therefore, we will consider both tranquilizers and hypnotics together. In keeping with modern prescribing practices, the focus will be on the use of benzodiazepines and related compounds—the class of tranquilizers that includes Valium, Xanax, and Halcion—and of buspirone (Buspar) with less attention given to the older less commonly used tranquilizers.

HISTORY

From the beginning, when alcohol was recorded as the first tranquilizer, society has been aware of the double-edged nature of calming agents. On one hand, they have the positive effects of helping people relax, loosening their inhibitions, and allowing for an easier time slipping into a peaceful sleep. On the other hand, when taken in too large a quantity, these same potions inhibit the capacity to work, make people clumsy, cause a sleepiness that is dangerous in some circumstances, and are potentially addictive with larger and larger doses being used to maintain a clinical effect. For some people, the goals of relaxation and sleep are replaced by the craving for the medication itself and all else fades into unimportance.

Over the last 125 years, the goal has been to discover a tranquilizer that would calm but not cause too much somnolence, that would be effective but not addictive, that would decrease physical tension but not cause clumsiness. From the discovery of chloral hydrate in 1869 to the barbiturates in 1903 to the nonbarbiturate sedatives such as meprobamate (Miltown) and finally to the benzodiazepines starting with chlordiazepoxide (Librium) in 1960 and diazepam (Valium) in 1963, each new class of medications was thought to achieve this goal of being the perfect tranquilizer. In general, although each new class of compounds (with the possible exception of the barbiturates) came closer to the ideal, they never came as close as initially hoped or touted. The non-barbiturate sedatives are slightly less addictive and less lethal in overdose than the barbiturates but are far from the nonaddictive "safe" medications initially promised. Benzodiazepines are relatively safe when taken in overdose, but are potentially addictive (although much less than their predecessors), can be dangerous when taken in conjunction with alcohol, and can cause significant impairment in physical and cognitive performance. Only buspirone (Buspar), released in 1986, seems to be devoid of the ill effects of all other tranquilizers. Unfortunately, though, it is not useful for inducing sleep, is ineffective when taken intermittently, and its efficacy in treating severe anxiety symptoms is doubtful. Its discovery, however, promises that new classes of antianxiety medications are on the horizon. Already, one recently released hypnotic, zolpidem (Ambien), exhibits somewhat different and more selective biological characteristics than its predecessors. Many of the anxiolytics in development show unique biological effects and are a far cry from "me too" drugs that mimic those agents already available. Some of the new tranquilizers not yet available are, like zolpidem, more selective than the benzodiazepines in their biological effects. Others, in contrast to most of the older drugs, are similar to buspirone in that they seem to work by affecting serotonergic function but do so via a variety of mechanisms. Over the next decade, at least some of these agents will undoubtedly be released. The search for the perfect tranquilizer continues.

BENZODIAZEPINES

Clinical Uses

The benzodiazepines are very commonly prescribed medications. Between 1 and 2 percent of adults use benzodiazepines regularly for one year or more while 11 to 15 percent of the population will use them at least occasionally over one year. However, for two-thirds of all users, the benzodiazepines are discontinued in less than one month (Salzman, 1993). Furthermore, benzodiazepine prescriptions have not increased lately, nor are they prescribed more in the United States than in other countries in Western Europe or in Canada (Shader and Greenblatt, 1993). Despite concerns about their ill effects, the widespread use of these medications accurately reflect their fundamental efficacy and safety when prescribed cautiously and knowledgeably. As examples, patients taking benzodiazepines tend to show high rates of emotional distress and psychiatric disorders while nonmedical uses of benzodiazepines have decreased over time (Woods, Katz, and Winger, 1995). Sadly, the confusion between appropriate use of benzodiazepines from the much less common inappropriate prescription and abuse has made many patients wary of taking these medications that might be very helpful to them (Kraupl-Taylor, 1989). Unwarranted hysteria surrounding benzodiazepines even led to the dreadful decision in 1989 in New York State making benzodiazepines a class of medications requiring triplicate prescriptions (required for controlled substances that are addictive and/or have street value). Because these prescriptions cannot be refilled on the telephone and require more paperwork for the physician, prescriptions for benzodiazepines subsequently decreased (consistent with the goals of the lawmakers). Unfortunately—and predictably—they were replaced by a marked increase in prescriptions in drugs like barbiturates and barbiturate-like drugs (e.g., meprobamate and chloral hydrate—see below) which are far more dangerous in overdose and are associated with greater physical dependence but do not require triplicate prescriptions. Serious tranquilizer overdoses consequently showed a marked increase (Schwartz, 1992; Weintraub, Singh, Byrne, Maharaj, and Guttmacher, 1991).

With rare exception, such as the occasional use of alprazolam for depression, the disorders for which the benzodiazepines are useful all involve heightened levels of arousal. Table 11–1 lists these disorders.

Insomnia—both primary (not due to any other disorder) and secondary—is frequently treated with benzodiazepines. These medica-

Table 11–1
Disorders for Which Benzodiazepines Are Useful

Disorder	Efficacy Rating
Insomnia	+++
Situational anxiety	+++
Generalized anxiety disorder	+++
Panic disorder	+++
Mania	++
Acute alcohol detoxification	+++
Acute catatonic episodes (of any etiology)	++
Acute agitation	++
Major depression	+

+++ = Definite efficacy
 ++ = Probable efficacy
  + = Possible efficacy

tions are most effective when taken on an occasional basis or for short periods of time. To diminish jet lag they are also frequently used to induce sleep on flights that involve crossing several time zones. Although some studies suggest that the hypnotic effect diminishes after one week or more of continuous use, clinical experience and a number of other studies indicate that some patients continue to sleep better on a chronic stable dose of medication for months and years. Whether this reflects an initial medication effect followed by a behavioral conditioning to the act of ingesting the pill ("When I take this pill, I know I will fall asleep more easily") or a prolonged pharmacological effect of the medication is unknown. The five benzodiazepines that are FDA indicated for insomnia are flurazepam (Dalmane), temazepam (Restoril), triazolam (Halcion), quazepam (Doral), and estazolam (Prosom). However, all agents in the class are likely to be effective for insomnia, and some, like diazepam (Valium) and alprazolam (Xanax), are probably more commonly prescribed for insomnia than some of the FDA-indicated agents. As will be discussed more below, the individual agents differ primarily in how quickly they act and how long their effects last.

Another common use of benzodiazepines is in treating situational anxiety. Probably the most common—and least studied—of these uses occurs when people keep one or two tranquilizer pills in their pocket to be used at a time of particular stress—at work, in a relationship crisis, or during a stressful day. Benzodiazepines are also often prescribed during the few weeks to months of a stressful situation, called adjustment disorder with anxiety in DSM-IV. When used in this way, all the benzodiazepines are likely to be effective, although alprazolam and diazepam seem to be the most popular.

Generalized anxiety, a more prolonged (months to years) anxiety disorder, is also very responsive to benzodiazepines. Here too, all the benzodiazepines are likely to be effective, although triazolam is virtually never used for this purpose because its actions are so brief. The long-term use (more than four months) of benzodiazepines for chronic anxiety is somewhat controversial (see below). However, many patients do indeed stay on low to moderate doses of tranquilizers for many years without developing tolerance to the effects of the medication (Rickels, Case, Downing, and Winokur, 1983). When used for chronic anxiety, optimal doses vary enormously.

Among the most well-documented effects of benzodiazepines is their efficacy in treating panic disorder. The bulk of the studies have focused on alprazolam (Xanax). Its immense popularity is, in large part, due to the impressive scientific and popular publicity it garnered during a series of studies on its antipanic properties (Ballenger et al., 1988). In the last few years, solid evidence has appeared documenting antipanic effects of lorazepam (Ativan), clonazepam (Klonopin), and, to a lesser extent, diazepam. It is likely, but not proven, that all benzodiazepines have antipanic properties. Benzodiazepine doses for panic are typically higher than those for generalized or situational anxiety.

Acute mania can be effectively controlled by benzodiazepines. Most of the research and clinical experience has centered on clonazepam, which is the most sedating medication of its type (Chou, 1991). Lorazepam has also been used with some success. Whether the antimanic efficacy of these two benzodiazepines extends to all medications of this class is unknown. There is no good evidence that benzodiazepines are effective by themselves as a preventive treatment in bipolar mood disorders.

Benzodiazepines are also prescribed in the acute detoxification from alcohol (Bohn, 1993). They will successfully diminish the acute withdrawal syndrome (including grand mal seizures) which can be severe at times and even, on rare occasions, life threatening. It is likely that all benzodiazepines would be effective for this purpose. Most commonly prescribed for alcohol detoxification are a long-acting agent—chlordiazepoxide—and two other agents—lorazepam and oxazepam—that are safer for those with liver disease.

Catatonic episodes, characterized by immobility, mutism, posturing, rigidity, negativism, stereotypical behaviors, waxy flexibility, and echolalia (repeating what was said by others) are well treated by lorazepam (Rosebush, Hildebrand, Furlong, and Mazurek, 1990). It is likely that other benzodiazepines are also effective although they have been less systematically evaluated (Hollister, Muller-Oerlinghausen, Rickels, and Shader, 1993). The benzodiazepines' ability to treat catatonia does not depend on the etiology of the episode.

Benzodiazepines are occasionally used to treat agitation both secondary to a variety of causes and adjunctively to antipsychotics in the treatment of acute schizophrenic episodes. Despite their adjunctive use in treating psychotic disorders, benzodiazepines do not have a primary antipsychotic effect.

Alone among the benzodiazepines, alprazolam has been shown effective in treating mild to moderate outpatient depression (Rickels et al., 1987). Despite the positive results of some large-scale research studies, most clinicians (myself included) consider alprazolam to be a weak second- or third-line option for treating depression. Doses of alprazolam used to treat depression are the same as those prescribed for panic disorder. No other benzodiazepine has been shown to share alprazolam's antidepressant effect, although the majority have not been tested. Many benzodiazepines are also prescribed as an adjunct to antidepressants in the treatment of acute depression. When used in this way the effect should be thought of as simply helping to calm the anxiety and agitation of acute depression and not as medications with any primary antidepressant effect.

Biologic Effects

As so often happens in pharmacology, the discovery of the benzodiazepines' clinical effects preceded the first clue as to their mechanism of action by many years. The modern understanding of these medications began in 1977 with the discovery of a specific receptor site on the surface of neurons to which all benzodiazepines seemed to specifically bind—in other words, a benzodiazepine receptor (Zorumski and Isenberg, 1991). That a group of related medications all shared a clinical and biological effect—in this case, decreasing anxiety and binding to a specific type of receptor—does not necessarily indicate a causal link between these two findings. More convincing was the discovery that the clinical potency of a benzodiazepine correlates highly with how tightly the medication binds to the receptor site (Hyman and Nestler, 1993). As an example, alprazolam, which is clinically effective in 1 mg doses, binds to the benzodiazepine receptor far more tightly than does diazepam, which is clinically effective in 10 mg doses. Furthermore, if the benzodiazepine receptor is blocked, benzodiazepines are no longer effective. Collectively, this was good evidence that the benzodiazepine receptor was the site mediating the medications' clinical effects.

The next link in the chain of understanding was the discovery that benzodiazepines enhanced the activity of GABA (gamma-aminobutyric acid), a widespread neurotransmitter in the brain that primarily exerts an inhibitory effect on neurotransmission (Paul, 1995). Further research demonstrated that the benzodiazepine receptor is a binding site on the larger $GABA_A$ receptor, a multi-subunit receptor complex that is the main GABA receptor in the central nervous system (CNS). ($GABA_B$ receptors are also present in the CNS, have been less well characterized than the $GABA_A$ receptor, and seem unrelated to the effects of benzodiazepines.) The $GABA_A$ receptor is composed of multiple subunits, each of which has its own subunits. Benzodiazepines probably bind to a site on the alpha subunit of the $GABA_A$ receptor. Another central component of the $GABA_A$ receptor is a channel through which chloride, an electrically charged particle, flows. Figure 11–1 shows a simplified version of this schematically (leaving out many of the subunits). When the chloride channel opens, chloride flow increases. This alters the electrical charge across the cell membrane, thereby making it more refractory to excitatory impulses. Thus, any chemical that increases chloride flow into the cell inhibits neurotransmission and "slows things down." Benzodiazepines are such chemicals: they increase chloride flow, but do so indirectly by increasing the sensitivity of the receptor for GABA itself. (The subreceptor to which GABA binds is located on the beta subunit.) For benzodiazepines to work, GABA must be available. This indirect effect of benzodiazepines on chloride ion flow and electrical activity may explain why overdoses with these medications are almost never lethal. In contrast, barbiturates, which seem to affect chloride flow directly even in the absence of GABA are extremely lethal in overdose.

Benzodiazepines also have multiple effects beyond those seen in decreasing anxiety. These include anticonvulsant properties, sedative (sleep-promoting) effects, and muscle relaxant properties. These diverse actions may be mediated either by benzodiazepine effects in different brain regions or by affecting slightly different $GABA_A$ receptor subtypes. If identical effects in different brain regions explain the diverse effects, it is hypothesized that the anticonvulsant effects of benzodiazepines are mediated by receptors in the cortex, the area controlling motor movements; their ability to cause muscle relaxation is likely due to their effects on spinal cord neurons. Sedating properties

Figure 11–1   GABA_ABenzodiazepine Receptor

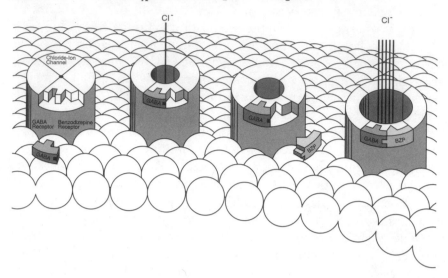

Legend: Cl = chloride
           BZP = benzodiazepine

Adapted from S. Paul (1987), *The Biochemical Basis of Anxiety,* Upjohn, Kalamazoo, Mich. Reprinted with permission of The Upjohn Company.

might be mediated by brain stem effects, while benzodiazepines' capacity to decrease anxiety probably occurs in the limbic system, the part of the brain that is primarily involved with the regulation of emotions.

Why would receptor sites exist that seem so specifically linked to a synthesized class of medications first released in the 1960s? It hardly seems likely that these receptors were the product of a thoughtful Creator who anticipated the synthesis of Valium or Xanax! What is more plausible, of course, is that the benzodiazepine receptor site is the target of a naturally occurring antianxiety agent—an endogenous Valium, as it were. Thus far, despite a number of proposed candidates and vigorous searching, this putative natural tranquilizer has yet to be discovered and synthesized. The search for this endogenous tranquilizer, however, is analogous to the search for and then discovery of the endorphins and enkephalins, the group of naturally occurring opioids whose effects are mimicked by exogenous opiates such as morphine.

A number of other compounds bind to the benzodiazepine receptor site but are associated with very different potential effects. Beta-carbolines are chemicals which bind to benzodiazepine receptors and, when given to animals and, in a very few experiments, humans), cause agitation, fright, and intense feelings of inner doom. Administering these compounds, which decrease chloride ion flow (the opposite of benzodiazepines), also blocks or reverses the effect of benzodiazepines (and vice versa). For this reason, they are called "inverse agonists" (although the term "active antagonists" might be more appropriate) (Insel et al., 1984).

Another group of compounds, called receptor antagonists, seem to bind to benzodiazepine receptors but have no intrinsic effect on anxiety or agitation at all. However, they will reverse both the antianxiety effects of benzodiazepines as well as the anxiety-producing effects of the beta-carbolines (Paul, 1995). The most likely explanation, as shown in Figure 11–2, is that these antagonists "fill" the receptor sites, thereby preventing the effect of any active compounds, but not causing any changes themselves. Benzodiazepine antagonists are useful in treating benzodiazepine overdose, but may precipitate acute withdrawal symptoms, similar to the effects of naloxone (Narcan), an opiate antagonist on opiate-dependent patients. Flumazenil (Romazicon), released in 1991, is such an agent. Between the agonists (the benzodiazepines

Figure 11–2   Benzodiazepine Receptor Agonist and Antagonist

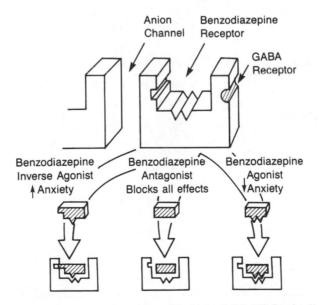

Adapted from T. R. Insel et al. (1984), *Archives of General Psychiatry, 41,* 741–750. Reprinted with permission.

themselves) and the antagonists lie compounds—called partial agonists—with activity midway between the two extremes. These medications bind to the receptor with partial effects, raising the possibility of
developing a tranquilizer which, because it is a partial agonist, might be
tranquilizing without causing sedation. Partial agonists are currently
being developed and tested.

Thus far, the types of anxiety models utilized in the research on
benzodiazepine receptors are most analogous to situational or generalized anxiety. How benzodiazepines effectively treat panic disorder is
not as well understood. They may work by increasing the effects of
GABA, which inhibits activity at the locus ceruleus, the area thought to
be centrally involved in panic attacks (see chapter 2 for details). Alternatively, since there are neural connections between the limbic system
(in which benzodiazepine receptors are found in high concentrations)
and the locus ceruleus, benzodiazepines' antipanic effects may be best
explained as indirect (Gorman, Liebowitz, Fyer, and Stein, 1989).

Choosing a Benzodiazepine

The thirteen benzodiazepines available for oral use are all equally effective in decreasing arousal and anxiety and in helping to diminish insomnia. Table 11–2 lists the currently available benzodiazepines and

Table 11–2
Benzodiazepines

Generic Name	Trade Name	Usual Dosage Range (mg/day)
Alprazolam	Xanax	0.5–4
Chlordiazepoxide[a]	Librium	10–100
Clonazepam	Klonopin	0.5–3
Clorazepate	Tranxene	7.5–60
Diazepam[a]	Valium	5–40
Estazolam	ProSom	1–2
Flurazepam	Dalmane	15–30
Halazepam	Paxipam	40–160
Lorazepam[a]	Ativan	1–6
Oxazepam	Serax	15–90
Quazepam	Doral	7.5–15
Temazepam	Restoril	15–30
Triazolam	Halcion	0.125–0.5

[a] Available in injectable form

their general dosage ranges. One additional benzodiazepine, midazolam (Versed), will not be considered further here since it is administered only intravenously as an anesthetic aid prior to surgery.

As with the antipsychotics, it is possible to classify the benzodiazepines into subgroups based on their chemical structure. In general clinical use, these subclassifications are not helpful. The important distinctions among the benzodiazepines that are well understood are how quickly they act and how long they last. Table 11–3 classifies the medications according to these criteria. Aside from these two known ways in which the benzodiazepines differ, a number of other factors are sometimes relevant in a psychopharmacologist's choice of one agent over another. These are the patient's potential for addiction, the drug's rate of redistribution from the brain to the rest of the body (see below), and the individual patient's past experience with these medications.

Speed of onset of action is sometimes, but not always, an important consideration. For instance, if the medication is prescribed to treat insomnia, it is relevant whether the problem occurs nightly (and can therefore be anticipated and treated preventively) or intermittently and unpredictably. In treating a symptom occurring occasionally, such as difficulty falling asleep, a rapid-to-intermediate-acting medication like flurazepam is preferable so that after taking the sleeping pill, the patient doesn't stare at the ceiling for an hour or more, waiting for the medica-

Table 11–3
Characteristics of Benzodiazepines

Generic Name (Trade Name)	Rapidity of Effect	Half-life (Rate of Elimination)
Alprazolam (Xanax)	Intermediate	Intermediate
Chlordiazepoxide (Librium)	Intermediate	Long
Clonazepam (Klonopin)	Intermediate	Intermediate–long
Clorazepate (Tranxene)	Rapid	Long
Diazepam (Valium)	Rapid	Long
Estazolam (ProSom)	Rapid	Intermediate
Flurazepam (Dalmane)	Intermediate	Long
Halazepam (Paxipam)	Slow	Long
Lorazepam (Ativan)	Intermediate	Intermediate
Oxazepam (Serax)	Intermediate–slow	Intermediate
Quazepam (Doral)	Rapid	Long
Temazepam (Restoril)	Intermediate	Intermediate
Triazolam (Halcion)	Intermediate	Short

tion to work. If the symptom is predictable, either slow- or fast-acting medications can be equally effective simply by taking the slower-acting pill earlier. Of course, in real life, it is easier for patients to take a sleeping pill a half hour before bedtime than one and a half hours before, at which time they may be away from home or unsure of when they will want to go to sleep.

An identical set of considerations applies in treating anxiety. The need for an occasional tranquilizer in times of particular stress suggests using a rapidly acting medication like diazepam. For the treatment of an ongoing anxiety state for a few weeks or longer in which the patient is taking a maintenance dose on a daily basis, speed of action is not important. In fact, more rapidly acting benzodiazepines may be at a disadvantage in these situations because they may produce more of the "rush" of sleepiness or spaciness that occurs at the peak of the medication's effects. A slowly acting medication such as oxazepam, therefore, might be preferable in treating ongoing anxiety, especially for those patients who are sensitive to the initial sedation of the benzodiazepines.

Rate of elimination from the body is the other major way in which the benzodiazepines differ. This property is commonly referred to as the half-life and is defined as the amount of time it takes for the blood level of the medication to decrease by half. The goal of the treatment will, in large part, determine the importance of the half-life. In treating insomnia, if the problem is in initiating sleep and the patient tends to be sensitive to side effects, a benzodiazepine that lasts a relatively short to intermediate length of time, such as triazolam or oxazepam might be preferable. Similarly, if the problem to be treated is anxiety around a short-lived situation such as a plane ride or in anticipation of an anxiety-provoking meeting, the use of short- or intermediate-acting benzodiazepines such as lorazepam or alprazolam would be preferable to longer-acting compounds such as clorazepate. But in treating ongoing anxiety lasting a few weeks or more, giving patients short-acting medications that may wear off within four to six hours will necessitate their taking a pill three or four times a day with the possibility of anxiety symptoms between doses. In these situations, the longer-acting benzodiazepines such as diazepam might be preferable. However, a potential disadvantage of using long-acting medication for an extended period of time—two weeks or longer—is that the blood levels of these medications gradually accumulate over time such that the level of diazepam in the bloodstream after three weeks of taking 20 mg daily is far higher than after three days on the same dose. For some patients, especially the elderly, this may predispose to greater somnolence and other side effects.

The half-life of the medication is also important in predicting possible withdrawal symptoms. (See below for an extended discussion of this topic.) By definition, the longer the half-life, the more gradually the drug will disappear from the body. With the long half-life benzodiazepines such as diazepam or clorazepate, this means a smaller chance of significant withdrawal symptoms because the medication "tapers itself" over many days. As will be discussed below, even with long-acting benzodiazepines, gradual tapering of the dose is frequently needed. With short or intermediate half-life drugs, such as alprazolam or triazolam, the quick drop in blood levels after a patient stops the medication is almost a guarantee of withdrawal symptoms unless the dose is decreased slowly. Since withdrawal symptoms reinforce the sense of needing medication both psychologically and biologically, their intensity is inherently linked with the addictive potential of any drug. Short half-life benzodiazepines, therefore, should be prescribed with greater caution to patients with potential addiction problems, especially to sedative-type drugs.

The considerations just noted, however, do not always fit with clinical experience. Other factors, some of which are still not well understood, also affect pharmacological activity. As an example, the effects of single doses of diazepam (Valium) do not necessarily continue for two to three days as one might expect from its half-life. The reason for this is that a major determinant of a benzodiazepine's clinical activity is not how much of the medication is in the body, but the amount of time it stays in the brain and available to the benzodiazepine receptors. A single dose of a medication that reaches the brain quickly—but leaves the brain quickly too—will have a clinically short duration of action even though it may stay in the fat and other body tissues for a long time thereafter (and be defined as having a long half-life). Diazepam, as an example of such a drug, is absorbed quickly and gets to the brain quickly, thus explaining its rapid onset of effect. But because it also then disappears from the brain rapidly, via distribution to other body tissues, its clinical effects may diminish even though its tissue levels remain substantial (Greenblatt, 1991).

Another important clinical consideration is that of tolerance. As discussed above, all benzodiazepines are both sedating (making the person sleepy) and tranquilizing (decreasing anxiety). With ongoing use of a benzodiazepine, tolerance develops more to the sedation than to the tranquilizing effect (Lucki, Rickels, and Geller, 1985). Thus, a medication that is effective but too sedating initially can, after days to weeks, continue to be effective with virtually no side effects. The development of tolerance explains why benzodiazepines that are slowly eliminated don't always show increasing side effects as the blood levels gradually increase over weeks of continual use. Even as the amount of the drug in the body increases, tolerance develops simultaneously, generally causing a decrease in side effects.

Despite all these considerations—rate of absorption, half-life, the shifting from brain to the rest of the body, the development of tolerance—in the final analysis, the benzodiazepines are more similar than different. How then should physicians in general, or psychiatrists pick a specific benzodiazepine for a particular patient? As with so many other medication choices, a patient's past experience with a particular drug should still be the most important determinant. If a patient has no prior experience with benzodiazepines, most psychopharmacologists will prescribe any one of three to five specific medications—usually one or two short half-life drugs and two or three of the longer-acting variety. I generally prescribe alprazolam and lorazepam as the former and diazepam and clonazepam as the latter, but one could easily substitute others with equal likelihood of a good effect.

Techniques for Prescribing

In treating intermittent anxiety, doses such as diazepam 5 mg, lorazepam 1 mg, or alprazolam 0.5 mg are generally effective, although individual sensitivities may necessitate slightly higher or lower doses. For insomnia, typical doses are flurazepam 15 to 30 mg, temazepam 15 to 30 mg, or triazolam 0.125 to 0.25 mg. Rapidly acting benzodiazepines (see Table 11–3) such as diazepam should be taken approximately 15 to 20 minutes before the desired effect. For intermediate drugs, 30 to 40 minutes are appropriate, while an hour may be needed for slow-acting medications like halazepam.

If benzodiazepines are being prescribed to decrease anxiety around the clock for days to weeks, most psychopharmacologists will start with a low dose and gradually increase over a number of weeks if needed. Typical initial doses would be diazepam 5 to 10 mg, lorazepam 1 to 2 mg, or alprazolam 0.5 to 1 mg. Doses should be increased by the equivalent of 5 mg of diazepam every four to five days if needed.

Except when treating insomnia, of course, most patients should be started on a divided dose regimen in the beginning of treatment, regardless of which benzodiazepine is being prescribed. The subset of patients being treated for generalized or situational anxiety (therefore requiring around-the-clock antianxiety effect) and who are sensitive to the sedative effects of benzodiazepines may be started on once-daily long-acting agents taken at bedtime. In these cases, the sedation will be maximal at night and the long-acting tranquilizer will gradually increase in efficacy over days. When benzodiazepines with short or intermediate half-life are prescribed, they should always be given in divided doses. Alprazolam, as a typical example, is generally taken three or even four times daily. Even with such short intervals between doses, many patients experience symptoms just before the next pill as a type of miniwithdrawal symptom (see below). Long half-life medications may be given once or twice daily with good effect.

Average effective antianxiety doses are 20 to 25 mg of diazepam or its equivalent. A patient's response in the first week of treatment is a good predictor of ultimate response (Downing and Rickels, 1987). Maximum improvement from the medication is generally seen within the first six weeks of treatment (Rickels, Case, and Downing, 1982). As noted above, tolerance to the tranquilizing effects—as opposed to the sedating effects—of the benzodiazepines is not common.

When an anxious patient does not respond to reasonable doses of a benzodiazepine, should the psychopharmacologist raise the dose further? If no side effects are evident and the patient is likely to respond—for example, when the medication is being prescribed for a short-lived stress-precipitated anxiety state—the answer is yes. Increased responses above diazepam 40 mg or alprazolam 4 mg daily for treating generalized anxiety are, however, unusual. For patients whose doses have increased to relatively high levels, have not responded, and have few or no side effects, benzodiazepine blood levels are available and may be helpful in selected cases. Unfortunately, the relationship between blood level and efficacy has been consistently shown only for alprazolam and only in treating panic disorder (Greenblatt, Harmatz, and Shader, 1993). Blood levels of other benzodiazepines can be measured but their interpretation is unclear and their clinical utility unproven. The vast majority of clinicians (myself included) do not use benzodiazepine levels in routine clinical work, relying instead on clinical observations to guide prescribing practices. If a therapeutic trial of one benzodiazepine is cut short by side effects, switching to another may be helpful. For instance, significant sedation soon after taking a dose of medication may be solved by switching to another benzodiazepine which is absorbed more slowly.

When treating panic disorder with benzodiazepines, the doses utilized tend to be higher than for anxiety. Since the bulk of the research experience has been with alprazolam, its antipanic dose is reasonably well established at 2 to 6 mg daily with initial doses generally 0.5 mg three times daily. My own experience and some recent clinical studies, though, suggest that many panic patients respond at 2 mg daily or less with fewer side effects than seen with higher doses (Lydiard et al., 1992). At any dose, the medication must be given multiple times during the day. Occasionally, much higher doses—up to 10 mg daily or more—are prescribed to treat panic. Initial and usual doses when alprazolam is prescribed to treat depression are the same as those for panic.

When clonazepam is used to treat acute mania, the doses prescribed range from moderate to prodigious—2 to 6 mg daily are common and 10 mg or more are used with regularity. Whether these high doses are more effective than moderate doses or reflect the pressure to do something to diminish the manic symptoms is unknown.

Benzodiazepine Withdrawal

The controversy surrounding the problem of withdrawing patients from benzodiazepines makes this an appropriate topic for discussion midway between techniques for prescribing and side effects since it encompasses both subjects. Therapist and psychopharmacologist alike must be aware of the realistic problems as well as the unwarranted publicity surrounding the discontinuation of benzodiazepines. Soon after the benzodiazepines were released, the first report of significant withdrawal symptoms appeared (Hollister, Motzenbecker, and Degan, 1961). Because that study utilized doses far in excess of what is usually prescribed, withdrawal symptoms from typical doses were initially thought to be unusual. Assuredly, the issue was underappreciated. More recently, there has been increased attention to the problem because of publicity in the lay press, the increasing use of shorter-acting benzodiazepines (with the likelihood of more intense withdrawal symptoms), and a series of excellent studies that carefully examined the topic.

Without question, the majority of patients taking benzodiazepines for any significant period of time will suffer withdrawal symptoms soon after stopping the medication. Yet in discussing the issue of benzodiazepine withdrawal, a number of important terms and concepts— abuse, tolerance, and dependence—must first be defined (Shader and Greenblatt, 1993). Abuse refers to the nontherapeutic use of drugs;

that is, the medication is taken for pleasure or intoxication (to get "high"), not to treat distressing symptoms. Tolerance is defined as a reduction of a medication's effects because of continued use, with the subsequent need to increase the dose to maintain the same effect. Dependence can be physical or psychological. Physical dependence implies that an objective, predictable withdrawal syndrome will occur after medication discontinuation. Psychological dependence describes the preference to take a drug rather than not take it. Psychological dependence has no clear relationship to tolerance, physical dependence, or even abuse.

If we utilize these definitions, benzodiazepines are infrequently abused, are generally not associated with tolerance to their therapeutic effect, but can cause physical dependence. Studies of nontherapeutic use of benzodiazepines indicate that the small group of patients likely to abuse benzodiazepines are those with histories of substance abuse with other drugs, especially other sedatives or alcohol. Consistent with this observation, in double-blind studies of drug preference, most individuals do not choose benzodiazepines over placebo unless they have a history of sedative or alcohol abuse (Woods, Katz, and Winger, 1995). Tolerance to benzodiazepines occurs with sedative effects (i.e., patients become less sleepy with continued use), whereas no tolerance is generally seen with the antianxiety effects of the medication as shown by the lack of escalating doses over months and years of use.

Finally, even though there is no doubt that benzodiazepines cause dependence to the extent that withdrawal symptoms are common with drug discontinuation, evaluating the seriousness of this problem is complicated by a number of factors. First, withdrawal symptoms and the return of the anxiety symptoms for which the medication was initially prescribed need to be distinguished—which is not always easy. Typically, it is thought that rapid-onset symptoms occurring within the first week after stopping the medication are due to withdrawal, whereas underlying anxiety emerges more gradually over a number of weeks. This is far from true for all patients and all situations, however, and overlap or confusion between the two conditions is common. Second, the effect of psychological dependence, especially given the high incidence of dependent personality in anxious patients, may magnify potential physical withdrawal symptoms. Third, it is important to distinguish mild withdrawal symptoms that may be no worse than one to three days of insomnia and irritability from more significant symptoms that are more disruptive. Finally, how the medication is withdrawn has an enormous impact on the difficulties the patient experiences. In most withdrawal studies, the benzodiazepine is stopped abruptly. Yet it is clear from everyday clinical experience (mine included) and the few studies that have examined the issue that tapering a benzodiazepine will diminish the severity of the withdrawal syndrome (Schweizer, Rickels, Case, and Greenblatt, 1990). There is virtually no clinical reason to abruptly stop a benzodiazepine. Patients, though, sometimes feel that the best way to stop using a drug is simply to go cold turkey. The resulting discomfort can be minimized if patient, therapist, and psychopharmacologist discuss these issues beforehand. In summary, to acknowledge that benzodiazepines can cause withdrawal symptoms is not tantamount to saying they are dangerous or that the psychopharmacologist, patient, or therapist is helpless if the medication should be stopped.

What common symptoms are seen when benzodiazepines are suddenly withdrawn? Table 11–4 lists them. As is obvious, the list com-

Table 11–4
Possible Symptoms of Benzodiazepine Withdrawal

Psychological:
  Anxiety
  Agitation
  Irritability
  Depressed mood
  Poor concentration, forgetfulness
Physical:
  Tremor
  Insomnia
  Loss of appetite
  Nausea, vomiting
  Sweating
  Tachycardia (fast heart rate)
Sensory:
  Depersonalization, derealization
  Hypersensitivity to light and/or sound
  Paresthesias (tingling)
Rare:
  Paranoia
  Severe depression
  Delirium/psychosis
  Grand mal seizures

prises a group of typical anxiety symptoms, both psychological and somatic, and some atypical sensory phenomena such as depersonalization, heightened sensitivity to sound, touch, or light, and perceptual distortions. Since these symptoms are sometimes seen in anxious patients before treatment, it is still not clear whether any of these are specific to withdrawal. There are sporadic reports of depression, paranoia, or in the most extreme and unusual cases, seizures. Fortunately, these are exceedingly rare. When they do occur, they are more likely with abrupt withdrawal of the more short-acting benzodiazepines such as alprazolam.

The time course of the withdrawal symptoms reflects the half-life of the benzodiazepine used. With long half-life drugs, the symptoms begin after twenty-four to thirty-six hours, peak at four to seven days, and subside in two to four weeks (Schweizer, Rickels, and Uhlenhuth, 1995). Abrupt withdrawal from short half-life drugs, on the other hand, can cause symptoms within six to twelve hours after the last dose with peak severity at two to four days and the symptoms subsiding in one to three weeks. There are some reports of rebound insomnia towards early morning when triazolam, the shortest-acting of the benzodiazepines, is taken in the beginning of the night (Kales, Soldatos, Bixter, and Kales, 1983).

It is difficult to predict the likelihood of withdrawal reactions from benzodiazepines. Estimates from various studies have ranged from 0 to 100 percent (!), reflecting both the varied definitions of withdrawal and the presence of risk factors that will affect the likelihood of these symptoms (Noyes et al., 1988). The more thoughtful studies indicate that more than 50 percent of patients taking benzodiazepines for an extended period of time (more than one year) will show at least some withdrawal symptoms even if the medication is tapered. (As noted before, however, many of these symptoms are mild and transient.)

Risk factors for withdrawal symptoms, shown in Table 11–5, can be divided into medication and patient predictors. For the first year of treatment, length of time on the medication predicts a greater likelihood of withdrawal symptoms. Even with long half-life drugs, withdrawal symptoms may be seen after as little as four weeks of use (Rickels, Fox, Greenblatt, Sandler, and Schless, 1988). No additional risk for withdrawal symptoms seems to occur after the first year of treatment (Rickels, Schweizer, Case, and Greenblatt, 1990). Short half-life drugs are associated with more severe as well as earlier withdrawal symptoms. As noted previously, abrupt discontinuation strongly predicts worse withdrawal symptoms and should always be avoided.

Table 11–5
Factors Predicting Benzodiazepine Withdrawal Symptoms

Medication predictors:
   Longer time on drug
   Short half-life
   Abrupt withdrawal (vs. tapering)
   High dose
Patient predictors:
   Current anxiety and depressive symptoms (before withdrawal)
   Personality factors—dependency traits
   History of alcohol or drug (especially sedative) abuse
   Past experience with benzodiazepines

Higher benzodiazepine doses are, not surprisingly, associated with greater likelihood and greater severity of withdrawal symptoms when the medication is withdrawn abruptly but not necessarily when a gradual tapering schedule is used.

Among the patient predictors for withdrawal symptoms, the most well-established are current symptoms and dependency traits. Both anxiety and depressive symptoms while on medication predict greater severity of withdrawal symptoms. Therefore, if possible, patients who are still symptomatic despite benzodiazepine treatment should be considered for other, more aggressive treatment to minimize symptoms prior to medication discontinuation. Dependency traits as a risk factor may simply reflect the fact that these patients have fewer coping skills and are intolerant of and afraid of any change in the way they feel. Earlier studies indicated that a history of drug/alcohol abuse and past experiences with benzodiazepines might also increase the likelihood of withdrawal difficulties.

Similar considerations apply to withdrawing benzodiazepines that have been prescribed for insomnia. Withdrawal effects may be seen quickly when short half-life drugs are discontinued. As when the benzodiazepines are used for anxiety, tapering is always preferred to abrupt discontinuation. With longer half-life drugs, rebound insomnia is typically seen three to four nights after the medication is withdrawn (Gillin, Spinweber, and Johnson, 1989). If withdrawn correctly, withdrawal effects, however, will often consist of no more than one to two nights of difficulty falling asleep.

Although it may sound as if discontinuing benzodiazepines is fraught with difficulties, for the majority of patients who do it *correctly* and with appropriate support and advice, it is not a major life trauma. Most important, educating and reassuring patients will help make the withdrawal much easier. Patients must know that the therapist and psychopharmacologist will work with them during the withdrawal period. They should anticipate that some anxiety or insomnia may be transiently experienced. It must be made clear that the speed of the tapering of the medication (since the benzodiazepines should *always* be tapered after any significant period of use) can always be slowed down if significant symptoms arise. Occasional doses of as-needed medication during the course of withdrawal should be allowed and not seen as a failure of will or character.

Table 11–6 lists the strategies for discontinuing benzodiazepines. The first set of strategies, as implied above, should be to slow the speed of the medication taper to slow or slower. With some patients, four to six months is not an excessively long time to gradually taper benzodiazepines. The first half of the tapering is typically more easily managed than the second, during which time the tapering schedule must often be slowed down further. Sometimes, however, no speed of tapering a short-acting benzodiazepine is effective in controlling withdrawal symptoms. In these cases, a number of other strategies may be helpful. The most common of these is switching to a long-acting benzodiazepine. The most popular of these switches is from alprazolam to clonazepam. This can be done over a few days to weeks since there is cross-tolerance between benzodiazepines (i.e., using one medication will prevent withdrawal symptoms of the other because they affect the same receptors in the brain). It is then much easier to taper the long-acting medication since the blood levels fluctuate much less within the course of a day and decrease so slowly over days. I have found this method helpful. However, because it is often difficult to ascertain the correct equivalent dose of the longer-acting medication for any indi-

Table 11–6
Strategies for Benzodiazepine Discontinuation

Slow taper
Slower taper
Switching to a long-acting benzodiazepine and then tapering
Adjunctive cognitive-behavioral therapy
Carbamazepine

vidual, the cross-over time (typically no more than a few days) is often characterized by transient withdrawal or sedation symptoms. Another helpful strategy is the adjunctive use of cognitive-behavioral therapy during the tapering period (Otto et al., 1993). Using this approach, the therapy utilizes interoceptive exposure and cognitive interventions targeted to discontinuation-related symptoms. For a few selected patients with whom the tapering has been unsuccessful, adding carbamazepine (Tegretol) just before tapering may be somewhat helpful (Klein, Colin, Stolk, and Lenox, 1994). Whether valproate, the other anticonvulsant mood stabilizer, might be similarly helpful is not yet established. Finally, both patient and clinician must remember that anxiety symptoms that return during a slow benzodiazepine taper may represent the reemergence of anxiety symptoms, not withdrawal effects. In these situations, treating the underlying anxiety with other agents, such as buspirone or tricyclics (which do not typically minimize withdrawal symptoms), may be beneficial.

> Linda's panic disorder had been successfully treated with alprazolam 1 mg three times daily. She experienced mild anxiety symptoms five hours after each medication dose until she took her next pill, but was otherwise symptom-free. Seven months later, a slow tapering of the medication was begun. Initially, she did well with the lower dose, eventually decreasing to 0.5 mg three times daily. At that point, lowering the dose, even at a rate of 0.125 mg every week, seemed to cause withdrawal symptoms. After three unsuccessful attempts to decrease the dose below 1.5 mg daily, alprazolam was switched to clonazepam over one week. During that time, Linda was alternately anxious and slightly sedated as the dose of the new medication was adjusted while the alprazolam was discontinued. After one week, however, Linda was taking 1.5 mg of clonazepam twice daily and experiencing no anxiety symptoms between doses. Over the next three months, clonazepam was decreased at a rate of 0.25 mg weekly until it was discontinued without the return of anxiety.

Other Side Effects

Table 11–7 lists the common side effects seen with the benzodiazepines. The most frequently observed of these relate to aspects of central nervous system depression. The single most common side effect is sedation to which there is significant accommodation over the

Table 11–7
Side Effects of Benzodiazepines

Common:
  Sedation
  Fatigue
  Ataxia (poor balance)
  Slurred speech
  Memory disturbances
  Psychomotor impairment
Rare:
  Intoxication
  Aggressive behavior
  Mania (with alprazolam)

first few days to weeks of treatment. Despite this, sedation is the side effect that most limits the use of higher doses of benzodiazepines. The extent of the cognitive and psychomotor effects with these medications is somewhat controversial.

Unquestionably, benzodiazepines can limit the ability to learn and recall new information (anterograde amnesia), especially around the time of peak sedation, which is typically one to two hours after ingestion (Greenblatt, Harmatz, Engelhardt, and Shader, 1989). With patients who use benzodiazepines on a long-term basis, the effect on memory is variable. Some studies have shown that patients who use low to moderate doses of benzodiazepines chronically (for many months or years) generally show no cognitive deficits except if tested during the one hour of peak sedation, implying that tolerance to the sedation may be linked to tolerance to cognitive side effects (Lucki and Rickels, 1986). Other evidence, however, suggests continued amnestic effects even after many years both in acquiring new knowledge and in some areas of recall. Whether triazolam causes greater memory impairment than other benzodiazepines is still unclear (Scharf, Fletcher, and Graham, 1988; Rothschild, 1992). Most importantly, however, the amnestic effects are completely reversible, disappearing after the medication is eliminated from the brain.

Soon after starting benzodiazepines, most patients will show diminished psychomotor skills (Taylor and Tinklenberg, 1987). The clinical importance of these effects is difficult to gauge, but the usual warnings to patients about driving a car or operating dangerous machinery are entirely appropriate. For most patients taking therapeutic doses of benzodiazepines on a maintenance basis, however, driving skills are not impaired (Salzman, 1993). (It is important to remember that untreated anxiety adversely affects driving skills.) When benzodiazepines are taken along with alcohol, sedation, cognitive, and psychomotor side effects are enhanced in an additive manner. Thus, one drink may feel like two (or one Xanax may feel like two) but no explosive potentiating effects (such as one drink feeling like six) occur.

Intoxication, aggressive behavior, and mania are unusual side effects that occur, albeit infrequently, with benzodiazepines. Intoxication is dose-related and should be understood in a manner similar to alcohol intoxication: a little bit will sedate, a lot will intoxicate. The presence of intoxication is a clear indication that the dose is too high and must be lowered immediately. Aggressive behavior or disinhibition has long been described as an occasional side effect of benzodiazepines. It is far less common than is supposed, probably occurring in less than 1 percent of patients treated with benzodiazepines (Dietch and Jennings, 1988). The evidence that it occurs more with one medication than another is unconvincing. Alprazolam may specifically precipitate manic episodes. It is unclear whether this is related to alprazolam's allegedly specific effect of alleviating depression. Finally, benzodiazepines can precipitate a depressive syndrome in a subset of treated patients.

Given these observations, how should therapists help counsel their patients on this issue? Because the majority of benzodiazepine prescriptions are written by primary care physicians, not psychiatrists, the therapist may be the only mental health professional involved. First, despite the potential withdrawal problems noted above, among all the psychotropic medications in current use, benzodiazepines are among the safest. Therefore, patients can be reassured that the evidence for safety and lack of tolerance to benzodiazepines' anxiolytic effects, even over years, is impressive. Second, if the benzodiazepine needs to be discontinued or if the patient desires a trial off the medication, the recommendations above will aid enormously in making this a relatively benign experience for all involved. If the primary care physician who has prescribed the medication is not familiar with the issues of benzodiazepine withdrawal, obtaining consultation with a psychopharmacologist experienced in these matters may be helpful. Third, since both anxiety and insomnia wax and wane in intensity over time, a patient's need for a benzodiazepine will also vary. Thus, if someone cannot stop the medication at one time, it is worth retrying at another time.

ZOLPIDEM

Zolpidem (Ambien), released in 1993, is the most recently released tranquilizer/hypnotic. Although related to the benzodiazepines, it is sufficiently different in both its biological effects and chemical structure to be classified separately. Zolpidem selectively binds to the benzodiazepine$_1$ receptor, in contrast to the benzodiazepines, which bind nonselectively to three receptor subtypes (Woods, Katz, and Winger, 1995). The clinical significance of the selective binding is not yet clear, but may explain zolpidem's lack of muscle relaxant and anticonvulsant properties.

Zolpidem has a rapid onset of action and a short half-life. It is marketed solely as a hypnotic and its efficacy as an antianxiety drug is untested. Typical doses are 5 to 10 mg before bedtime. A common side effect is drowsiness, with dizziness, headache, and nausea occasionally reported. Although purported not to be associated with withdrawal reactions, these have already been described in case reports (Cavallaro, Regazatti, Covelli, and Smeraldi, 1993). Most clinicians perceive zolpidem as clinically similar to triazolam—an effective short-acting rapid onset hypnotic, but whose capacity for withdrawal symptoms is still unclear.

BUSPIRONE

Buspirone (Buspar), the other first-line antianxiety agent aside from the benzodiazepines, is completely unrelated to all previous tranquilizers including the benzodiazepines. First released in 1986, it represents the only original antianxiety agent released in the last thirty-five years. Buspirone is also the first of many compounds developed as anxiolytics (and the only one currently available) that diminish anxiety through serotonergic activity as opposed to those whose mechanisms of action are through the benzodiazepine receptor and/or GABA. (I am excluding the SSRI antidepressants in this discussion, which are effective for some forms of anxiety and presumably work via serotonergic effects.)

Clinically, the predominant use for buspirone is in treating generalized anxiety disorder. In most but not all of the initial studies, buspirone was as effective as benzodiazepines in decreasing anxiety (Sussman, 1994). Anxious patients previously treated with benzodiazepines may be less likely to respond to buspirone (Olajide and Lader, 1987). Buspirone's onset of action is clearly slower than that of the benzodiazepines, with four weeks needed for a full response, although positive effects are often seen by the end of the first week.

In contrast to the benzodiazepines, buspirone is ineffective when taken on an occasional basis and is virtually nonsedating. The advantage to this, of course, is that patients taking buspirone rarely complain of feeling drugged or "spacy" in the way they often do with benzodiazepines. The drawback is that buspirone cannot be used to treat acute situational anxiety (no one carries a Buspar in his pocket in case of a stressful day!) or insomnia.

Other than in its use in generalized anxiety disorder, buspirone has been evaluated in treating a number of other disorders (Schweizer and Rickels, 1994). (See Table 11–8.) It is ineffective in treating panic disorder. There is some evidence that buspirone may have some efficacy in treating most of the other anxiety disorders including social phobia, post-traumatic stress disorder, and obsessive compulsive disorder, but not sufficiently to be considered a first-line agent for any. In treating obsessive compulsive disorder, it is almost always prescribed as an adjunctive treatment with inconsistent efficacy. Similarly, in treating depression, buspirone shows some efficacy both as a primary treatment and in an adjunctive role (Joffe and Schuller, 1993; Rickels, Amsterdam, Clary, Puzzuoli, and Schweizer, 1991). Unfortunately, it has not been systematically compared to other antidepressants and has been typically evaluated in patients with depression with prominent anxiety. Buspirone is never used as a first-line agent for depression.

A final use of buspirone is in treating agitated or aggressive behavior in patients with brain disorders such as Alzheimer's disease or other

Table 11–8
Pharmacological Uses of Buspirone

Disorder	Efficacy Rating
Generalized anxiety disorder	+++
Social phobia	+
Obsessive compulsive disorder	+
Post-traumatic stress disorder	+
Major depression	+
Aggressive behavior in brain-disordered patients	++

+++ = Definite efficacy
++ = Probable efficacy
+ = Possible efficacy

dementias, or children with developmental disabilities. Unfortunately, it has never been evaluated in treating aggressive behavior in non–brain disordered patients.

Buspirone's mechanism of action predominantly reflects its effect on the serotonin-1A receptor (Coplan, Wolk, and Klein, 1995). It does not significantly affect either GABA, the inhibitory neurotransmitter, or the benzodiazepine receptor site. The specific manner in which buspirone's clinical effects are mediated is still obscure due to multiple effects of the drug on the serotonin-1A receptor. In some ways, buspirone increases serotonergic function, while in other ways, serotonergic activity seems to be diminished. This reflects two complex phenomena. First, serotonin-1A receptors are located both presynaptically and postsynaptically (see chapter 2 for details). The effect of stimulating the presynaptic receptor is to inhibit serotonin function while stimulating the postsynaptic receptor has the opposite effect. Second, buspirone is classified as a partial agonist (at least at the postsynaptic receptor), meaning that it has less than a full effect. Overall, then, buspirone's clinical activity is the sum of a variety of effects, some of which are contradictory.

Starting doses of buspirone are 5 mg twice daily, with increases of 5 mg approximately every four days. Average daily doses are 20 to 25 mg, although some patients will do best on 60 mg daily. In treating depression, buspirone doses tend to be higher, typically ranging between 40 and 90 mg daily. Buspirone should always be given in at least two or three divided doses, since it has a short half-life and because of increased side effects one to two hours after the ingestion of a large single dose.

As noted in chapter 4, however, there is a general sense among most psychopharmacologists (myself included) that buspirone is inferior to benzodiazepines in treating most anxious patients. It seems to be prescribed far more for the milder anxiety syndromes seen in primary care practices than for psychiatric patients. The reason for the disparity between clinical experience and research studies in which buspirone is consistently effective is unclear, but it may reflect inadequate dosing or difficulty in waiting the two to four weeks for the drug to work. Additionally, many patients treated with buspirone have taken benzodiazepines in the past and may expect sedation (seen with benzodiazepines but not with buspirone) as part of an antianxiety drug.

Why then is there so much interest in this drug? The answer lies in its side effect profile: the problems it doesn't cause that benzodiazepines do. More than any other single factor, the key attraction of buspirone is that it has no potential for addiction or dependence. Because buspirone lacks an immediate clinical effect, it also has no intrinsic reinforcing properties and is therefore at no risk for abuse. Because of this, buspirone may have a unique niche in treating anxious alcoholics (for whom benzodiazepines are relatively contraindicated) (Kranzler et al., 1994).

Buspirone also causes no withdrawal syndrome, even when discontinued abruptly after months of continual treatment (Rickels et al., 1988). Because it is not sedating to any significant degree, buspirone does not cause any decrease in either cognitive or psychomotor skills, which may translate clinically into fewer problems while learning new information and greater safety when driving a car. Moreover, in contrast to the benzodiazepines, it does not show additive sedating or discoordinating effects when taken with alcohol. Thus, one alcoholic drink with buspirone feels like one alcoholic drink.

The most common side effects of buspirone are nausea, dizziness, and occasional headaches. Side effects seem worst one to two hours after taking the medication and then generally subside. As a rule, though, buspirone is extremely well tolerated.

NONBARBITURATE SEDATIVES AND HYPNOTICS

Chronologically released midway between the barbiturates and the benzodiazepines were a group of diverse compounds that were commonly prescribed to treat anxiety and insomnia in the late 1950s and 1960s. These medications include meprobamate (Miltown), used primarily as a tranquilizer, and ethchlorvynol (Placidyl), glutethimide (Doriden), methyprylon (Noludar), ethinamate (Valmid), and methaqualone (Quaalude). The latter five were primarily considered hypnotics, although Quaaludes were frequently taken as a recreational drug in the late 1960s and 1970s. (Because of the widespread abuse with Quaaludes, it was withdrawn from the market and is now unavailable in the United States.) Initially, these drugs were thought to be a major advance over the barbiturates in both lack of addictive qualities and safety in overdose. Unfortunately, they were neither to any significant degree. They are addictive, with the capacity to cause severe withdrawal symptoms, and are lethal if taken in overdose. Because of this, once the benzodiazepines were released and became more widely used, the nonbarbiturate sedatives faded in popularity, as they should have. Currently, there is no good reason to prescribe any of these medications as a first-line drug for anxiety or insomnia unless the patient, usually older, has used it safely and effectively without problems in the past. Otherwise, these medications should be left to the history books.

The oldest hypnotic (other than alcohol), available since 1869 and still used with some regularity, is chloral hydrate (Noctec). Because its half-life is relatively short, it has some utility as a sleep-inducing agent in doses of 1 to 2 grams. It is not nearly as safe as many people assume, with the possibility of a lethal overdose if only 5 to 10 times the therapeutic dose is ingested. Chloral hydrate can also produce physical dependence as exemplified by the number of people addicted to it early in the century.

BARBITURATES

The barbiturate sedatives and hypnotics dominated the treatment of anxiety and insomnia from the early part of this century until twenty-five years ago. There are still some medical and psychiatric uses for the barbiturates. Phenobarbital is commonly prescribed for the treatment of seizure disorders while some short-acting types, such as thiopental (Pentothal) are used as anesthetics. Amobarbital (Amytal) has long been used to help diagnose catatonic states. Patients in catatonic states who are given amobarbital intravenously will often "wake up," respond to questions appropriately, and give information on their thought processes (which often include psychotic experiences.) Once the drug wears off, the patient typically lapses back into catatonia. Thus, the technique is much more helpful diagnostically than therapeutically. Because catatonic states seem to be less common than in the past, this use of barbiturates is now unusual. Similarly, amobarbital is used, albeit rarely, as a "truth serum" to recover repressed memories after traumatic events. As with its use in catatonic states, the medication seems to decrease the frozen state of either repression or catatonia by causing short-lived relaxation. Unfortunately, the veracity of memories recovered in this manner is clinically and medicolegally suspect. This technique should therefore be used cautiously and sparingly, if at all. The last current use of barbiturates is to sedate an acutely agitated inpatient who is behaviorally dangerous. Even in this way, however, amobarbital has generally been replaced by lorazepam which is similarly effective but safer.

In the treatment of anxiety and insomnia, barbiturates have appropriately fallen into disfavor since the introduction of the benzodiazepines. A number of different barbiturate preparations—amobarbital, burabarbital (Butisol), mephobarbital (Mebaral), pentobarbital (Nembutal), and secobarbital (Seconal)—are still available. They are highly addictive, cause severe and potentially fatal withdrawal syndromes, and are easily fatal if taken in overdose. As with the nonbarbiturate sedatives, the only reason they are prescribed at present is for the rare patient who has used them in the past with success and does not need them on a regular basis.

L-TRYPTOPHAN AND MELATONIN

Certainly the most natural sleep-inducing agent is l-tryptophan, an essential amino acid that is ultimately converted to the neurotransmitter serotonin. Because of its nonprescription status, pharmaceutical firms have had no incentive to fund research on l-tryptophan and there are few good studies on its efficacy and safety. It does seem to be an effective hypnotic, generally in doses of 1 to 5 grams, although it may not be quite as effective as the benzodiazepines (Hartmann, 1977). If taken in excessive quantities, it is safe and causes neither physical dependence nor withdrawal symptoms. Its major drawbacks are high cost and large pill size. Unfortunately, l-tryptophan was removed from the market in 1990 because of severe and sometimes fatal allergic reactions, called the eosinophilia-myalgia syndrome. Most of these reactions were found to be caused not by l-tryptophan itself, but by impurities present in one manufacturer's batch (Belongia et al., 1990). Yet l-tryptophan is still unavailable, except as part of multi–amino acid preparations.

More recently, melatonin, a hormone secreted by the pineal gland, has developed a reputation as an effective hypnotic. (Given its role in regulating the body's response to light/dark cycles, it may also aid in diminishing jet lag.) Unfortunately, given the paucity of good research into such issues as optimal dosage, likelihood to cause side effects, especially when taken at the greater than physiologic doses in which it is sold, and long-term effects, melatonin's proper place among available hypnotics is unclear.

ANTIHISTAMINES

Medications such as hydroxyzine (Atarax or Vistaril) and diphenhydramine (Benadryl) are antihistamines that are primarily used in the treatment of allergic conditions. Because they are also sedating, they are occasionally used as hypnotics or, more rarely, as daytime antianxiety agents. They are more sedating than tranquilizing and not nearly as effective as benzodiazepines. However, they show no capacity to be addictive and are therefore occasionally prescribed for alcoholics for whom the risk of addiction to other tranquilizers is high. Other than drowsiness, the major side effects of the antihistamines are anticholinergic effects such as dry mouth, constipation, urinary hesitation, and possibly confusion if taken in too high a dose, especially by an elderly patient. Many of the over-the-counter sleeping aids contain antihistamines.

CLONIDINE

Clonidine (Catapres) was initially prescribed as a treatment for hypertension. However, because its mechanism of action is to decrease the activity of norepinephrine in the central nervous system, it has been investigated in the treatment of a variety of psychiatric conditions. Its most well-documented psychiatric use is in diminishing withdrawal symptoms from opiates, such as heroin (Bond, 1986). Although it decreases the adrenergic hyperactivity seen in opiate withdrawal, it is less effective in diminishing insomnia, muscle aches, and drug craving. Another established use for clonidine is in the treatment of Tourette's disorder, the childhood syndrome characterized by tics (see chapter 8) (Coffey, Miguel et al., 1994). A third, more recent use of clonidine has been in treating children with attention deficit/hyperactivity disorder (ADHD). Clonidine may be most effective for those ADHD children with motorically aggressive and impulsive behaviors, and/or those with comorbid tics (Green, 1995). It is rarely prescribed for treating panic disorder and generalized anxiety. Although it seems to be beneficial for some patients, its therapeutic effects are limited by sedation, hypotension (low blood pressure), fatigue, and the development of tolerance to its antianxiety effects (Uhde et al., 1989). When prescribed for adults, it is started at a dose of 0.1 mg twice daily, increasing every two to four days up to 0.6 to 0.7 mg daily. Higher doses than these are unlikely to yield greater benefit.

BETA-BLOCKERS

Beta-blockers are a group of medications used in general medicine for a variety of disorders, including angina, hypertension, and migraine headaches, that are also effective psychopharmacological agents. The most commonly prescribed beta-blockers in psychiatry are propranolol (Inderal) and atenolol (Tenormin). With the possible exception of their use in performance anxiety, they are not first-line drugs for psychiatric disorders. Nevertheless, they are often useful.

Three different anxiety disorders are sometimes treated with beta-blockers. For many years, either propranolol or atenolol has been prescribed for performance anxiety (Liebowitz, Gorman, Fyer, and Klein, 1985). Because performance anxiety is both intermittent and predictable, the medication is typically prescribed on an as-needed basis. When used for generalized anxiety, propranolol is less effective than the benzodiazepines and is therefore rarely used as a first-line agent. Propranolol may be more effective in diminishing the physical symptoms of anxiety, such as fast heartbeat and sweaty palms, than the psychological and subjective components. Similarly, propranolol is probably effective for only a small group of patients with panic disorder and far inferior to the other available treatments (Noyes, 1985).

More common is the use of beta-blockers to decrease medication side effects characterized by excessive movement. Tremors induced by lithium and by the more stimulating antidepressants are effectively treated by propranolol on either an as-needed basis or with continual use. Propranolol also successfully decreases akathisia, the motor restlessness caused by antipsychotic agents (Fleischhaker, Roth, and Kane, 1990). For this purpose it is prescribed either alone or in combination with anticholinergic medications.

Propranolol is intermittently prescribed to treat aggressive outbursts associated with a variety of disorders, including dementias, personality disorders, and disinhibition secondary to brain injuries (Haspel, 1995). Less commonly, beta-blockers are prescribed for treatment-resistant schizophrenia (typically administered in extraordinarily high doses) (Lader, 1988).

The presumed mechanism of action of beta-blockers is by decreasing some of the effects of the neurotransmitter norepinephrine, through blocking the beta-adrenergic receptor. (As noted in chapter 2, each neurotransmitter has a number of different receptor types.) All conditions for which the beta-blockers are helpful are characterized by some degree of heightened arousal, either physical or psychological. What is not clear is whether these medications work in the central nervous system, at the nerve endings throughout the rest of the body, or both.

Doses of the beta-blockers depend on the disorder being treated. For performance anxiety, taking propranolol 20 to 40 mg or atenolol 50 mg one hour before the anxiety-producing event is sufficient. In treating panic or generalized anxiety, propranolol 40 mg is typically prescribed, given in two to four divided doses, gradually increasing by 40 mg every four days up to 160 mg. Doses for treating either lithium-induced tremor or akathisia tend to be lower, typically 20 to 60 mg daily, with half the dose given every twelve hours.

The most common side effects of the beta-blockers are lightheadedness, dizziness, and fatigue (Noyes, 1985). It is generally thought that the sluggishness/fatigue symptoms are more common with beta-blockers that cross into the brain more easily, such as propranolol. Depressive symptoms have been reported to occur with propranolol, especially at doses over 100 mg daily.

IN THE FUTURE

Medications that are being actively investigated as anxiolytics reflect the more recent understanding of the biology of anxiety and the diversity of ways to decrease it. In reviewing the tranquilizers of the future, however, it is important to remember that many agents look promising early in development. Only a small number ultimately get released, due to a number of factors. Some are shown to be associated with toxic side effects; others show less efficacy than hoped for, while others are not released because they are unlikely to fill a specific niche and will not be profitable. Thus, the exact future of any of the compounds mentioned here is unknown.

One series of antianxiety compounds currently being evaluated are benzodiazepine partial agonists which, as noted above, bind to the benzodiazepine receptor but with less than full effect. Theoretically, this results in less sedation, less dependence, and fewer psychomotor effects. Agents of this class include abecarnil, bretazenil, and zopiclone.

A second class of investigational agents are those related to buspirone by being serotonin-1A partial agonists. No one agent of this class seems to be near release.

The third class of promising antianxiety agents are serotonin-3 antagonists, some of which are already available. Ondasetron (Zofran), already available as an antiemetic (to decrease nausea and vomiting), is the most actively investigated of these medications.

12

Antipsychotics

IN 1952, the treatment of schizophrenia and other psychotic disorders shifted course forever when chlorpromazine (Thorazine) was demonstrated to be effective in dramatically decreasing psychotic agitation. Within a few years, it became clear that chlorpromazine could significantly decrease psychotic thinking with or without agitation. With these discoveries, the road to transforming what had been a group of hospital-based disorders into outpatient disorders with only intermittent hospitalizations was opened. From the 1950s until 1990, over a dozen other antipsychotic drugs were developed and released, all of which are as effective as chlorpromazine for treating psychotic states. Unfortunately, none demonstrated greater efficacy than chlorpromazine. Once the initial glow of the antipsychotics waned, it became obvious to clinicians and researchers alike that these medications were simultaneously invaluable and inadequate. In treating schizophrenia, the most severe of the psychotic disorders, although psychotic symptoms were controlled in the majority of patients, other disabling symptoms were less affected. In addition, psychotic relapses, although diminished by antipsychotics, still occurred with regularity in treated schizophrenic patients. Furthermore, the side effects associated with the antipsychotics became more apparent with continued use. These included both acute side effects that caused subjective discomfort and were associated with medication noncompliance, and tardive dyskinesia, the potentially irreversible movement disorder caused by the long-term use of antipsychotics.

Then, in 1990, when clozapine was released as the first antipsychotic that differed biologically and clinically from all other agents, the second era of antipsychotic medications began. With other atypical antipsychotics either already released or likely to be available within the next decade, much of the sense of stalled progress in the treatment of psychosis has been replaced by modest hope and optimism.

HISTORY

Prior to 1952, no medications available in Western medicine had any major effect in treating either the profound agitation or the psychotic thinking of schizophrenia. (Interestingly, before this time, in India the rauwolfia plant had been successfully used to tranquilize patients suffering from mental disorders. In fact, the word tranquilizer was first used to describe the effect of the active ingredient of rauwolfia, reserpine, later marketed as the first antihypertensive and notable for causing depression in some patients) (Bein, 1970). Before then, insulin coma, cold packs, and electroconvulsive treatment (ECT) were the only treatments available.

Chlorpromazine was first investigated as a potentially sedating and hypothermic (decreasing temperature) medication for use in surgery (Deniker, 1970). Following the documentation of chlorpromazine's efficacy in schizophrenia, a number of similar compounds were released, all of which had similar antipsychotic properties. This was hardly surprising since the new compounds were first synthesized by altering the structure of chlorpromazine slightly and testing for similar effects. Other antipsychotics that were not structurally similar to chlorpromazine were tested because of their similar biological and behavioral effects in animals. Some of these antipsychotics, though, had notably different side effects. As an example, haloperidol, first released in Europe in 1958, was noted to be far less sedating than chlorpromazine but also caused far more Parkinson's disease-like side effects, such as stiffness and restlessness.

Unfortunately, the testing of new compounds based on similarity to older ones in either chemical or clinical effects frequently results in a generation of "me too" drugs that do not offer new approaches in pharmacotherapy. This was the case in the field of schizophrenia research where antipsychotics were screened in animal models for their ability to cause dopamine-blocking effects similar to existing medications. Interrupting this trend, and offering a genuinely new option, clozapine was released in the United States in 1990. Accidentally discovered in the 1950s while searching for a benzodiazepine-like tranquilizer, clozapine was found to be an effective antipsychotic that was relatively devoid of typical antipsychotic side effects. Then, following the deaths of a number of clozapine-treated patients in Finland in 1975 because of agranulocytosis (lack of white blood cells to fight infection), clozapine was less aggressively investigated. However, the positive experience generated by the earlier trials and general dissatisfaction with conventional antipsychotics resulted in further research. These later studies indicated that, compared to conventional antipsychotics, clozapine was more effective in treatment-resistant psychotic patients, was associated with a unique side effect profile, and had very different neurotransmitter effects. This latter point helped spur further investigation into other agents that did not simply mimic the dopamine-blocking effects of conventional antipsychotics but had more complex activities affecting dopamine and serotonin in a variety of ways, similar to clozapine. The ongoing second era of antipsychotics is dominated by investigation into these new medications that are qualitatively distinct from the older agents, promising fewer side effects, better patient compliance, and enhanced efficacy. The use of the newer antipsychotics for disorders other than schizophrenia is in its infancy, but will be an inevitable direction of clinical research in the next decade.

CLINICAL USES

The use of the term *antipsychotics* and not *antischizophrenics* correctly suggests these medications' broad pattern of clinical efficacy. (These medications are also called neuroleptics, a word coined by the early French researchers meaning "that which takes the neuron.") They are at least somewhat helpful in treating any disorder in which psychotic thinking is prominent. For schizophrenia, in which the psychotic symptoms are central, neuroleptics are vital. For other disorders in which psychotic thinking plays a lesser role, these medications can be useful but generally in a more adjunctive role. Antipsychotics are also beneficial in some disorders in which overt psychotic thinking is not present. The best example of this is nonpsychotic mania. The exact mechanism of action by which antipsychotics effectively treat nonpsychotic disorders is not known but presumably relates to some combination of dopaminergic and serotonergic effects. Table 12–1 lists the disorders for which antipsychotics are most appropriately prescribed.

Schizophrenia is unquestionably the most important and most common disorder for which antipsychotics are prescribed. In groups of patients, all antipsychotics except clozapine are equally effective in treating schizophrenia, although there are numerous anecdotes of one medication being more effective than the others in a particular individual (Kane and Marder, 1993). As noted above, clozapine is more effective than other antipsychotics for treatment-resistant schizophrenia (Kane, Honigfield, Singer, Meltzer, and the Clozaril Collaborative

Table 12–1
Disorders for Which Antipsychotics Are Useful

Disorder	Efficacy Rating
Schizophrenia	+++
Schizoaffective disorder	++
Mania	+++
Psychotic depression	++
Borderline personality disorder	++
Dementia, including Alzheimer's disease	+
Tourette's syndrome	++
Drug-induced psychoses	+

+++ = Definitive efficacy
 ++ = Probable efficacy
  + = Possible efficacy.

Study Group, 1988). The antipsychotics show clear efficacy in both treating an acute schizophrenic episode, causing a marked decrease in psychotic experiences such as delusions and hallucinations, as well as reducing diffuse and loose thought processes. They are also very effective in decreasing relapse rates of schizophrenia when they are prescribed as a maintenance treatment (Gilbert, Harris, McAdams, and Jeste, 1995). Chapter 5 provides more details on these effects.

Schizoaffective disorder is also commonly treated with antipsychotics (Keck, McElroy, Strakowski, and West, 1994). In acute schizoaffective disorder, bipolar type, the antipsychotics may be prescribed alone but frequently are combined with mood stabilizers. Schizoaffective disorder, depressed type, is typically treated with antipsychotics in conjunction with antidepressants, although antipsychotics are sometimes prescribed alone. All antipsychotics are likely to be effective in treating schizoaffective disorder. Recently, increasing numbers of patients with refractory schizoaffective disorder are being successfully treated with clozapine (Frankenburg and Zanarini, 1994).

Acute mania is another condition for which antipsychotics are frequently prescribed. Haloperidol is probably the most commonly prescribed neuroleptic for mania, in part because its relative lack of sedation allows higher doses before somnolence becomes a problem. Because of this, acutely manic patients in hospital are frequently treated with astonishingly high doses of haloperidol. Since there is no evidence that very high doses are better than moderate doses, the high doses mostly reflect the need to do something—anything—to diminish the symptoms of an acute frenzied mania. All neuroleptics are likely to be effective in treating acute mania.

Warnings abound in the psychiatric literature about the risks of using antipsychotics in the maintenance treatment of bipolar disorder, primarily because of the possibility of tardive dyskinesia (Sernyak and Woods, 1993). Nonetheless, there are some patients who need maintenance neuroleptics along with a mood stabilizer like lithium for the optimal control of symptoms. Unfortunately, other patients are treated with maintenance antipsychotics without first being tried off the medications following the acute episode. Antipsychotics should be prescribed for maintenance treatment in bipolar disorder only after unsuccessful attempts have been made to discontinue the drug and other treatments have been considered.

Antipsychotics are frequently used to treat psychotic depression (major depressive episode with psychotic features in DSM IV) typically in combination with an antidepressant since this combination is the most effective pharmacotherapy (Spiker et al., 1986). Because the risk of tardive dyskinesia is very small during the first six months of antipsychotic treatment, this is not a major concern in treating an acute depression.

Over the last decade, a number of studies have demonstrated the efficacy of antipsychotics in treating patients with borderline personality disorder (Gitlin, 1995a). The majority of these studies show that antipsychotics diminish anxiety, depressed mood, hostility, and the transient psychotic symptoms occasionally seen in these patients. The doses prescribed are significantly lower—typically 20 to 50 percent of the usual dose—compared to those given to overtly psychotic patients with schizophrenia and/or mania. A variety of antipsychotics have been used in these studies, suggesting that all are likely to be equally effective. The antipsychotic is often prescribed when the patient is experiencing a time of either overwhelming affect, increased behavioral outbursts (such as self-mutilation, suicidal gestures) that are seemingly uncontainable by psychotherapeutic means alone, or when the patient is becoming fragmented under stress. The usual warnings about tardive dyskinesia apply, thereby suggesting the more intermittent short-term use of antipsychotics in these patients.

Demented patients, such as those with Alzheimer's disease, can be helped somewhat by the judicious use of antipsychotic medications (Raskind, 1995). They are prescribed for two reasons. The first is to diminish the paranoia, delusions, and hallucinations that are sometimes seen in these patients. When used in this way, the antipsychotics, if prescribed carefully and in low dose (and sometimes very low dose), may be helpful. The second reason is to control behavior in an agitated, difficult-to-manage patient. Unfortunately, the efficacy of neuroleptics in treating demented patients for either of these reasons is modest and the dangers—sedation, falls resulting in broken hips, usual antipsychotic side effects, and tardive dyskinesia—are substantial. Doses used are often excessive and attempts to stop the antipsychotic medications are uncommon. When antipsychotics are used in treating demented patients, the high-potency types such as haloperidol (Haldol) are preferred in order to avoid the excessive sedation seen with lower-potency agents. The antipsychotics have no effect on the core cognitive dysfunction of the dementia or on the progression of the disease.

Antipsychotics are the most common pharmacological agents used in the treatment of Tourette's syndrome, a disorder typically arising in childhood and characterized by tics and other involuntary movements as well as obsessive and compulsive symptoms and attention deficit symptoms in some patients (Coffey et al., 1994). Among the antipsychotics, haloperidol and pimozide (which is rarely prescribed except in Tourette's syndrome) are used the most, although fluphenazine may also be prescribed. The doses prescribed are tiny compared to typical antipsychotic doses. Unfortunately, even at low doses, the usefulness of the medications is limited by both side effects and partial responses. Tardive dyskinesia is a risk with long-term use of the medication, especially since Tourette's is unquestionably a lifelong disorder and the treatment needs to be considered in terms of years. The risk is mitigated somewhat by the low doses prescribed and the possibility of intermittent therapy.

Occasionally, antipsychotics are used in the treatment of drug-induced psychoses (Grinspoon and Bakalar, 1986). Most commonly, the medication is prescribed to decrease the psychotic symptoms of drug-induced psychoses caused by phencyclidine (PCP), LSD, or amphetamines. If psychopharmacological treatment is needed (and preferentially, the patient should be treated without medications), antipsychotics can be helpful. The nonsedating, low anticholinergic medications, such as haloperidol or fluphenazine are preferable because they will have the fewest side effects that may interact with the effects of the initial drug. There is some controversy about prescribing antipsychotics to treat PCP-induced psychosis, but they are commonly used. Antipsychotics should *not* be used for treatment of withdrawal syndromes from drugs such as benzodiazepines, barbiturates, or alcohol, even though psychotic symptoms may arise.

Finally, antipsychotics are occasionally prescribed in the treatment of profound generalized anxiety. This is not a generally recommended approach, especially since other antianxiety agents that do not cause tardive dyskinesia are available. Additionally, anxious patients become easily psychologically dependent on medication and changing them to another drug may be very difficult.

BIOLOGIC EFFECTS

The central scientific observation which ultimately led to the dopamine hypothesis of schizophrenia is that all effective conventional antipsychotics decrease the activity of the neurotransmitter dopamine. Furthermore, the older antipsychotics all decreased dopamine activity in the same way—by blocking the dopamine receptor. (There are other ways to decrease dopamine activity. For instance, reserpine works by depleting the dopamine stores in the neuron, not by dopamine blockade.) With the discovery of multiple dopamine subreceptors, it became clear that the specific blockade of the dopamine-2 (D_2) receptor was the important factor in antipsychotic activity (Seeman, 1992). (See chapter 2 for more details.) Of course, the truth of these two central findings—that all antipsychotics are antidopaminergic and that these medications are effective in decreasing psychosis—does not necessarily imply a causal link between them. This is comparable to the observation that until recently all cyclic antidepressants caused dry mouth; yet the mechanism of this side *effect*—anticholinergic blockade—is unrelated to the antidepressant effect of the medications. A more impressive piece of evidence suggesting that the dopamine blockade is related to a medication's capacity to decrease psychosis is that the clinical potency of a neuroleptic (i.e., how many milligrams are necessary to cause a clinical effect) is highly correlated with its affinity for the dopamine receptor (which in turn is a measure of how effectively it blocks dopamine) (Creese, Burt, and Snyder, 1976). Thus, a neuroleptic that is weaker in blocking dopamine may require 600 mg to exert a clinical effect whereas a more powerful dopamine blocker may show the same effect with only 5 mg.

These initial observations hid a number of major flaws in simplistically linking successful treatment of psychotic disorders—especially schizophrenia—with D_2 blockade. First, the discovery of multiple receptor subtypes has led to the observation that blockade of other dopamine receptor subtypes is also associated with antipsychotic activity, casting doubt on the specific importance of the D_2 receptor. Second, the dopamine blocking effect occurs quickly, yet the clinical effects emerge gradually over a number of weeks. This is analogous to a similar flaw in the monoamine hypothesis of depression and the mechanism of action of antidepressants. (See chapters 2 and 9.) Third, in the treatment of schizophrenia, conventional antipsychotics are inadequate drugs with many patients showing breakthrough psychotic symptoms despite treatment and negative symptoms that are poorly treated. If psychosis and schizophrenia were specifically associated with excessive dopamine, conventional antipsychotics should be more effective than they are.

Finally and most importantly, the emergence of the atypical neuroleptics has forced a major change in the dopamine hypothesis since the biochemical effects of these medications on D_2 and other receptors differ markedly from conventional agents. Whereas conventional neuroleptics have their most consistent effects on D_2 blockade, atypical agents have relatively weak D_2 blockade and stronger effects on D_1 and D_4 blockade as well as serotonin blockade. Moreover, the atypical agents—clozapine, risperidone, and others which will be released over the next few years—differ from each other almost as much as they do from conventional agents, thereby precluding easy generalizations (Gerlach and Casey, 1994).

Much of the research on the mechanism of action of the atypical antipsychotics has focused on clozapine because of its unique clinical effects and unusual side effect profile. It is still unclear which combination of clozapine's biological effects—low D_2 blockade, high D_1 and D_4 blockade, and high serotonin-2 blockade— are most relevant to its clinical effects. Of interest, many atypical neuroleptics that block the serotonin-2 receptor—clozapine, possibly risperidone, and ritanserin (which will probably not be released in this country)—seem to have an enhanced capacity to ameliorate negative symptoms of schizophrenia (Carpenter, 1995). Here too, however, a simple one-to-one correlation between serotonin-2 blockade and efficacy in treating negative symptoms is premature.

The conventional antipsychotics' ability to block dopamine also explains their most characteristic side effects—the extrapyramidal symptoms and tardive dyskinesia. As discussed in chapter 2, one of the areas that utilize dopamine as a neurotransmitter is the nigrostriatal tract—an area that is central in the regulation of movement. It is known, for instance, that Parkinson's disease, which is structurally characterized by destruction of the nigrostriatal dopamine neurons, manifests symptoms similar to those seen as side effects of antipsychotics. The best current treatment for Parkinson's disease is l-dopa which is metabolized into dopamine and substitutes at least partially for the loss of naturally occurring dopamine. Thus, the extrapyramidal symptoms are sometimes correctly called pseudoparkinsonian symptoms or drug-induced Parkinson's symptoms.

Some of the other side effects seen with antipsychotics are caused by the effect of these medications on neurotransmitters other than dopamine (Richelson, 1984). All antipsychotics block dopamine and are therefore able to cause dopamine-blocking side effects. Yet haloperidol causes far more akinesia than does chlorpromazine. The explanation for this is found in the relative capacity of each antipsychotic to also block acetylcholine (i.e., to have anticholinergic activity). The regulation of movement as discussed above is best explained by the balance of activity between dopamine and acetylcholine and not by dopamine activity alone. Thus, increasing dopamine or decreasing acetylcholine will result in the same clinical effect. For instance, prior to the discovery of l-dopa, the most common medications used to treat Parkinson's disease were anticholinergic medications (which are still being used today). All antipsychotics block acetylcholine—but each to a different degree. An antipsychotic with low anticholinergic activity, such as fluphenazine, will cause a great many parkinsonian side effects whereas chlorpromazine, with its strong anticholinergic activity, is relatively devoid of these side effects.

Although not completely understood, the different side effect profiles of the atypical neuroleptics reflect their unique effects on neurotransmitters. Clozapine's exceedingly low rate of extrapyramidal symptoms (EPS) reflects not only its low D_2 and high anticholinergic effects, but also the effect of serotonin-2 blockade on diminishing dopamine blockade itself (Huttunen, 1995). Additionally, clozapine may have a selective effect in blocking D_2 receptors in the limbic area of the brain (where antipsychotic effects are presumably mediated) compared to the nigrostriatal area (where movements are regulated and extrapyramidal side effects are mediated), thereby causing antipsychotic activity with a relative paucity of EPS.

The positive effects of the conventional antipsychotics in treating the disorders (other than schizophrenia) listed above can be understood by their ability to decrease psychosis, arousal, and excessive movements. Whether psychosis is present or not, mania is certainly characterized by increased arousal which can be diminished by antipsychotics. Similarly, the capacity of these medications to have beneficial effects with borderline personality patients in times of crisis or fragmentation can be understood as decreased arousal or psychosis or both. Antipsychotics are effective in Tourette's syndrome in large part because of their ability to reduce movements, possibly in the same area that is involved in Huntington's and Parkinson's diseases.

Risperidone and clozapine have just recently been prescribed for nonschizophrenic disorders, often with excellent results. Given the different biochemical profile of these newer medications, if the initial positive results are borne out in future observations, it may further aid in our understanding of how antipsychotic medications are helpful in such a diverse group of disorders.

Among the drug-induced psychoses, the effect of the antipsychotics in reducing symptoms is best understood for stimulants such as cocaine and amphetamines. These drugs exert their clinical effects by releasing and blocking the reuptake of dopamine and norepinephrine. Therefore, dopamine blockers are extremely effective in decreasing the symptoms of amphetamine psychosis. PCP is less well understood. It unquestionably has some dopamine-like activity similar to amphetamines, but it has a host of other biochemical effects as well. Dopamine blockers are therefore less reliably effective in treating PCP psychoses compared to amphetamine-induced states. Although LSD is thought to exert its effects primarily through serotonergic mechanisms, it also enhances dopamine activity as well. A general effect on diminishing arousal may be the best current explanation for the capacity of the antipsychotics to treat PCP and LSD psychoses.

CHOOSING AN ANTIPSYCHOTIC

Table 12–2 shows the currently available antipsychotics, their trade names, and general dosage ranges. As noted above, with the exception of clozapine they are all equally effective for treating most psychotic states.

The first and simplest system for classifying antipsychotics distinguishes between conventional neuroleptics (which includes the vast majority of the currently available agents) and the novel or atypical neuroleptics, of which only two—clozapine and risperidone—are currently available. The distinction of conventional vs. atypical antipsychotic divides the neuroleptics by presumed mechanism of action: D_2 blockade vs. the more complicated effects of atypical agents. As noted above, however, this classification will quickly become obsolete in the future when other atypical agents are released, since they themselves differ from each other in their biological effects.

A second and important classification system, shown in Table 12–2,

Table 12–2
Antipsychotics[a]

Generic Name (Trade Name)	Usual Dosage Range (mg/day)
Low Potency	
Chlorpromazine[c] (Thorazine)	100–600
Mesoridazine[c] (Serentil)	50–300
Thioridazine (Mellaril)	100–600
Middle Potency	
Loxapine[c] (Loxitane)	10–100
Molindone (Moban)	10–100
Perphenazine[c] (Trilafon)	8–64
Thiothixene[c] (Navane)	5–50
Trifluoperazine[c] (Stelazine)	5–50
Trifluopromazine[b,c] (Vesprin)	—
High Potency	
Droperidol[b,c] (Inapsine)	—
Fluphenazine[c] (Prolixin)	2–30
Haloperidol[c] (Haldol)	2–30
Novel Antipsychotics	
Clozapine (Clozaril)	200–600
Risperidone (Risperdal)	2–16
Long-Acting Injectable	
Fluphenazine (Prolixin Decanoate)	6.25–25 every two weeks
Haloperidol (Haldol Decanoate)	25–100 every four weeks

[a]Procholperazine (Compazine) and pimozide (Orap) are also antipsychotics but are virtually never used to treat psychotic states.
[b]Droperidol and trifluopromazine available *only* as an injectable medication for inpatients.
[c]Available in short-acting injectable form.

divides conventional neuroleptics into subgroups based on their potency (the number of milligrams needed for therapeutic efficacy) and side effect profiles. (For a variety of reasons, the atypical neuroleptics cannot be classified using this system.) Those in one group, called the low-potency antipsychotics, cause a great deal of sedation and result in relatively few extrapyramidal symptoms (EPS). Others, grouped as high-potency, are prescribed in small doses, are relatively nonsedating, and frequently cause EPS. Still others, of course, are in the middle. Since high-potency antipsychotics are similar to each other, as are the low-potency drugs, it is not necessary to be familiar with all the antipsychotics. Typically, a skilled psychopharmacologist will be very familiar and experienced with three or four conventional neuroleptics and use the others only rarely. I, for instance, prescribe thiothixene and perphenazine a great deal as a middle-potency medication, acknowledging that trifluoperazine would work just as well with the same general side effects.

Another not very useful classification divides the conventional antipsychotics by their chemical structures, since they belong to a number of different chemical classes, one of which has three subclasses. Knowing which medication is an aliphatic phenothiazine (chlorpromazine) and which is a thioxanthene (thiothixene) may make for polysyllabic sentences but will not be of help in making practical clinical decisions. Ignore these classifications.

Many of the commonly prescribed antipsychotics are available in short-acting injectable forms, typically administered intramuscularly (IM) to patients who are acutely psychotic, dangerous, and/or refuse oral medications. Neither of the atypical agents is available in an intramuscular preparation. As a general rule, when given intramuscularly, the antipsychotic dose is half the oral dose for the same desired clinical effect since IM medication is not metabolized as quickly.

The two available long-acting injectable preparations are appropriate therapeutic options only in the maintenance treatment of schizophrenia. These medications are usually administered deep in the buttocks (less commonly in the arm) and work by releasing the antipsychotic gradually over many weeks. The long-acting antipsychotics are listed in Table 12–2 with their approximate dosage ranges.

In order to decide which antipsychotic to prescribe, the most important considerations are the patient's past experience and potential side effects. Patients who hate haloperidol because they experienced terrible side effects when they took it previously should be given a different antipsychotic. If, for instance, the side effect was severe EPS, a lower-potency drug such as trifluoperazine or thiothixene can be prescribed. If side effects are not the reason for the patient's aversion to a particular medication (as might be the case if the negative feelings about medication are a displacement from his feelings of shame about being psychotic and hospitalized the year before), a different medication that is pharmacologically similar can be employed. A reasonable substitute for haloperidol might be fluphenazine which is, in many ways, indistinguishable. If weight gain has been a significant problem with antipsychotics in the past, molindone, which is least likely to cause this side effect, can be prescribed.

Atypical Antipsychotics

Atypical or novel antipsychotics can be broadly defined as those medications that effectively treat psychosis without the typical extrapyramidal side effects that are consequences of strong D_2 blockade. All atypical agents currently available or likely to be released in the near future share some combination of D_1, D_4, and serotonin-2 blockade with variable effects on D_2.

Risperidone is the most recently released of the atypical antipsychotics. Risperidone's efficacy is at least the equal of the conventional neuroleptics, with some studies showing a somewhat superior efficacy, especially in treating negative symptoms (Marder and Meibach, 1994). Unfortunately, the design of these studies makes these conclusions less than definitive. However, compared to conventional agents, in typically prescribed doses, risperidone is unquestionably associated with fewer extrapyramidal symptoms such as akinesia and akathisia. In contrast to clozapine, risperidone is not associated with life-threatening blood dyscrasias and blood monitoring is not required with its use. Therefore, in many ways, risperidone seems destined to become *the* first-line antipsychotic medication, similar to how the SSRIs have come to dominate the antidepressant world within a few years of their release. Yet, as with the SSRIs only a few years after their release (risperidone will have been available in the United States for just over two years when this book is released), there is a need for more clinical experience before risperidone's place can be more clearly defined. As an example, it is still unknown how frequently psychotic patients who have failed to respond to an adequate trial of a conventional neuroleptic (as opposed to those who cannot tolerate the older agents) will respond to risperidone. Thus, its utility in treating treatment-resistant patients is unknown. Moreover, risperidone does have side effects (see below), albeit fewer than those seen with conventional antipsychotics, that may interfere with some patients' ability to take it regularly. Finally, risperidone is far more expensive than conventional agents, introducing another complication for some patients. For now, then, risperidone should be considered a most promising new antipsychotic and should unquestionably be considered for those patients who have either not responded adequately to conventional agents or find their side effects bothersome.

In contrast, clozapine, the other available atypical antipsychotic, has achieved a more clearly defined role in treating psychosis. Because it confers the risk of life-threatening agranulocytosis (see below for details), clozapine is *never* prescribed as the first antipsychotic. The general recommendation is that clozapine should be considered for those patients who have not responded adequately to two different antipsychotics at reasonable doses for at least six weeks each. It should be considered not just for treatment-resistant schizophrenia but in treating any disorder requiring an antipsychotic and that has been poorly responsive to other agents. These include schizoaffective disorder, bipolar disorder, psychotic depression, and others (Frankenburg and Zanarini, 1994). It should also be strongly considered for those patients who are either intolerant of at least a few neuroleptics or have socially disabling tardive dyskinesia.

Because weekly blood tests are mandatory components of its treatment, clozapine can only be considered for cooperative patients who are willing to participate in a demanding therapy. Furthermore, adding the cost of blood monitoring to the cost of the medication itself makes clozapine staggeringly expensive, requiring insurance that covers its use for the majority of patients treated. However, the potential benefit is that clozapine has been clearly demonstrated as effective in a substantial percentage of those patients who have not responded adequately to other antipsychotics (Kane et al., 1988; Breier et al., 1994). Its efficacy in schizophrenia is seen in diminishing both psychotic symptoms and, in many patients, negative symptoms. For those patients whose illness has required multiple hospitalizations, clozapine may be associated with lower health care costs since the expense of the treatment is more than balanced by the savings associated with fewer days in hospital (Meltzer et al., 1993).

Many other atypical neuroleptics, each with a slightly different biological and side effect profile, are undergoing active investigation and a few may be released within the next five years. Because a number of the most promising candidates from even two years ago have now been withdrawn from consideration for a variety of reasons (e.g., remoxipride will not be released because it causes blood abnormalities without providing the kinds of clearly demonstrated benefits of clozapine that justify the risk), it is difficult to anticipate which specific medications will be available in the near future. The most likely agents, however, are olanzapine, sertindole, seroquel, and ziprasidone. Like clozapine and risperidone, all four investigational antipsychotics block serotonin-2 receptors with variable effects on D_1 and D_2 receptors. They also all seem to be associated with fewer extrapyramidal side effects compared to conventional antipsychotics (Meltzer, 1995). Some preliminary evidence suggests possible enhanced efficacy of some of these newer agents in treating negative symptoms. None have thus far been associated with blood dyscrasias.

TECHNIQUES FOR PRESCRIBING

Although except for clozapine, they are all equally effective, the antipsychotics are not equipotent. In order to solve the problem of discussing the different doses needed for equivalent responses, a uniform potency system had to be established. Since chlorpromazine was the first antipsychotic released, it was arbitrarily used as the reference drug and all other antipsychotics were compared to it. Thus, in the discussion of doses, I will occasionally refer to chlorpromazine-equivalents (CPZ-E), which is the number of milligrams of chlorpromazine equivalent to the dose of that particular antipsychotic. Table 12–3 shows the approximate potency equivalence among antipsychotics. Because of its unique role in treating treatment-resistant patients, it is not meaningful to include clozapine in this comparison. In discussing doses, this section will focus on using antipsychotics for schizophrenia. Use of these medications for treating other disorders will be described at the end of the section.

When treating acute schizophrenia with antipsychotics, the evidence is clear that optimal response is seen with a daily dose of not more than 700 mg CPZ-E (Baldessarini, Cohen, and Teicher, 1988). For most patients, this translates to optimal daily doses of haloperidol 10 to 15 mg, thiothixene 20 to 30 mg, or risperidone 4 to 8 mg. Despite this, many patients are treated with far higher doses which are not only not helpful but may ultimately cause a decreased response. (See discussion on "clinical window" below.) A reasonable way to start treatment with an acutely psychotic schizophrenic patient is by prescribing a daily dose of 200 mg CPZ-E, such as haloperidol 5 mg, thiothixene 10 mg or risperidone 2 mg. Usually, this is given initially in two or three divided doses, although the antipsychotics have long half-lives and each dose lasts for far longer than twenty-four hours. Divided doses in the initial stages of treatment may utilize the tranquilizing/sedating effects

Table 12–3
Antipsychotic Dosages Equivalence[a]

Generic Name (Trade Name)	Dosage Equivalence
Low Potency	
Chlorpromazine (Thorazine)	100
Mesoridazine (Serentil)	50
Thioridazine (Mellaril)	100
Middle Potency	
Loxapine (Loxitane)	10
Molindone (Moban)	10
Perphenazine (Trilafon)	10
Thiothixene (Navane)	5
Trifluoperazine (Stelazine)	5
High Potency	
Fluphenazine (Prolixin)	2.5
Haloperidol (Haldol)	2.5
Atypical Antipsychotics	
Clozapine (Clozaril)[b]	—
Risperidone (Risperdal)	1.5

[a]In chlorpromazine-equivalents (the number of mg of each drug equal to chlorpromazine 100 mg)
[b]Antipsychotic equivalence for clozapine is not meaningful.

of these medications which are separate from their antipsychotic effect. The dose can then be raised to the final dose over the next few days to two weeks if the patient does not begin to improve. Once the patient is stabilized on a consistent dose, the medication should be taken once daily at night. Since the effects of antipsychotics occur gradually over numbers of weeks, not dissimilar to the effects of antidepressants, there is little rationale for changing doses very frequently except, of course, to decrease side effects. If a patient is having a particularly agitated day early in treatment, an as-needed extra dose of the antipsychotic or the addition of a low-dose benzodiazepine tranquilizer can be given. To raise the daily dose with every increase in symptoms early in the course of treatment is to doom the patient to high dose treatment. This will cause more side effects but will not decrease the psychosis any faster.

Although the warnings about polypharmacy are generally correct—that there are very few reasons to combine two or more medications of the same class—there is one clinical situation in which the simultaneous use of two antipsychotics can be helpful. If a patient is gradually improving on a nonsedating antipsychotic, such as fluphenazine, but is still suffering from insomnia, it is a reasonable option to also prescribe a low dose of a sedating antipsychotic at bedtime, such as chlorpromazine 50 mg for a period of days to weeks.

Unfortunately, there are no good guidelines as to the "correct" psychopharmacological strategies to be used when a patient shows a poor response to an adequate trial of an antipsychotic at an appropriate dose. Raising the dose to much higher than 700 CPZ-E is virtually always considered. Although groups of patients will not generally respond, an occasional patient may. It is important, though, that if the higher dose is not clearly more effective than the lower dose, it should be lowered to its original level. Another important option is switching to an injectable antipsychotic in case the patient is surreptitiously not ingesting the medication or is metabolizing it unusually quickly. Switching to an atypical neuroleptic (for now, risperidone) if a conventional agent is the first antipsychotic prescribed or, conversely, from risperidone to a conventional neuroleptic is another reasonable option. No data exist as to the success rate of this approach. Switching from one conventional agent to another may also be considered but is generally ineffective (Kinon et al., 1993).

Finally, as noted above, those patients who are truly unresponsive to at least two neuroleptics given for six weeks each and those who could not tolerate multiple neuroleptics should be considered for a clozapine trial. Clozapine should be started at a dose of 12.5 to 25 mg twice daily, increasing gradually to 300 to 500 mg daily over two to five weeks.

When switching antipsychotics from one subtype to another—for example, from a conventional agent to risperidone or from any agent to clozapine—it is vital that the transition be accomplished slowly over many weeks, not days. Rapid switching of antipsychotics over days is frequently associated with dramatic relapse, partly related to the withdrawal of a partially effective medication before the new one has had time to take effect.

If maintenance, preventive treatment is appropriate, the appropriate doses used are only slightly less than those needed for acute antipsychotic treatment. The best recent estimate is that optimal prophylaxis will occur when the maintenance dose is between 300 and 600 mg CPZ-E (Baldessarini et al., 1988). As discussed in more detail in chapter 5, there may be important risk/benefit decisions to be made even within this range, with higher doses decreasing the number of exacerbations and relapses but at the cost of subtle, typically unrecognized side effects that have an adverse effect on quality of life. It would be helpful if we could just lower the dose of maintenance medication until symptoms reappear and know that this is the threshold dose. However, since the effect of maintenance treatment is primarily preventive, the dose could be lowered to subeffective levels and the relapse might not occur for many months, thereby preventing any simple understanding of a minimum effective dose.

It may be useful to think of a "therapeutic window" to help conceptualize the relationship between dose and response for both acute and maintenance treatment but especially for the latter. Figure 12–1 shows this visually. Unfortunately, blood levels of antipsychotics are neither reliable nor meaningful enough to be used clinically. The only exception to this may be clozapine, for which blood levels above 350 to 400 ng/ml are associated with a better response. Because of the overall poor relationship between plasma level and therapeutic response, Figure 12–1 substitutes dose for blood level. For each patient, at some point on the curve, raising the dose will make the patient worse, gener-

Figure 12–1   Dose/Response Relationship for Antipsychotics in Schizophrenia

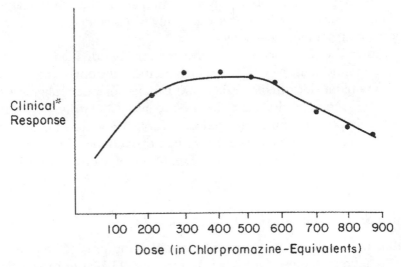

Clinical* Response

Dose (in Chlorpromazine-Equivalents)

*-Measured by symptoms in acute treatment of lack of relapse in maintenance treatment

ally not by increasing psychosis but by increasing depression or lack of motivation or anxiety or emotional withdrawal. It is vital for all therapists who treat schizophrenic patients to look for evidence of the toxic effects of treatment since they are usually more subtle than the therapeutic effects.

All of the statements made above apply equally when antipsychotics are prescribed for schizoaffective disorder, mania, or psychotic depression. Because of the astonishing energy seen in hospitalized manic patients, prodigious doses of antipsychotics are often prescribed, sometimes up to 3,000 mg CPZ-E (or haloperidol 60–70 mg) or more. Patients with borderline personality are usually treated with lower doses, typically in the range of 50 to 200 mg CPZ-E. Antipsychotic doses used to treat Alzheimer's patients are much smaller than those noted above. It is not unusual to see therapeutic benefit (acknowledging the limits of that benefit) at 10 to 50 mg CPZ-E. Similarly, Tourette's patients are treated with haloperidol doses of 0.5 to 5 mg daily (20–200 mg CPZ-E).

SIDE EFFECTS

The difficulties of evaluating and treating the side effects of antipsychotics are notorious. Not only are the side effects subjectively extremely distressing at times, but some of them are difficult to distinguish from the psychopathology of the disorders themselves. An added problem is that schizophrenic patients may have a particularly hard time describing side effects, especially when acutely psychotic and experiencing somatic delusions.

Antipsychotic-induced side effects can be divided into three groups: (1) the acute side effects which include dystonias, the common extrapyramidal side effects (EPS), and the neuroleptic malignant syndrome; (2) nonneurological side effects; and (3) tardive dyskinesia, which only occurs with prolonged use. Table 12–4 classifies the most common side effects typically seen with antipsychotics. Table 12–5 lists the antipsychotic classes by their likelihood of causing each of the major side effects.

Acute Side Effects

Within the group of acute extrapyramidal symptoms (EPS) are dystonic reactions, akinesia, akathisia, and tremor. The latter three side effects mimic the classic symptoms of Parkinson's disease although the

Table 12–4
Side Effects of Antipsychotics

Acute side effects
  Dystonic reactions
  Akinesia, akathisia (and tremor)
  Neuroleptic malignant syndrome
Common non-neurological side effects:
  Sedation
  Anticholinergic effects
  Postural hypotension
  Weight gain
Other non-neurological side effects:
  Sexual dysfunction
  Photosensitivity
  Gynecomastia (breast swelling)
  Retinal pigmentation (causing permanent change in vision) occurs only with
    thioridazine in doses over 800 mg daily
  Hypersalivation occurs with clozapine only
  Seizures (especially with clozapine)
  Agranulocytosis (low white blood cell count) occurs with clozapine only
Tardive dyskinesia

---

tremor is seemingly less common or milder than in typical Parkinson's disease. The prevalence of acute side effects from neuroleptics varies widely from a few percent to 90 percent, depending on the medications used, the doses prescribed, and the vulnerability of the population treated (Casey, 1993). For all EPS, the key to treatment is recognizing the symptoms as side effects from the medication and not from the psychosis, depression, or other disorders. Unrecognized neuroleptic side effects are a major cause of poor outcome and noncompliance. Additionally, the best predictor of those patients who are at highest risk for EPS is a history of these side effects when treated with antipsychotics in the past (Keepers and Casey, 1991).

Dystonic Reactions

Typically within hours to days after the beginning of antipsychotic medication, some patients will experience sudden muscle tightening, typically in the neck and/or jaw. These reactions are very frightening but rarely dangerous. They are most likely to occur in young men and in those patients taking high-potency antipsychotics (Casey, 1993).

Table 12–5
Antipsychotic Classes and Their Likelihood
to Cause Common Side Effects

Medication Class

Generic Name (Trade Name)	Side Effects			
	Extrapyramidal Symptoms (EPS)	Sedation	Anticholinergic Effects	Postural Hypotension
Low Potency	+	+++	+++	+++
Chlorpromazine (Thorazine)				
Thioridazine (Mellaril)				
Mesoridazine (Serentil)				
Middle Potency	++	+ to ++	++	++
Loxapine (Loxitane)				
Molindone (Moban)				
Perphenazine (Trilafon)				
Thiothixene (Navane)				
Trifluoperazine (Stelazine)				
High Potency	+++	+	+	+
Haloperidol (Haldol)				
Fluphenazine (Prolixin)				
Novel Antipsychotics				
Clozapine (Clozaril)	0	+++	+++	+++
Risperidone (Risperdal)	+	+ to ++	+	++

+ = Minimal
++ = Moderate
+++ = Severe

Another acute dystonic reaction is called an oculogyric crisis, in which the eyes involuntarily look toward a certain direction, typically up. If patients are instructed to look elsewhere, they can, but their eyes will gravitate back to their original position when distracted. Both the classic muscle dystonia and the oculogyric reactions can be treated quickly and effectively with diphenhydramine (Benadryl, a common antihistamine) or benztropine (Cogentin). If the dystonia is very disturbing, these antidote medications can be administered either intramuscularly or intravenously. When given intravenously, the dystonia may vanish within 30 seconds to a minute. The prophylactic use of anticholinergic medications, such as benztropine will prevent these reactions to a substantial degree (Arana, Goff, Baldessarini, and Keepers, 1988). Dystonia may occur more than once in the beginning of treatment but almost never thereafter.

Akinesia

Akinesia is the most common and most important EPS. The word literally means "without movement." In its most obvious state, akinesia is characterized by a decrease in spontaneous movement. A patient with akinesia will exhibit fewer of the natural movements that all of us spontaneously exhibit, such as crossing our legs, scratching ourselves, shifting positions in chairs, and showing random spontaneous facial expressions. When walking, akinetic patients will have less arm swing than normal, may shuffle, and will look generally stiff. The terms "masked facies" and "wooden appearance" are often used to describe these patients. When people say that someone looks like a "mental patient," they are frequently referring to medication-induced akinesia.

The description of akinesia has thus far concentrated on physical side effects. A more important group of akinetic side effects are those related to psychological symptoms such as lack of motivation and spontaneity, diminished range of affect, even lack of spontaneous thought (Van Putten and Marder, 1987). These are similar, if not identical, to some of the core features of schizophrenia—the negative symptoms. The difficulty in making an accurate diagnosis when the side effects of the treatment mimic the symptoms of the disorder being treated becomes even more pointed when trying to distinguish between post-psychotic depression and akinesia. Compounding the difficulty is the possibility of having both or all three of these potentially identical-looking syndromes—akinesia, negative symptoms, and depression. It is sometimes necessary to prescribe antiparkinsonian medications at relatively high doses as a diagnostic tool: if the symptoms are relieved, they were probably due to akinesia. If not, they were either negative symptoms or depression.

In understanding akinesia, it is helpful to remember that dopamine blocking, which is assuredly the cause of akinesia, occurs not only in the areas of the brain that regulate movement, but in areas that are involved with affect and cognition too. It should not be surprising, therefore, that in some patients, the side effects can manifest themselves in cognitive/affective slowing as well as physical slowing. In the book *Awakenings*, Oliver Sacks describes patients with post-encephalitic Parkinson's disease who existed in a frozen state for decades until they were given l-dopa (Sacks, 1983). Descriptions of their internal experiences during those years and the changes (some good, some not) after taking l-dopa help to make clear the role dopamine may play in psychological variables such as will and motivation.

Akinesia typically emerges gradually within days to a month after starting a neuroleptic with older patients at highest risk to develop it. Among conventional antipsychotics, the high-potency agents are the most likely to cause akinesia. This assuredly reflects the anticholinergic effects of the low- and middle-potency agents which partially protect against the development of akinesia. Compared to the conventional antipsychotics, the novel antipsychotics are characterized by far lower rates of akinesia: clozapine almost never causes it, and risperidone is associated with low rates of akinesia up to 6 mg daily. Above this dose, the rate of akinesia and other EPS gradually rises, probably reflecting increasing D_2 blockade at the higher doses (Marder and Meibach, 1994).

Akinesia can be treated in three ways. The most common method is to prescribe antiparkinsonian medications—either anticholinergics or amantadine (see below for details on doses)—which are very effective. Another successful approach is to lower the medication dose. If possible, this is undoubtedly the wisest strategy. Sometimes, however, the side effects disappear coincident with the disappearance of therapeutic effects, thereby precluding this strategy. The third possibility is to switch to a different antipsychotic which causes less akinesia, such as lower-potency agents or risperidone.

There is no consensus as to whether antiparkinsonian medication should be prescribed preventively in the beginning of antipsychotic treatment. The advantage, of course, is the prevention of dystonias, akinesias, and other EPS. But the antiparkinsonian medications confer their own risk of side effects such as dry mouth and constipation. For most acutely psychotic patients who are treated with at least moderate doses of middle- or high-potency neuroleptics, it is prudent to begin prophylactic antiparkinsonian drugs. EPS can be very unpleasant, and it is best to prevent patients from disliking a medication (and then refusing to take it) that may be very helpful to them. Those patients treated with either low-potency antipsychotics, risperidone, or clozapine should not routinely be given prophylactic antiparkinsonian drugs since they are less likely to be needed. In those cases in which prophylactic antiparkinsonian drugs are not prescribed (e.g., outpatients on low-to-medium doses of antipsychotics), patients should be informed about the side effects that may emerge. Sometimes, outpatients are given a prescription for the antidote medication to be taken in case these side effects occur.

Conflict also exists as to whether patients on maintenance antipsychotics need to remain on antiparkinsonian medications. Although some patients can be withdrawn from their antiparkinsonian medication during maintenance treatment without the re-emergence of akinesia, a great many cannot (Manos, Gkiouzepas, and Logothetis, 1981). My own experience is that cavalierly stopping medications like benztropine during the maintenance phase of antipsychotic treatment causes an increase in symptoms, both psychological and physical, in many patients. It is appropriate to attempt to withdraw antiparkinsonian medications occasionally. This should be done gradually and with patient, therapist, and psychopharmacologist looking for clinical changes.

Akathisia

Akathisia (literally meaning not sitting) is the other very common EPS (Sachdev and Loneragan, 1994). Although it is not as socially disabling as akinesia, akathisia is typically more uncomfortable. In its classic form, akathisia is described as a motor restlessness in which patients exhibit increased numbers of fidgety, purposeless movements. These movements typically include crossing and uncrossing the legs, rubbing the thighs repeatedly while seated, or shifting position in a chair an unusual number of times. In more severe akathisia, patients will shift continually from foot to foot while standing or seem to walk in place (Van Putten and Marder, 1987). These fidgety movements are typically done unconsciously; if they are pointed out, patients will stop the movement transiently and then resume it when distracted. Patients who exhibit the typical restless movements of akathisia but without any subjective feelings of discomfort are sometimes described as having pseudoakathisia.

Since the movements of classic akathisia are observable and differ somewhat from classic manifestations of anxiety, they are relatively easy to diagnose. What is more difficult to diagnose are the akathetic symptoms manifested purely by subjective feelings. Patients may complain of feeling jittery, restless inside, or wired, in the absence of external fidgeting. They may describe feeling unable to relax or not being able to get in a comfortable position when they try to sleep. In an extreme form, patients will note an "indescribable tension." For some of these patients, the subjective discomfort is so painful as to be associated with suicide attempts, noncompliance, and psychotic exacerbation. Even an extremely astute clinician with a great deal of experience with schizophrenic patients and antipsychotics would be hard pressed to distinguish definitively between subjective akathisia and anxiety/agitation. Further complicating the clinical picture, akathisia arises at variable times through the course of neuroleptic treatment, from within hours after the first dose to weeks later. An even more muddled situation arises when the patient is experiencing both anxiety *and* akathisia.

The cause of akathisia is not understood. Although dopamine blocking is thought to be implicated, it is likely that other biochemical systems are also involved. High-potency neuroleptics are more likely than low-potency agents to cause akathisia. As with akinesia, clozapine rarely causes akathisia, while risperidone causes it infrequently at lower doses. The same general treatment strategies used for akinesia are also helpful for akathisia—lowering the antipsychotic dose, using antidote medications, and switching antipsychotics. Antiparkinsonian drugs, however, are more effective for akinesia than for akathisia. Because of this, two other medications are sometimes prescribed to decrease akathetic symptoms. First, the group of medications known as beta-blockers, commonly used for hypertension, angina, and migraine headaches, have been shown to be effective for akathisia. Seemingly, the most effective is propranolol (Inderal) which, unfortunately, is also the most likely to cause lethargy and fatigue (Fleischhacker, Roth, and Kane, 1990). Propranolol can be used by itself or in conjunction with antiparkinsonian agents. Benzodiazepines such as diazepam and lorazepam, and clonidine, a sedating antihypertensive, are the other two types of medications that are sometimes effective in diminishing akathisia. Neither beta-blockers nor benzodiazepines are effective in treating akinesia.

Neuroleptic Malignant Syndrome

The least common and most dangerous of all neuroleptic-induced side effects is the neuroleptic malignant syndrome (NMS), the hallmarks of which are fever and muscle rigidity, typically in combination with mental status changes (e.g., confusion, stupor) and tachycardia (fast pulse). Neuroleptic malignant syndrome typically, but not exclusively, occurs soon after beginning antipsychotic treatment or after raising the dose. All neuroleptics have been reported to cause NMS, including risperidone and clozapine. The use of higher doses of neuroleptics, especially when the dose is rapidly increased, is associated with greater risk of NMS (Keck, Pope, Cohen, McElroy, and Nirenberg, 1989). The exact cause of neuroleptic malignant syndrome is unknown, although decreased dopamine transmission seems central. Once the diagnosis is made, the antipsychotic must be stopped immediately. Medical hospitalization is mandatory. General treatment approaches include decreasing temperature, keeping the patient well hydrated, and treating any intercurrent infections. If these measures are not sufficient, a number of medications have been used with some success. These include dantrolene which decreases muscle rigidity, bromocriptine or amantadine (both of which increase dopamine), and benzodiazepines. Without treatment using at least one of these specific medications, up to 20 percent of cases of NMS are fatal, a figure which is reduced to less than 9 percent with specific pharmacotherapeutic approaches (Sakkas, Davis, Janicak, and Wang, 1991). If further antipsychotic treatment following recovery is needed—as it often is—it is imperative to wait at least two weeks and, possibly, to use a low-potency antipsychotic (Rosebush, Stewart, and Gelenberg, 1989).

Non-Neurological Side Effects

The most common nonneurological side effects seen with antipsychotics are sedation, anticholinergic symptoms, postural hypotension, and weight gain. These side effects are caused by the interactions of the medications with nondopamine neurotransmitter systems, such as norepinephrine, histamine, and acetylcholine. In this way, they are similar to the tricyclic antidepressants which cause many of the same side effects. The most common nonneurological side effect is sedation. In general, the higher-potency antipsychotics, such as fluphenazine and haloperidol, are the least sedating although molindone is notably less sedating than other middle-potency medications. Among the atypical neuroleptics, risperidone is moderate in its sedating capacity, while clozapine is markedly sedating. There is some accommodation to the sedation but it is rarely complete. Thus, a patient who is initially very sedated from a specific antipsychotic may get less sedated over a period of time, but it may always be somewhat of a problem.

Like the tricyclic antidepressants, the antipsychotics can cause a cluster of side effects referred to as anticholinergic. These include dry mouth, constipation, urinary hesitation, blurry vision, and possible memory dysfunction. There is an inverse relationship between an antipsychotic's capacity to cause EPS on one hand and anticholinergic side effects on the other (Richelson, 1984). This is understandable since the major treatment for EPS is anticholinergic medication. It is as if some antipsychotics have their own built-in antidote, thereby preventing EPS but causing a great deal of dryness.

Postural hypotension refers to a drop in blood pressure upon standing up or shifting from lying to sitting. The antipsychotics most likely to cause this are the low-potency compounds and clozapine.

Weight gain can be a terrible problem with all antipsychotics except molindone. Clozapine may be more associated with weight gain than other antipsychotics. The etiology of weight gain is unknown, although appetite stimulation seems to play at least some part in it.

Sexual dysfunction of all kinds is also seen with any of the antipsychotics. Thioridazine is unusual in its capacity to cause retrograde ejaculation in men, in which the ejaculation is directed inward towards the bladder instead of toward the penis.

A number of other side effects are sometimes seen with antipsychotics (see Table 12–4). Photosensitivity, characterized by an increased sensitivity to the sun's effects, makes patients more likely to become badly sunburned. Because of this, many patients must wear sunblock, especially during the summer and in very sunny climates. Chlorpromazine is more likely to cause this side effect than are the other antipsychotics.

Clozapine's side effect profile differs substantially from those of the other antipsychotics. It is similar to the low-potency compounds in the frequency with which it causes sedation, constipation, and postural hypotension. In contrast, however, clozapine produces increased salivation. More than the other antipsychotics, clozapine is also associated with grand mal seizures, occurring in up to 10 percent of patients treated over four years (Devinsky and Pacia, 1994). One clozapine-induced seizure does not preclude further treatment but is usually handled by either lowering the dose or adding an antiepileptic medication.

The most important and dangerous side effect of clozapine, which limits its use except in treatment-refractory patients, is its capacity to cause agranulocytosis, seen in just under 1 percent of those treated, and characterized by a marked decrease in white blood cells that puts the patient at risk for life-threatening infections (Alvir, Lieberman, Safferman, Schwimmer, and Schaaf, 1993). Even with weekly blood monitoring, twelve patients have died in the first four years since clozapine was released in the United States (Kane, 1995a). Those at greater risk for agranulocytosis are older patients and women. As a consequence, clozapine can be prescribed only in conjunction with a mandatory program of weekly blood counts, so that if agranulocytosis occurs, it is discovered quickly—and the medication stopped. Because the risk of clozapine-induced agranulocytosis decreases after the first six months of use, many other countries require blood counts less frequently than on a weekly basis after that time. In the United States, however, weekly monitoring is currently required on a continuous basis.

Tardive Dyskinesia

Tardive dyskinesia (TD) is the most feared of all neuroleptic-induced side effects. And yet, it is not as dangerous as neuroleptic malignant syndrome, not as unpleasant as akathisia, generally not as socially disabling as akinesia. But all of these other side effects will assuredly disappear if the antipsychotic is discontinued. Tardive dyskinesia is the only side effect that is potentially irreversible. It is this visual spectre— of spending a lifetime with progressively worsening twitching and grimacing—that provokes the greatest fear of TD. Despite the validity of the fear—TD is a potentially irreversible disorder and may be progressive—its prognosis is far more variable than is usually appreciated by patients and clinicians alike.

TD's manifestations are varied. In the most common type, the increased movements primarily involve the face. Tongue thrusting, chewing movements, lip smacking, and eye blinking are typical. Another common version is characterized by movements of the extremities described as choreoathetoid (literally dancing without position or place). The fingers move in repetitious writhing patterns that are often extremely subtle. More severe types of TD involve the respiratory muscles, causing grunting or odd breathing patterns, or truncal dyskinesias in which the torso moves in thrusting motions. Fortunately, this last type is exceedingly unusual.

In all the TD variations, the movements are involuntary. Usually, patients will not even be aware of them. If they are pointed out, patients are typically able to suppress the movements voluntarily for a while. The movements get worse with anxiety or stress and disappear during sleep.

Less commonly, other neuroleptic-induced tardive (occurring late in the course of treatment) movement syndromes can occur. The expression of these disorders, such as tardive dystonia and tardive akathisia, is similar to the acute, nontardive types, except in their timing and potential irreversibility after neuroleptic withdrawal. Optimal treatment of these TD variants is unclear, but medications used are the same as for the acute syndromes.

It is difficult to estimate the exact prevalence of TD in patients on antipsychotics. Reasons for this include the varying definitions of TD, its waxing/waning quality, differences in the population studied, the capacity of neuroleptics to acutely suppress the movements they are causing, and so on. Rates of TD across studies range from 3 to 62 percent, with a mean of 24 percent (Yassa and Jeste, 1992). Also, some schizophrenic patients have TD-like movements not related to their medication treatment. Loose-fitting dentures, common in the elderly, will cause oral movements similar to TD. Moreover, observers in the pre-neuroleptic era described movements seen in a number of schizophrenic patients that were identical to those of TD (Fenton, Wyatt, and McGlashan, 1994). Because these movements were associated with high rates of both negative symptoms and intellectual impairment, it is assumed that they express part of the core neuropsychiatric pathology of certain schizophrenic subtypes.

TD never occurs immediately upon exposure to antipsychotics. The risk for developing its starts after a few months of treatment. The usual estimate is that the rate of new cases of TD is approximately 4 to 5 percent per year for the first five years of treatment, after which the rate of new cases per year decreases (Kane, 1995b). Older age is the single most consistent risk factor for developing TD. Other risk factors include gender (with females having higher rates) and having a non-schizophrenic diagnosis (e.g., a mood disorder).

Among medication variables, the most important risk factor is time (at least for the first five years, beyond which the effect of time is less clear). A longer time on neuroleptics is associated with higher risk of TD. Surprisingly, higher neuroleptic doses are not necessarily associated with higher TD rates. Nonetheless, virtually all psychopharmacologists assume that lower doses decrease the risk of TD to some degree. All conventional neuroleptics confer an equal risk of TD. Clozapine seems to be associated with TD only rarely if ever (Kane, Woerner, Pollack, Safferman, and Lieberman, 1993). Because it has been available for a relatively short length of time, the TD risk associated with risperidone is unknown. Theoretically, it should confer a lower risk at low dose

(6 mg daily or less) with higher TD rates at higher doses. Prescribing short "drug holidays" (stopping the antipsychotic for a few days to weeks at a time intermittently) does not decrease the risk of TD.

The most common hypothesis of TD is that it occurs because of the effect of chronic dopamine blockade in creating supersensitive dopamine receptors (Casey, 1995). It is known that when a receptor is blocked on a chronic basis (as, for instance, dopamine receptors are with the long-term use of antipsychotics), it becomes supersensitive—that is, it overreacts to whatever stimulation it receives. Thus, the acute dopamine blockade that causes akinesia (decreased movements) can, over a long time, cause tardive dyskinesia (increased movements). However, the dopamine receptor supersensitivity hypothesis is both oversimplified and inconsistent with a number of clinical and research findings. The correct explanation for TD is surely more complex and will reflect the contributions of other neurotransmitter systems in the development of abnormal involuntary movements.

The most important recent finding about TD concerns its natural history. As noted above, everyone's major fear was that not only was it irreversible but that it was progressive, that it would get worse over time. Thankfully, that is true in only a minority of cases. Even patients who stay on neuroleptics despite TD because of relapses when the antipsychotic is withdrawn will often either show an improvement or no change in the movements over the ensuing years (Gardos et al., 1994). Additionally, the severity of TD within an individual on a constant neuroleptic dose can be remarkably variable, with the movements getting worse, getting better, disappearing occasionally, and then reappearing again. For patients who can successfully lower their antipsychotic dose or discontinue the medication altogether, improvement or disappearance of the movements, even after years, is common (Glazer, Moore, Schooler, Brenner, and Morgenstern, 1994).

Even after decades of research, the proper management of tardive dyskinesia is still unclear. Without question, the most important treatment is prevention: antipsychotics should be prescribed for more than three months only for patients whose need for them is clear and well documented. Of course, since there are no treatments even remotely as effective as antipsychotics for chronic schizophrenia, the risk for TD is frequently unavoidable in these patients. Earlier use of clozapine would likely decrease TD risk; its other side effects, however (see above), preclude this as a preventive strategy. The second strategy is to use the lowest dose of medication possible. Once TD is diagnosed, the need for maintenance antipsychotics should be reevaluated. If the antipsychotic is discontinued, the TD will typically worsen temporarily as a result of the cessation of dopamine blockade (called withdrawal dyskinesia).

If the TD is mild to moderate, the patient, psychotherapist, and psychopharmacologist can discuss all risks and benefits fully and may decide together to continue treatment as is, since the risks of being off antipsychotics may be far greater than the potential social disability of the TD movements. In this decision, the variable course of TD even with neuroleptic continuation is an important factor. If antipsychotics need to be continued but the movements are significant and treatment is necessary, a remarkable array of possible treatments exist. As frequently occurs, this reflects the less than optimal efficacy of all these approaches. Paradoxically, raising the neuroleptic dose will suppress the movements since this will increase the dopamine blockade and thereby diminish the amount of dopamine available to the receptor. At the same time, though, it may simultaneously increase the risk for more long-term movements. Other treatment alternatives include beta-blockers such as propranolol, stimulants, cholinergic agents (lecithin, choline, and deanol), clonidine, benzodiazepines, valproate, verapamil, and buspirone. None are consistently effective (Gardos and Cole, 1995). A recent treatment that has gained some support is vitamin E. Theoretically, antipsychotics increase the production of potentially toxic free radicals in the basal ganglia, the area that regulates movements. The antioxidant effects of vitamin E might decrease and neutralize the toxic effects of these free radicals. Controlled studies indicate that vitamin E is safe, well tolerated, and provides a consistent but modest effect in decreasing TD movements (Dabiri, Pasta, Darby, and Mosbacher, 1994).

ANTIPARKINSONIAN MEDICATIONS

Because antiparkinsonian medications are so important in the ongoing treatment with antipsychotics, it is worth looking at the specific choice of medications available. Table 12–6 shows the names, classes, and typical dose ranges of the antiparkinsonian medications. The anticholinergic medications are the most commonly prescribed antiparkinsonian drugs. They are all probably equally effective although benztropine and trihexyphenidyl are the most popular. Trihexyphenidyl is a potentially abusable drug, possibly because of its mild stimulant effect. All of the anticholinergic drugs share the same side effects, such as dry mouth, constipation, urinary hesitation, blurred vision, and decreased memory

Table 12–6
Antiparkinsonian Medications

Generic Name (Trade Name)	Dosage Ranges (mg/day)
Anticholinergics	
Benztropine (Cogentin)	2–6
Trihexyphenidyl (Artane)	4–15
Biperiden (Akineton)	2–8
Procyclidine (Kemadrin)	7.5–20
Diphenhydramine (Benadryl)	25–100
Dopaminergic	
Amantadine (Symmetrel)	100–300

that are seen with other medications (such as the low-potency antipsy-chotics or some of the tricyclic antidepressants) with anticholinergic effects. If too high a dose of these medications is taken or if there are additive effects when they are combined with other medications that have their own anticholinergic effects, anticholinergic toxicity can result. This might be the case, for example, in a patient who is being treated simultaneously with chlorpromazine, benztropine, and amitriptyline for schizoaffective disorder, depressed type. Further, since many over-the-counter sedatives and cold remedies contain anti-cholinergic compounds, the patient could add to the risk without knowing it. Anticholinergic toxicity may be manifested by confusion, overt psychosis with visual hallucinations, incredibly hot dry skin, and very dilated pupils. (In the Renaissance, atropine, which causes signifi-cant anticholinergic effects, was used by women for the much desired and admired effect of dilated pupils, thus giving rise to the nickname for atropine—belladonna [beautiful woman].) If anticholinergic toxic-ity is present, all anticholinergic medications must be discontinued.

The only antiparkinsonian drug that is not anticholinergic is aman-tadine which is also used as an antiviral medication. It does not cause anticholinergic side effects, but in my experience is less effective than the anticholinergics. Because it is a dopamine agonist, it can aggravate psychotic thinking. Fortunately, this is rare.

13

Electroconvulsive Therapy (ECT); Stimulants

BOTH ELECTROCONVULSIVE THERAPY (ECT) and stimulants are in-frequently used treatments in modern psychiatry that are often thought of as dangerous, to be used only in desperate situations—and maybe not even then. Inappropriate use of both has certainly occurred, more in the past than recently. As with so many treatments, however, a therapy that is used incorrectly—with the wrong patients or for the wrong reasons—does not accurately reflect the qualities of the treat-ment but the need for care in its use. ECT and stimulants are impor-tant options that can be very effective in specific clinical situations. ECT, in fact, is potentially lifesaving. Although it is technically not a medication, of course, and is used predominantly with psychiatric in-patients, ECT is often considered as a treatment option for severe mood disorders. Yet because of its past abuses and the intensity of feel-ings it engenders, myths, half-truths, and accurate observations about ECT are usually presented in equal proportion when it is discussed. It is therefore vital that all therapists have at least some knowledge of ECT, its appropriate uses, and its side effects.

ECT

First used in the late 1930s, ECT is among the oldest biologic treat-ments in psychiatry still currently utilized. Starting with the premise that schizophrenia (dementia praecox as it was then called) and epilepsy were rarely seen together and might therefore be antagonistic, early researchers induced grand mal seizures in schizophrenic patients and noted some clinical response. Initially, the seizures were provoked with medications. Using electric currents to cause seizures began in 1938 and gradually replaced the medications because the new tech-nique was more reliable and controllable. It also became apparent at that time that those with severe depressions were most responsive to this new treatment. Because antidepressants, lithium, and antipsy-chotics had not yet been discovered and other effective biologic treat-

414

ments for severe psychiatric disorders simply did not exist, ECT quickly became a popular treatment—and an overused one. Despite increasing safety in its use (the risk of fractures, for example, has been virtually eliminated through the administration of short-acting muscle paralyzing medications), ECT fell into increasing disfavor because of its use and abuse as a means of behavioral control and not as a treatment of specific disorders. Several studies over the last twenty years, however, have helped reestablish ECT as an important option for severe mood disorders and in a few other clinical situations. There is no evidence that ECT is currently used to treat the underprivileged. Rather, those patients most likely to receive it are white, voluntary patients who are covered by private insurance and not by state-subsidized insurance (Thompson and Blaine, 1987). Other than race, demographic factors predicting greater ECT use are being female (probably due to the higher rate of depression in women) and being older (presumably due to ECT's excellent safety profile in medically ill patients and higher levels of medication intolerance in the elderly) (Thompson, Weiner, and Myers, 1994).

Clinical Uses

With a few uncommon exceptions, the proper use of ECT is in the treatment of major mood disorders. Table 13–1 shows the disorders and clinical situations for which ECT should be considered. All forms of major mood disorders (including all subtypes of major depression, bipolar depression, mania, and mixed states, but not including milder mood disorders) should be considered highly responsive to ECT (Fink, 1994). ECT may have a specific advantage in treating acute delusional depression in which patients are not only severely depressed but also show clear evidence of mood-congruent delusions. The case for ECT in these patients is strengthened by their relatively poor response to antidepressants (Kroessler, 1985). Unipolar and bipolar depressions are equally likely to improve with ECT (Black, Winokur, and Nasrallah, 1986). In contrast to earlier observations, melancholic (or endogenous) depressions do not show a better response to ECT compared to nonmelancholic depressions (Prudic, Devanand, Sackeim, Decina, and Kerr, 1989). Milder depressive conditions such as dysthymic disorder and adjustment disorder with depressed mood are thought to be unresponsive to ECT.

Acute mania is also responsive to ECT (Mukherjee, Sackeim, and Schnur, 1994). Since other less disruptive treatments for mania, such

Table 13–1
Disorders and Situations for Which ECT is Beneficial

Psychiatric Disorder or Situation	Efficacy Rating
Delusional depression	+++
Major depression	+++
Mania	+++
Major depression, unresponsive to antidepressants	++
Catatonia (from any cause, either psychiatric or medical)	++
Schizophrenia	+
Severe mania or depression during pregnancy	+
Depression in the context of severe medical illness	+

+++ = Definite efficacy
 ++ = Probable efficacy
  + = Possible efficacy

as mood stabilizers, are also available, ECT is infrequently used for this purpose.

Among the most common uses of ECT is in the treatment of depressed patients who have been unresponsive to antidepressants or who cannot tolerate adequate doses because of side effects. Although ECT is effective in medication-resistant patients, it is probably less effective in these patients, compared to those who have not failed at least one medication trial (Prudic, Sackeim, and Devanand, 1990). No consensus yet exists as to how many medication trials should be attempted before ECT is used. This issue is especially relevant now given the multiple antidepressant classes from which to choose. As an example, is ECT appropriate after a depressed patient fails to respond to one tricyclic? Or is failure to respond to an SSRI, a tricyclic, and an MAO inhibitor necessary? Typically, the decision is made on the basis of individual factors such as the clinical urgency of the situation.

A less common but effective use of ECT is in treating catatonic syndromes of any etiology (Fink, 1990). Catatonia is a psychomotor syndrome characterized by motor immobility, such as stupor or waxy flexibility, excessive purposeless motor activity, extreme negativism or mutism, bizarre posturing, echolalia (parrot-like repetitions of words said by others), and echopraxia (repetitive imitations of the movement of others). Catatonic symptoms may be seen in schizophrenia, mania, and severe depression as well as in neurological disorders.

Finally, acute schizophrenia is sometimes treated effectively with ECT. Because antipsychotics are very effective for these same patients,

ECT is rarely, if ever, given as a first treatment for acute schizophrenia. Possible predictors of a good response may be acute onset, and the presence of affective or catatonic features (Sackeim, Devanand, and Nobler, 1995). Chronic schizophrenia is thought to be unresponsive to ECT.

Two clinical situations for which ECT can be helpful are severe mood disturbances in patients with special medical needs, such as pregnant women or those with severe medical problems. Given the potential risk of fetal malformation from the use of medications to treat pregnant women, particularly in the first trimester when the most sensitive aspects of fetal growth occur, ECT is sometimes considered to treat severe mania or depression. In mania, frenzied activity and inattention to safety may pose a great risk to the fetus, while anorexia and risk of suicide are fetal risks in depression. (See chapter 8 for discussion of using biological treatments in pregnancy.) Because the medications used in ECT induction last no more than minutes (see below), they are less likely to be of risk than many pharmacological agents used for treating mood disorders, all of which cross into the placenta and are taken on a daily basis. With minimal alterations in the actual technique of the treatments, ECT is probably safe for both mother and fetus (Nurnberg and Prudic, 1984).

Similarly, depressed patients with medical problems for whom the side effects of antidepressants are dangerous or intolerable are candidates for ECT. Because the more recently released antidepressants such as the SSRIs, bupropion (Wellbutrin), and venlafaxine (Effexor) generally cause fewer side effects than the older ones, however, a trial of at least one antidepressant is usually undertaken before ECT is seriously considered.

Mechanisms of Action

Two central statements regarding ECT's mechanism of action can be made: First, its positive effects are related to the electrical seizure caused by the ECT, and not to the magic of the ritual involving anesthesia or from the simple passage of electricity through the brain. Second, despite decades of research into its biochemical actions and attempts to link these with those of antidepressants or other medications, the biological mechanisms by which ECT exerts its therapeutic effects are unknown.

Concerns that ECT's efficacy was due to a placebo or suggestion effect have been laid to rest by a series of double-blind studies comparing real and "sham" ECT. In these studies, patients receiving sham

ECT were given all the procedures of ECT—anesthesia, electrodes applied to the head, and so on—except that no current was passed and no seizure occurred. Without question, real ECT is more effective than sham ECT (Janicak et al., 1985). These studies and the observation that ECT worked just as well when anesthesia and muscle-relaxants were introduced (compared to the earlier more frightening and dangerous techniques in which patients were conscious until the time of the actual treatment) also refuted the belief that ECT's effectiveness was related to the sense of punishment or regression induced by the procedure.

Another early concern was that the "mind-scrambling" effect of ECT as exemplified by memory loss (see below) was the essential therapeutic ingredient. This is unlikely to be so, since memory deficits do not correlate with therapeutic response (Sackeim, 1994). Furthermore, the recent changes in ECT techniques have resulted in less memory loss without a diminishment in therapeutic efficacy.

The therapeutic effects of ECT are inherently linked to the induction of an electrical seizure in the patient, completely analogous to a spontaneously occurring seizure in an epileptic. The differences between an epileptic patient's seizure and that induced by ECT are due to the anticipated, controlled nature of the latter. During ECT, because of pretreatment with muscle relaxants, there are no muscle contractions, and because of control of breathing by the attendant anesthesiologist or nurse-anesthetist, oxygenation continues safely. In the seizures of epilepsy, both muscle contractions and lack of oxygen are potential problems.

Passing a current through the brain while blocking the creation of an electrical seizure makes ECT clinically useless, implying that it is not the current that mediates the efficacy but the seizure that is important. Consistent with this, if the amount of electricity given during an ECT treatment is insufficient, producing an incomplete seizure (termed a "missed seizure"), it is less effective. Yet the exact relationship between the electrical seizure and the therapeutic effect of ECT is more complicated than previously thought. Both the placement of the electrodes (unilateral vs. bilateral, see below) as well as the intensity of the electrical stimulus affect the efficacy of the ECT (Sackeim et al., 1993). Low-dose (of the electrical stimulus) unilateral ECT is a relatively ineffective treatment despite clear documentation of full seizures. Thus, the electrical seizure should be thought of as necessary but not sufficient for ECT to be clinically effective. The biological factors that mediate the greater efficacy with bilateral electrode placement and higher intensity of the electrical stimulus are currently unknown.

Biochemically, the effects of ECT on a variety of neurotransmitters—including those thought to be involved in mood regulation, such as norepinephrine, serotonin, and dopamine—have been investigated repeatedly. To sum up a whole body of literature, the known effects of ECT on neurotransmitters do not yield a consistent pattern of results and certainly do not help elucidate its mechanism of action (Mann and Kapur, 1994; Sackeim, Devanand, and Nobler, 1995).

Techniques of Administration

First and foremost, if the patient is competent to understand the nature of the procedure, ECT should only be given after fully informed consent, typically after far more extensive discussion than for any other procedure in psychiatry. Each state has slightly different regulations regarding the informed consent procedure and how to proceed with a legally incompetent patient. Overall, however, the vast majority of abuses of the past have been eliminated. Some hospitals even provide videotapes for patients and their families that serve to educate and demystify ECT.

ECT should be administered only by those psychiatrists specifically trained and knowledgeable in its use. Although it is administered predominantly to inpatients, it can be used with outpatients who have friends or family who can drive them to and from the hospital for treatments and stay with them for the rest of the day. Because it avoids the high cost of inpatient psychiatric hospitalization, outpatient ECT has been increasingly utilized recently. For outpatient ECT to be considered, however, the patient must not exhibit other clinical needs that would suggest the need for inpatient hospitalization such as significant suicidality or the inability to eat or care for self.

The specific number of ECT treatments given to an individual patient for a complete course of therapy varies. Typically, six to twelve treatments are effective, although some severely ill patients may require up to twenty. In the United States, ECT is typically given three times weekly, making a total course of therapy last between two and four weeks for the majority of patients (in England, twice-weekly treatment is the norm with somewhat fewer total treatments given than in the United States [Scott and Whalley, 1993].) The number of treatments should be determined purely by the patient's response, with the end-point being clinical remission or a plateau of response. Despite a lack of data supporting the technique, some psychiatrists give one or two extra treatments after maximum benefit has been achieved in order to prevent early relapse.

As befits a treatment that depends on a mechanical device, a number of technical considerations will affect the quality of the ECT treatment. The four important considerations are the type of electrical stimulus delivered, the placement of the electrodes, the dose of the stimulus administered, and the frequency of treatments.

Most hospitals in the United States now deliver ECT using a brief pulse stimulus (as opposed to the old method of a sine wave stimulus). The brief pulse requires less electricity to be given to provoke the seizure and is therefore associated with fewer cognitive deficits (Weiner, Rogers, Davidson, and Squire, 1986).

The second important decision is whether to use bilateral (on both sides of the head) or unilateral (with the current delivered to the non-dominant, right hemisphere of the brain) electrode placement. In both circumstances, seizures will occur. Without question, unilateral ECT causes less acute post-ECT disorientation and fewer memory deficits. For many patients, however, it may be less effective (Sackeim et al., 1993). Therefore, a common strategy is to start with unilateral treatment, switching to bilateral after five or six treatments if no improvement is seen.

The third technical consideration is the dose of electricity given, usually described in relation to the patient's seizure threshold, defined as the minimum dose that will cause the necessary seizure. Thus, the dose can be described as just above the seizure threshold (low dose) or suprathreshold doses (high dose, typically 150 to 250 percent above the threshold). For unilateral ECT, low dose is clearly less effective than high dose. With bilateral ECT, the efficacy rates are similar (Sackeim et al., 1993). However, low dose is associated with fewer cognitive side effects, analogous to unilateral vs. bilateral ECT.

Finally, as noted above, the ECT treatments are typically given in a twice- or three-times-weekly schedule. Twice-weekly treatment is associated with similar response rate and less cognitive impairment compared to three-times-weekly treatment (Lerer et al., 1995). However, three ECT treatments per week may cause a more rapid remission of symptoms. Therefore, if rapid remission is an important factor, three-times-weekly treatments may be preferred.

Before treatment, patients always receive some sort of medical evaluation, with each hospital requiring different tests. General screening blood tests are usual as is an electrocardiogram. Sometimes, back X-rays (to note the presence of old fractures) are taken. Medications that interfere with seizures, such as benzodiazepines or anticonvulsant mood stabilizers are reduced in dose or discontinued.

On the morning of an ECT treatment, the patient has usually fasted for eight to twelve hours. Atropine, a medication that minimizes a transient slowing of the heart rate from ECT, is sometimes given. After being taken into a room that is specifically equipped for the ECT procedure, an intravenous line (IV) is inserted through which the patient is given methohexital, a very short-acting barbiturate that induces sleep virtually immediately. Then succinylcholine, a muscle relaxant that prevents the actual physical manifestations of the seizure, is given. During this time, blood pressure and electrocardiogram monitoring is continual while the patient's breathing is insured by the use of a breathing bag and mask handled by the anesthesiologist or anesthetist. The electrodes are then placed on the patient's two temples for bilateral treatment or on the right temple and near the middle of the head for unilateral ECT. After the current is delivered, monitoring for the actual presence of the seizure is done through a variety of means, the most precise of which is the electroencephalogram (EEG, or brain wave test). Since succinylcholine blocks the muscle twitching, there may be no physical evidence that a seizure is occurring. Following the ECT treatment, the patient is observed, first in the recovery room and then on the ward. Patients awaken gradually within minutes to an hour after the procedure.

A successful course of ECT should always be followed by continuation treatment to prevent relapse, analogous to the treatment of mania or depression following clinical remission from antidepressants or mood stabilizers (American Psychiatric Association, 1990). (See chapter 3 for discussion of continuation treatment.) It is likely that all antidepressants and lithium are effective for some patients as continuation treatment after ECT. Unfortunately, relapse rates after successful ECT treatment are relatively high despite antidepressant continuation treatment (Sackeim, et al., 1993). Moreover, relapse rates are highest among those patients who were treated with ECT because of nonresponse to antidepressants (as opposed to those who had ECT because of medical reasons or clinical urgency) (Sackeim et al., 1990). Because of the frequent relapses, a number of patients are given continuation ECT in which patients are given a treatment every two weeks initially, decreasing to approximately once a month. Because patient acceptance of continuation ECT is understandably poor, it is rarely considered unless there have been multiple relapses after ECT despite antidepressant treatment. Similarly, some patients with recurrent depression (or less commonly, bipolar disorder) whose episodes cannot be prevented by other modalities are given once-monthly maintenance ECT for extended periods of time. No study has yet systematically evaluated the efficacy of continuation and/or maintenance ECT.

Side Effects

Although ECT, as currently practiced in the United States, is not a completely safe procedure, it is a far cry from the early days in the 1940s and 1950s when it was genuinely dangerous. At that time, mortality rates from ECT were significant—one per thousand—and rates of major complications, most commonly fractures, occurred in up to 40 percent of those treated (Consensus Conference, 1985). With the advances in ECT techniques—the use of anesthesia, muscle relaxants, and better control of breathing and oxygenation—the dangers have diminished dramatically. At present, mortality rates are the same as those associated with the use of short-acting barbiturate anesthetics, and fractures have been virtually eliminated. Cardiovascular changes from the procedure are a significant risk only for those who have preexisting cardiac problems. However, even when ECT is administered to older patients with cardiac histories, the procedure is safer than in the past, with few major complications (Rice, Sombrotto, Markowitz, and Leon, 1994).

The major side effects of ECT of current concern to patients and psychiatrists alike are those related to cognition. Seizures in general, and ECT treatments specifically, have clear adverse effects on cognition and memory. The most predictable of these is a post-ECT confusional state that increases with the number of treatments given, bilateral rather than unilateral placement, the type of waveform used (pulse vs. sine wave) and intensity of the electrical stimulus (dose). Patients awaken from the ECT with confusion and possibly disorientation to time, place, and/or situation which lasts between minutes and a few hours in the vast majority of patients.

Of more concern are the effects of ECT on memory. Both anterograde memory (the ability to learn new material) and retrograde memory (the ability to retrieve previously acquired material) are affected (Sackeim, 1992). As with the acute confusional effects, memory problems increase with more treatments, higher electrical dose, and with bilateral (vs. unilateral) treatments. During the time in which ECT is given and typically for a few weeks thereafter, anterograde memory is decreased in most patients. This deficit gradually diminishes and a return to normal capacity to learn new information is generally evident by two months in most patients and by six months in almost all patients.

Retrograde memory deficits are also maximal right after ECT, improving gradually over weeks to many months. Memory for recent events is disrupted more than those related to the distant past. Thus, two weeks after the last ECT treatment, a patient may remember events occurring years before but not what happened two months before. By six months after ECT, the more recent event is likely to be retrievable. Remembering specific events that occurred just prior to the ECT treatments or during the time of the hospitalization, however, may be permanently lost. Overall, within a few months after ECT, cognitive function is consistently improved compared to pre-ECT measures, assuredly due to the improvement in depression and the diminution in mood-related cognitive deficits (Sackeim et al., 1993).

Despite the studies that have documented the conclusions just presented, many patients complain that, following ECT, their memory is not as good as it had been previously. A variety of possibilities exist to explain these complaints (Squire, 1985). The most obvious is that the tests used to assess memory function are simply not sensitive enough to document these complaints. Also, it may be that because of the disruption of memory around the time of the ECT, a feeling of discontinuity of experience is translated as memory deficit. Having a time of memory impairment may additionally sensitize patients to normal memory gaps which are then interpreted as secondary to ECT. The effects of recurrent depression on memory may also play a part in these complaints for some patients.

Finally, many patients have heard that ECT causes permanent brain damage. The animal studies that purport to show brain damage have induced far greater numbers of seizures, and in some cases continuous seizures, than are used with ECT. Additionally, ensuring the delivery of oxygen to the brain during seizures, which may be a vital factor in preventing brain damage and is done routinely in modern ECT, is ignored in animal studies. Ongoing work in this area continues, but for now, the evidence is consistent that ECT does not cause permanent brain damage (Coffey, 1994).

To summarize the current knowledge about the risks of ECT: (1) In contrast to its use in the past, ECT is now a medically safe procedure in which the risk of serious medical complications is very low. (2) Transient confusion predictably occurs but is never a long-term problem. (3) Around the time of the ECT, the ability to learn new material and to retrieve old memories is unquestionably disrupted, but these effects disappear in the overwhelming majority of patients within a few months at most. Some patients, however, continue to complain of memory problems for months and years that cannot be explained by our current knowledge.

STIMULANTS

Similar to ECT, stimulants are among the oldest biological treatments in psychiatry, having been first developed more than fifty years ago, initially as a treatment for asthma. Amphetamines were prescribed (or obtained on the black market), in extraordinary quantities between the 1940s and 1970. The most common reasons for their use during those years were to enhance energy and alertness, promote weight loss, and less frequently to treat depression. Once the dangers of amphetamine abuse became clear to the medical community and to the general society, the production and prescription of stimulants markedly declined. Over the last few years, the pendulum has swung again and stimulant prescriptions for legitimate psychiatric reasons have increased. (They are also prescribed by other physicians as appetite-suppressing drugs for weight loss and in treating narcolepsy, a neurological disorder characterized in part by excessive sleepiness.) Unfortunately, a number of psychiatrists refuse to prescribe them in any circumstance because of their abuse potential and because of the government's scrutiny of prescriptions written for the two most common stimulants, d-amphetamine and methylphenidate.

Clinical Uses

The three major uses for stimulants in psychiatry are in the treatment of attention deficit/hyperactivity disorder (ADHD), depressive disorders, and apathy/fatigue syndromes seen in patients with AIDS or those with serious medical illnesses.

For patients with ADHD, both children and adults, stimulants are the mainstay of treatment. The evidence for efficacy in children is clear and beyond dispute for both methylphenidate (Ritalin) which is the most commonly prescribed stimulant and dextroamphetamine (Dexedrine). Pemoline (Cylert) is also effective, although possibly less so than the other two. Evidence from controlled studies on the use of stimulants for adults with ADHD is less impressive, but this may reflect the greater difficulty in making the diagnosis and/or the presence of associated conditions (such as drug and alcohol abuse) that complicate the disorder.

Increasingly, stimulants are used to treat depression. Certainly they are never appropriate first treatments for clear, uncomplicated major depressive disorder. The two major uses of stimulants for depression are: (1) as single agents for those depressed patients who either did not respond to or could not tolerate the effects of antidepressants; and (2) as adjunctive agents, added to an ineffective or partially effective antidepressant. It is not currently possible to predict which depressed patients will respond to a stimulant, although most psychopharmacologists are less likely to choose this approach with very anxious patients. No controlled studies exist examining the use of stimulants as adjunctive agents. Nonetheless, virtually all psychopharmacologists have treated at least a few depressed patients who have shown clear antidepressant responses to adjunctive stimulants. Stimulants seem to be effective when added to antidepressants of all classes. Except in rare circumstances, however, stimulants should not be added to MAO inhibitors because of safety considerations. (See chapters 3 and 9 for more details.) Responses to stimulants for depression are typically seen within a few days.

Patients with apathetic, depressive syndromes, not all of whom meet criteria for major depressive episode, are also commonly treated with stimulants (Rosenberg, Ahmed, and Hurwitz, 1991). As with their use as adjunctive agents, the response to stimulants in these patients is rapid, typically within a few days of initiating treatment, and the response is frequently dramatic. Stimulants are also prescribed with benefit to patients with cognitive and affective symptoms related to AIDS (Angrist et al., 1992; Fernandez and Levy, 1994).

Mechanisms of Action

Stimulants seem to exert their major effects on brain biology by increasing the functional activity of the catecholamines (see chapter 2), dopamine and norepinephrine. They cause the immediate release of dopamine from the neuron and may also block its reuptake, further increasing its availability (Chiarello and Cole, 1987). Similar, although less consistent, effects are seen with norepinephrine. The result of these actions is that stimulants typically produce increased arousal, decreased fatigue, and a heightened ability to concentrate. Their ability to cause euphoria is inconsistent, as are their effects on increased motor activity (Rapoport et al., 1980). Stimulants reliably decrease appetite and increase pulse rate, effects that are somewhat dose-related.

Techniques of Administration

Table 13–2 lists the stimulants used for the disorders previously noted with their typical dosage ranges for both adults and children. (Other amphetamine-like agents such as phentermine, diethylpropion, and phendimetrazine are available in generic and many trade name brands but are prescribed almost exclusively as appetite suppressants.) d-Amphetamine and methylphenidate are very similar in their therapeutic and side effects. They are both short-lived, lasting between two and five hours, and are equally effective, although individual patients occasionally prefer one or the other. d-Amphetamine is prescribed at somewhat lower doses than is methylphenidate to achieve the same effect. Because both stimulants are so brief in duration, they are often prescribed two to four times daily. Both medications are available in sustained-release forms which, unfortunately, are not always released as gradually as one would want, thereby limiting their usefulness. Initial doses for stimulants in treating both child and adult ADHD are 5 mg twice daily for methylphenidate and 2.5 to 5 mg twice daily for d-amphetamine. Because the effects are seen rapidly, often within the first day, dose adjustments can be made relatively quickly, typically

Table 13–2
Stimulants

Generic Name	Trade Name	Usual Dosage Range (mg/day)
d-Amphetamine	Dexedrine Dexedrine spansules (sustained release)	5–60
Methylphenidate	Ritalin Ritalin-SR (sustained release)	10–100
Pemoline	Cylert	18.75–150
d-Methamphetamine	Desoxyn	5–40

every two or three days. When prescribed for depression, especially for the medically ill, the lowest possible dose, such as 2.5 mg of methylphenidate, is often prescribed first. Dose adjustments are then made carefully on the basis of the initial response.

Compared to the other two stimulants, pemoline is slower in onset of action and longer in duration. It is also not quite so effective as the other two. Improvement at any dose will be seen more gradually, typically over days to a week. Because it lasts longer, pemoline has a distinct advantage in being effective when given only once daily, typically in the morning. Initial doses of pemoline are 18.75 or 37.5 mg, increased after a number of days or a week by 18.75 mg at a time. (It is not clear why pemoline tablets are available in these unusual potencies.) Reflecting its lesser capacity for abuse, pemoline prescriptions are not scrutinized by government regulatory agencies as are those for d-amphetamine and methylphenidate.

Tolerance to their therapeutic effects with the need for higher doses is generally not seen when stimulants are used to treat ADHD. The extent of tolerance when stimulants are prescribed for depression is extremely variable but seems to be higher than for ADHD.

Side Effects

The most common side effects from stimulants are, as expected, related to overstimulation. These include anxiety, irritability, insomnia, headaches, decreased appetite, weight loss, as well as increased pulse and blood pressure. Since the side effects are typically dose-related, they usually diminish if the dose is decreased. Also, tolerance often develops to a number of these side effects, specifically insomnia, the pulse/blood pressure effects, and the diminished appetite. When prescribed for the depressed medically ill, stimulant side effects rarely cause clinically significant problems. When taken in high dose for an extended period of time, stimulants can precipitate an acute paranoid psychosis.

When either methylphenidate or d-amphetamine is prescribed for children, other side effects may be seen. The most important of these are their effects on height. Children taking stimulants show a small (average of less than one inch) decrement in height. If, however, stimulants are withdrawn during adolescence, a growth rebound occurs with the children's final height the same as others (Gittelman-Klein and Mannuzza, 1988). If the medications are withdrawn over two summers, the small decrement in height disappears (Gittelman-Klein, Landa, Mattes, and Klein, 1988). The concern, then, is for those children who continue stimulant treatment throughout adolescence without interruption because of ongoing ADHD symptoms.

Other side effects commonly seen with children are crying spells, lethargy, dysphoric mood, nausea, and abdominal discomfort. Children with Tourette's syndrome, a tic disorder (see chapter 8), may have an exacerbation of their symptoms.

Pemoline causes liver inflammation in an occasional patient, necessitating infrequent checks of liver function.

The final problems with stimulants concerns their potential for abuse. Without doubt, both methylphenidate and d-amphetamine are abusable drugs. For that reason, they need to be prescribed with caution. However, drug abuse and dependence occur as an interaction between a drug and an individual with a particular vulnerability for abusing drugs. Thus, cavalierly prescribing Dexedrine to a former "speed freak" who complains of distractibility is simply not comparable to administering the same medication to a 58-year-old compliant, treatment-refractory patient with depression. In other words, stimulants are useful with the right patients at the right time, but can be dangerous when prescribed unwisely.

SECTION

FIVE

14

The Split Treatment Model

Interactions Between Psychotherapy and Pharmacotherapy

M ORE AND MORE OFTEN, therapeutic tasks for patients with psy-
chiatric/psychological disorders are shared by two professionals,
the psychotherapist and the pharmacotherapist. Although the interactions between psychotherapy and pharmacotherapy are themselves
worthy of discussion, splitting the two treatment modalities adds other,
often unexplored factors. The first half of this chapter describes psy-
chotherapy/pharmacotherapy interactions and theoretical aspects of
what is best described as split treatment; the second half is devoted to
the more practical issues of finding a psychopharmacologist and working within the split treatment model. Because virtually no research on
these topics has been done, in the discussion I rely primarily on clinical
observations, theoretical concerns, and practical suggestions.

EARLY MODELS, EARLY PROBLEMS

If split treatment simply means two professionals performing different
therapeutic functions, it is not new. In psychoanalytically oriented hospitals, more in the past than recently, the therapist/analyst would treat
the patient in intensive psychotherapy while another physician would
be responsible for giving or withdrawing passes, setting behavioral limits, occasionally prescribing medications, and interacting openly with
the nursing staff on issues of the patient's behavior. The goal of this
split was to avoid disrupting the intimacy or trust of the primary therapeutic relationship by segregating psychoanalysis from other aspects
of therapy which were considered of lesser importance and theoretical
interest. Thus, even though the therapy was split, no attempt was made
to integrate the two treatments.

This legacy of keeping therapies pure and eschewing more integra-
tive approaches to treatment was equally apparent when biological
therapies emerged in the 1960s. Early psychopharmacologists dis-

played the same tendency for dichotomous thinking as had psycho-analysts, but in reverse. Medication treatments for the more "biologi-cal" disorders, such as bipolar disorder and schizophrenia, were thought to be sufficient for maximal improvement, and psychotherapy was relegated to a minor place, at best. As an example, following the es-tablishment of lithium as helpful in treating bipolar disorder, many bi-ologically oriented psychiatrists naively thought that bipolar patients had no psychological problems and therefore no need for psychother-apy. Patients supposedly took their lithium, had their doses adjusted, their blood drawn, and otherwise led symptom-free normal lives. Little attention was paid to the impact of stressful events or personality vari-ables on these patients' mood disorders and lives. The overly simplistic psychoanalytic model had been replaced by an equally simplistic med-ical model.

With this tendency to dichotomous thinking, notions that patients might suffer from difficulties that were both biological *and* psychologi-cal and might therefore benefit from multimodal treatment were lack-ing. Thus for patients with marked rapid mood swings, the question posed might be whether they suffered from narcissistic pathology (a "psychological" disorder) or cyclothymia as a variant of bipolar disor-der (a "biological" disorder)—but rarely both. With these unimodal formulations, combined treatment was rarely considered. Whatever its other faults, the series of DSMs, beginning with DSM-III, published in 1980, attempts to avoid this dichotomous approach to psychopathol-ogy. The multiaxial format of DSM-III, III-R, and IV (see chapter 1 in this book) effectively forced readers to think about multiple simulta-neous disorders. Thus, the clinician wondering if a patient's mood in-stability was evidence of cyclothymia or of narcissistic personality disorder could now conceptualize both disorders existing simultane-ously—and consider multiple treatments. Similarly, a multiaxial approach encouraged clinicians to pay attention to the complex interactions be-tween life events (Axis IV), personality variables (Axis II), and the course of Axis I disorders. For example, in evaluating and treating bi-polar disorder, personality disorders and stresses can affect the course of the mood disorder while the bipolar disorder may cause psycho-logical difficulties. Both the triggers of the mood episodes and the psychological scars resulting from them may be amenable to psycho-therapeutic intervention in addition to, not instead of, pharmaco-therapy.

Aside from the narrow unimodal models of psychopathology, the other major obstacle to the development of split treatment was a series of fears and prejudices that evolved between psychiatrists and the growing numbers of nonphysician therapists. In large part, these fears resulted from the competition between the two professions for status in the community as well as from the different fees charged. Therapists feared that a consulting psychiatrist might denigrate the therapist's competence and then steal the referred patient by providing psychotherapy as well as psychopharmacological consultation. Psychiatrists were worried that their position at the top of the psychotherapeutic hierarchy was being threatened and therefore placed great emphasis on the different training received by nonphysician therapists. Furthermore, as malpractice suits became a greater source of concern, some psychiatrists felt an increased need for control of the patients with whom they were involved. The split treatment model was a direct threat to control. For example, if a patient in split treatment committed suicide during a time when the patient was in intensive psychotherapy but in maintenance pharmacotherapy (and therefore seeing the psychopharmacologist infrequently), some pharmacotherapists feared that, as a member of the treatment team, they might be held liable for the outcome. Their possible liability might be heightened had the patient overdosed on the prescribed medications. Ignored in these scenarios, of course, was the importance of mutual respect and trust between the two professionals and the need for them to work *together* and not in isolation from each other.

Marked shifts in the financing of health care as well as recent demands for more efficient psychological/psychiatric treatments have further heightened the tensions between nonmedical and medical mental health professionals. In a number of states, some organizations representing clinical psychologists have pushed for state legislation allowing their members prescription privileges, a move that is (not surprisingly) vigorously opposed by organized psychiatry. Moreover, the increasing domination of mental health care by managed care companies with their emphasis on lowering costs has left those psychotherapists who charge more (such as psychiatrists) out of the referral loop, or forced them to accept marked fee reductions, causing great resentment. Finally, as part of the overall movement towards briefer, less expensive, and more focused psychotherapies, there continues to be a shift away from psychoanalysis (or intensive psychoanalytically-oriented psychotherapy). Because psychoanalytic institutes have been traditionally dominated by psychiatrists (albeit less so recently), fewer psychotherapy patients are being seen by psychiatrists.

The result of all of these changes has been that more practitioners are competing for smaller and more precious pieces of the clinical pie—and these changes are likely to be irreversible. Inevitably, the alterations in the referral patterns and financing of mental health care cause conflict, resentment, and anxiety. With the new models of mental health care still in evolution, it is impossible to prepare for the future with as much certainty as any of us would like. Yet, just as two individual professionals treating the same patient need to work in a coordinated manner for optimal clinical outcome, medical and nonmedical mental health professionals must do the same. The split treatment model is unlikely to disappear in the foreseeable future, and is very likely to emerge as a dominant model of mental health care. For the best care of our patients as well as for the survival of all mental health professionals, it behooves all clinicians to be skilled in this model.

PSYCHOTHERAPY/PHARMACOTHERAPY INTERACTIONS: THEORETICAL ISSUES

Among the more important concerns for therapists considering having a patient participate in both psychotherapy and medication treatment are those related to the hypothetical negative interactions between the two modalities, whether utilized by one practitioner or two. Of most concern to therapists is that drug therapy will have negative effects on psychotherapy. Specific concerns include the following (Klerman, 1991):

1. Medication use could undermine psychotherapy by promoting an antitherapeutic attitude (negative placebo effect) in both therapist and patient. In this view, taking medication fosters dependency and passivity. It subtly promotes a stance in which the patient waits to be "fixed" by external magic, be it medication or the therapist, thereby discouraging the mutual exploratory active mode that is characteristic of good psychotherapy.
2. Medication-induced reduction of symptoms reduces the motive for continuing patient treatment. Most therapists would agree that an "optimum" level of distress is needed for most successful therapies. If the level is too high, the patient will become overwhelmed; if it is too low, motivation will decrease and defenses will help seal over the underlying problems without resolving the conflict, thereby making it likely that the same problems will arise at a later time. Because successful pharmacotherapy diminishes symptoms/ distress, there is a concern that the patient will then not be sufficiently motivated to continue to explore underlying issues and

will terminate therapy prematurely. A further theoretical concern is that the symptom relief seen with pharmacotherapy will lead to symptom substitution, again without any resolution of underlying problems.

3. The introduction of possible medication treatment may produce an altered sense of self in a psychotherapy candidate and provoke a variety of negative feelings in the patient (see below). In terms of its meaning for the therapy, some patients may interpret the suggestion of medication evaluation as implying that they are not appropriate for "pure" psychotherapy and that they are less interesting than other patients. It can be seen as a failure of their capacity to work through issues by themselves, without the crutch of drugs.

As hypotheses, these concerns are individually valid. Medication treatment can have these negative effects with some patients. As pharmacotherapy becomes more popularized in the lay media, more patients are presenting to mental health professionals with the inner conviction that their lifetimes of dysphoria and poor interpersonal relationships are chemical in origin; what they need, they seem to say, is to have their chemical imbalances fixed. The vignettes describing personality "transformations" in *Listening to Prozac* (Kramer, 1993) exemplify the fantasies of many patients. Without question, this attitude and a fixation on chemical imbalances as the sole cause of one's misery would indeed undermine any psychological therapies.

Fortunately, this kind of rigid thinking is unusual in the majority of patients. If, in the course of a good psychotherapy, medication is introduced, the psychodynamic meaning of taking pills, of its transference implications, of its possible effects of promoting passivity are all issues that can and should be explored in the treatment. Furthermore, these concerns have been examined, albeit sporadically, in a number of studies (Conte, Plutchnik, Wild, and Karasu, 1986; Beitman, 1988). Whether treating patients with mood disorders, anxiety disorders, or schizophrenia using combined treatment, the evidence can best be summarized as follows: (1) There is no consistent evidence that psychotherapy and psychopharmacology when used together are less effective than either treatment alone; neither a negative placebo effect nor symptom reduction as a motive for discontinuing psychotherapy is found. (2) Combined therapy is as effective or more effective than either treatment alone. Of course, neither the patients treated in these studies nor the types of structured psychotherapies used are necessarily compara-

ble to that of community practice. As such, these studies may not adequately address the concerns of some therapists. Nonetheless, until
conflicting evidence is presented, it should be assumed that pharmacotherapy does not diminish the effects of psychotherapy.

THERAPEUTIC SPLIT MODEL

The concerns about psychotherapy/pharmacotherapy interactions discussed are relevant whether the therapies are provided by one or two
professionals. When the two treatments are split, there is another series
of considerations. These can be most easily explored by describing the
advantages and disadvantages of a therapeutic split treatment model.

Advantages of the Split Model

1. The therapeutic split keeps the psychotherapy focused on psycho-
    logical issues. If medications are introduced in the course of an on-
    going psychotherapy, it can be disruptive to the already established
    themes and patterns of therapist/patient interaction. Especially in a
    psychodynamic therapy that encourages fantasies, dreams, projec-
    tions, and explores transference distortion, asking about side ef-
    fects and discussing medication dosage adjustments may distract
    both the patient and the therapist from the psychotherapeutic
    work. Even in a more supportive psychotherapy, a discussion of
    the events of the previous week or strategies to handle an interper-
    sonal problem can be sidetracked by a focus on medication con-
    cerns. In a therapeutic split model, the psychopharmacologist can
    evaluate the efficacy of the medication, and explore side effect is-
    sues consistently without fear of disrupting the therapy while the
    therapist can defer most of the medication questions to the psy-
    chopharmacologist. This can be especially useful when a patient
    has a somatic focus and side effects become a paramount issue.
    Depressed, somatically preoccupied patients can spend astonish-
    ing amounts of time in therapy dwelling on complaints of consti-
    pation, dry mouth, dizziness, and fatigue, with the attendant
    paralysis in addressing psychotherapeutic issues. With a split
    model, the "medication visit" can be the designated forum for dis-
    cussing symptoms and side effects. If the therapist and psy-
    chopharmacologist establish a good working relationship, the
    patient's somatic concerns can be contained effectively, allowing
    more psychotherapeutic work to be accomplished.

2. Similarly, the therapeutic split allows for the different interviewing styles to be used most effectively. The structured, fact-based questions of a medication visit (How well are you sleeping? Are you experiencing any dizziness? Is your mood worse in the morning?) is obviously different from the less directive and more open-ended approach of psychodynamic psychotherapy or the more event-focused approach of supportive therapies. Switching back and forth between the directive medical model style and the less structured psychotherapeutic models as would be inevitable if a single practitioner were doing both treatments might be confusing to the patient and retard a productive working rhythm of psychotherapy.

3. The therapeutic split model may help in the management of an overwhelming or unmanageable transference/countertransference relationship. Patients with both severe personality disorder (usually narcissistic or borderline) and a concomitant mood disorder, either unipolar or bipolar, are seemingly becoming more common in clinical practice. Managing patients with severe borderline disorder is difficult enough, but when Axis I biological instability is also present, the ensuing chaos can be overwhelming and sometimes unmanageable. The impulsivity of bipolar disorder can heighten the potential self-destructiveness of these patients, while psychomotor retardation and depressive fatigue can exacerbate their emotional isolation and despair. In these instances, having two professionals working together can minimize the therapeutic exhaustion that so commonly interferes with the treatment of these patients. This is especially relevant currently, since for many patients a lack of inpatient insurance precludes hospitalization. Even those patients with insurance are typically hospitalized for only brief periods of time given the short lengths of stay in psychiatric inpatient settings. In these situations, the ongoing presence of more than one professional may be vital in managing the multiple therapeutic crises.

Brenda was an exhausting patient. At age 41, she had been in psychotherapy for almost twenty years for treatment of her severe borderline personality, with self-mutilation, chronic rage, erratic performances at work, and chaotic relationships. The intensity and unremitting nature of her psychopathology and of the overwhelming hostile, dependent transferences that were typical of her psychotherapies often culminated in her therapists feeling overwhelmed and depleted. At these times, either through a conscious resignation from the case or through unconscious countertransference behaviors that made the therapy unworkable, Brenda would be pushed out of psychotherapy and would begin again with a new therapist. Because of her chronic dysphoria that was clearly based in her personality disorder, the presence of a superimposed major depressive disorder and the possibility of adjunctive antidepressant treatment was difficult to ascertain. Nonetheless, a psychopharmacological consultation was ultimately obtained. Over the next four years, despite a minimal response to a variety of medications, Brenda continued to see both her therapist and the pharmacotherapist. The two professionals communicated regularly during this time with much clarification of potential splitting issues and even more mutual commiseration. During this time, it became clear that the presence of a colleague allowed each to tolerate what would have been intolerable if working alone. The therapy proceeded slowly with the psychopharmacologist providing a once monthly visit, medication management, an occasional time when the negative transference would temporarily switch to him, and a source of support to both Brenda and her therapist.

4.   Splitting the two treatments allows the patient to be seen simultaneously via the microcosmic, intensive observations of the psychotherapist as well as the more macrocosmic, broad view of the pharmacotherapist. Therapists working with patients in intensive psychotherapy one to three times weekly will naturally focus on links between the material being presented and the patients' mood. It is remarkably easy for them to miss possible cyclical changes in mood that vary, as an example, by the season of the year. Seasonal patterns would be more easily discovered if the patient were seen once a month in a setting that focused more on symptom patterns and not on psychodynamic issues.

Roberta was being treated by a psychiatrist experienced in psychopharmacology with a combination of psychotherapy and medication for narcissistic personality disorder and atypical depression. Because of her increasing depressive symptoms, antidepressants were prescribed at a time when the focus of the therapy was on the dependent relationship the patient maintained with her husband. Within a month, Roberta was markedly less depressed, made plans for a new career, and decided to separate from her husband. Her changes were decisive, even bold, and out of character for her. Two months later, it became clear to both patient and psychiatrist that she was experiencing a pharmacological hypomania, and that many of the changes she made were impulsive and difficult to sustain. Had a second professional who was not involved in the psychotherapeutic issues been prescribing the antidepressants, it is far more likely that he would have noted the hypomania precipitated by antidepressants and intervened to diminish the impulsivity earlier.

Donna was being seen in weekly psychotherapy for severe narcissistic personality disorder and atypical depression. Her psychiatrist, who saw her for both therapy and medication, prescribed an MAO inhibitor as a maintenance treatment. Despite the success of the antidepressant in decreasing depressive responses to rejection, the patient still experienced frequent short-lived mood swings that were easily understandable as psychodynamically based in her narcissistic pathology. Following a series of major stressors in a relationship and at work, these mood swings intensified. The patient was ultimately fired from her job because of emotional instability. A second opinion was obtained at that time, and the pattern of a rapid-cycling Bipolar II disorder that had emerged over the previous six months was diagnosed. Lithium was prescribed with clear benefit, although narcissistic mood swings persisted.

In both these cases, the simultaneous presence of two types of mood swings—"biological"/bipolar as well as psychological/narcissistic—made accurate diagnosis difficult. The psychodynamic pathology so dominated both the overall clinical picture and the content of the therapeutic hour that the emergence of the more severe bipolar mood swings was not diagnosed in either case as early as it might have been. Had the split treatment model been used, it is more likely that the hypomania in the first case and the bipolar mood swings in the second would have been diagnosed sooner and appropriate treatment instituted earlier.

5. The split model is often less expensive than seeing a psychiatrist alone. Initially, the split treatment costs more because of the initial medication consultation and the relatively frequent number of medication visits when doses are being adjusted. Over time, however, the number of medication visits generally decreases to one visit every few months. Since psychiatrists tend to charge more than other therapists, the split treatment ultimately saves money. It is this cost savings that has made the split model increasingly utilized in managed care settings or in comprehensive health care plans. Additionally, for those patients with indemnity insurance (in which no restrictions are placed on the care provider the patient sees), insurance companies often reimburse medication consultations and their follow-up visits at the medical rate, typically 80 per-

cent of usual and customary charges, far more than the rather meager psychotherapy insurance reimbursements.

Disadvantages of the Split Model

The core disadvantage of the therapeutic split model is the dichotomous nature of the treatment and its effect on retarding the development of an integrated view of the self. This difficulty may be manifested in a variety of ways:

1. The split model may foster resistance to one or the other modalities of treatment. Separating medication treatment from psychotherapy by time, place, and person (i.e., going to different offices at different times to see different professionals) undermines the spirit of an integrated but multimodal treatment. It becomes easier for patients to dismiss psychotherapeutic needs ("the antidepressant will make me all better, so talking about my relationships is a waste of time") or medication needs ("I know I've had three psychotic episodes but now I'm working on the roots of my problems in therapy and I'll never get sick again"). Although similar resistances can occur with just one treating professional, the split is easier when two separate individuals are involved.

2. The split model can exacerbate the splitting seen in patients with primitive defenses. Narcissistic and borderline patients tend to split a single therapist into an omnipotent and a devalued object over the course of treatment. With two treating professionals, the tendency to split them into good and bad objects is heightened. This can result in the psychopharmacologist being seen as the malevolent, withholding, distant bad object who spends too little time with the patient and "throws pills" at him while the therapist is seen as the caring, engaging, soothing good object. Conversely, the therapist can be seen as the ineffectual, soft, and incompetent bad object while the psychopharmacologist is seen as the powerful, effective keeper-of-the-magic. Because these stereotypes frequently reflect the professionals' unconscious biases, a split between the two professionals can easily occur, with either one (or both) unconsciously undermining the treatment of the other.

Robert was in twice weekly psychotherapy with Dr. C for his narcissistic personality and in maintenance lithium treatment with Dr. D for cyclothymia. Both were very competent professionals whose styles differed. Dr. C was soft spoken and worked within a psychodynamic framework. Dr. D, on the other hand, was a very talkative clinician who was wary of any approaches reminiscent of classical psychoanalysis but had always worked well with patients in psychotherapy and respected Dr. C's work. As Robert's psychotherapy focused on his anger at various parental figures throughout his life, he began to complain about his therapist to Dr. D. He expressed concern that Dr. C stayed silent at times when he, Robert, was feeling helpless and needed some guidance or reassurance. He expressed appreciation that Dr. D carried a beeper and was more available than his therapist. Dr. D's more open approach, he said, helped him feel more grounded and let him deal better with the world. Although initially Dr. D encouraged Robert to speak directly with his therapist, he was becoming increasingly sympathetic to Robert's complaints about his therapy. He considered suggesting to him that he should seek therapy either with himself or with a more reality-oriented therapist. His feelings made him uneasy and he called Dr. C to clarify the situation. Not surprisingly, Dr. C related that Robert had actually been making unrealistic demands in the therapy, insisting that his therapist see him whenever he wanted and not require him to come to his regularly scheduled appointments, that he lower his fee (for no particular reason), and so on. In retrospect, it was clear that when Robert had complained about his therapist, Dr. D had unconsciously encouraged it because of his own concerns about psychoanalytic techniques. Once the two therapists talked, Dr. D was able to resume a more neutral stance with Robert and the potential for a serious therapeutic rift subsided.

3. The split model can retard the patient's ability to integrate various aspects of himself—the biological/psychological, heredity/environment, mastery-through-understanding/mastery-through-medication dichotomies. Having experiences such as manic episodes, psychotic depressions, or panic attacks and being able to integrate these as part of oneself without being defined by them ("I have bipolar disorder" vs "I am bipolar"), or having them overwhelm all other aspects of identity is difficult. The goal should be to integrate these experiences yet hold them slightly apart to be able to examine, understand, and deal with them realistically. Seeing two professionals—"one for my mind and one for my brain" creates a very real obstacle to this type of integration.

4. The limited interaction between the psychopharmacologist and the patient can become a frustrating experience for both. Patients may bring up important material that needs to be explored psy-

chotherapeutically in the midst of a (typically) short medication visit. Since the patient is in therapy with someone else, the pharmacotherapist is always forced to suggest that the patient explore the issue elsewhere, promoting feelings of rejection. Of course, if the patient consistently brings tantalizing psychodynamic material to the pharmacotherapist while the psychotherapy is at a standstill, this may indicate that the patient is frightened of these issues and brings them up only in settings where they cannot be explored.

5.   In the split model, it is more difficult to deal with the issues surrounding the potential for suicide and the possibility of overdosing on the prescribed medication. If the psychopharmacologist gives a six-week supply of medication to a stable patient who then becomes suicidal two weeks later, it is the therapist (who has not prescribed the medication) who must then think of how many pills the patient has, whether the patient is safe with the pills at home, and so on. Although theoretically, a shared therapeutic responsibility promotes a more coordinated team approach for both professionals, it also makes it easier for this kind of vital information to "slip through the cracks" to the detriment of patient care.

PSYCHODYNAMICS OF PSYCHOPHARMACOLOGY

Having a therapist suggest the possibility of a medication consultation, seeing a separate professional, and taking pills to alter the way in which one thinks or feels are all parts of an interaction that may have powerful meanings to a patient—meanings that are rooted in individual sensitivities, past experiences, and transference distortions. Reactions may vary, from extremely positive to sufficiently negative to cause a disruption in therapy. In order to integrate the consultation procedure into the psychotherapy, therapists must be prepared to explore patients' reactions and be alert to covert responses that may be expressed in the days or weeks following the initial discussion. Even though the use of medications for psychological/psychiatric disorders is increasingly accepted (especially for depressive disorders), the response to the suggestion of a medication consultation often yields rich understandings about the patient's inner life and can be used fruitfully in psychotherapy. Patients' feelings can be divided into responses to the therapist, to the psychopharmacologist, and to the medication itself.

The simple suggestion of a psychopharmacological consultation may provoke a wide range of powerful feelings. Some patients may experience it as a rejection, that their therapist doesn't want to work with them; some may think that they are crazy or that their problems are too overwhelming for their therapist. (Of course, at times, it may be true that the consultation expresses an overwhelmed feeling on the therapist's part or the concern that the patient cannot be contained by talking therapy alone.) Others may feel narcissistically wounded, that they are not good enough for "pure" psychotherapy and that they've let the therapist down. They may interpret the suggestion as reflecting the therapist's impatience or dissatisfaction with the patient's progress. All of these reactions are rooted in the patient's own self-concept and past experiences with others. As an example, a patient who feels that his parents pushed him away whenever he revealed his inner concerns would be more likely to experience a suggestion for a consultation as a repetition of the earlier parental rejection. Working through these feelings will be useful, not only for the outcome of the consultation, but for the psychotherapy itself.

Responses to the psychopharmacologist may also reflect a combination of realistic appreciation of the physician as well as transference distortions of parental figures. The transference is especially powerful for father figures in view of the societal role physicians have always played. This may in large part determine whether the pharmacotherapist is perceived as warm and nurturing, a figure who will soothe the suffering of the patient with his medications, or as a distant, controlling figure who cares little for the patient's inner life but is simply interested in manipulating behavior through pills. A split transference often develops with the maternal therapist and paternal pharmacotherapist perceived according to the patient's childhood memories. This transference configuration is enhanced with the common situation of a female therapist and a male pharmacotherapist.

Finally, the pills themselves can provoke powerful feelings. Medication may be viewed as a form of control by an external power with subsequent feelings of rage and inner helplessness. If a patient has had previous episodes of psychiatric disturbance treated with psychotropic medications—for instance, recurrent depressions treated with antidepressants—pills may also symbolize the disorder previously treated and may evoke strong feelings of disappointment, denial, or anger. Similarly, a patient whose mother was psychiatrically disturbed and was treated with medication will often see taking medications as tantamount to becoming the hated crippled parent. Conversely, if the patient's own past experience with caregivers or psychopharmacologist has had some positive aspects to it, medications can be thought of as a source of support. At times, pills can become powerful transitional objects with a needed ability to soothe during periods of potential fragmentation (Adelman, 1985).

More recently, a new set of fantasies, associations, and expectations about the pills themselves have emerged as part of the intense debate surrounding serotonergic antidepressants and the book *Listening to Prozac* (Kramer, 1993). (See chapter 7 for further discussion.) The two most common fantasies have been that patients taking these medications could reasonably expect personality transformations into new selves, and that these drugs could be routinely used as "cosmetic psychopharmacology," such that patients could become better than well with extra alertness, assertiveness, confidence, and more. Inherent in these pharmacological rescue fantasies are the underlying themes of passivity and magic. These themes are especially relevant when, as is increasingly common, patients themselves suggest a pharmacological consultation.

Understanding and working through these potential distortions—both positive (especially the rescue fantasies) and negative—can be extremely useful in itself, and can also aid enormously in better compliance with treatment. It is important to remember, however, that some of the reactions to individual pharmacotherapists may be rooted in realistic appraisal of the manner in which they treat patients. A patient sensitized to issues of paternal distance and rejection will have an even more difficult and probably unhelpful experience with a distant pharmacotherapist. Knowing a patient's individual sensitivities and working with a psychopharmacologist with some psychological mindedness can make the difference between a successful consultation and a failure.

PATIENT EDUCATION

Among the more unfortunate legacies of the medical model in psychiatry is the tradition of treating patients like helpless young children, incapable of understanding the nature of their problems and too fragile to be told "painful truths." This has led to the all-too-frequent situation of expecting intelligent, clear-minded adults to take their medication compliantly without explanations as to what disorder is being treated, why the medication is being prescribed, what positive effects might be expected, and what side effects should be looked for. Among the many consequences of this paternalistic (in the worst nineteenth-century sense) attitude are patient passivity, patient fear, and retardation in the development of the type of healthy cognitive mastery that strengthens the therapeutic partnership between patient and physician. Moreover, treating patients as children is likely to diminish compliance. Patients who understand the nature of the disorder being treated and the treatment offered are more likely to work productively in an active collaboration. This may result not only in better compliance but in improving the overall outcome of treatment (Cochran, 1984).

The tradition of prescribing medication for psychiatric problems and disorders is recent; acceptance of these medications by society in general is even more recent. As such, patients come to a psychopharmacological consultation with a varied set of truths, half-truths, fantasies, and misconceptions. The fantasies relating to the serotonergic antidepressants and their effects on personality noted above are prime examples of these. Therefore, among the tasks inherent in psychopharmacological work is the need to explain to patients the nature of the disorder for which medication may be prescribed and the rationale for treatment. The exact amount of information will differ between patients, based on their desire and capacity to understand the information. Additionally, patients may want and need different amounts of information at different times during treatment. For instance, the optimum amount of information given to a profoundly depressed suicidal patient who has limited ability to concentrate is less than should be given to that same patient when he is no longer suicidal, beginning to emerge from the depression, and able to think clearly. Furthermore, if at a later time the patient is considering the pros and cons of maintenance treatment, additional information must be provided.

Patients derive information about psychiatric medications from a variety of sources. What is difficult is acquiring accurate information from reliable sources. Too frequently, patients and psychotherapists alike obtain information from articles in the lay press describing the wonders—or evils—of the new medications. These articles typically distort the information to be consistent with the slant of the story. For education to be helpful, the information must be accurate and understood in its proper context.

A number of books or booklets are currently available that offer clear and readable explanations of the nature of psychiatric disorders and current treatment options. My own feeling is that these books can be extremely helpful but only as adjunctive educational tools. The primary mode of communicating knowledge should still be verbal. Direct discussion is preferable because it allows flexibility in the language used and the amount of detail presented. In addition, the physician is available for clarifications and answering questions. Most importantly, these discussions help establish the therapeutic partnership between the psychopharmacologist and patient.

The main issues that need to be addressed with the patient (and the referring therapist) are:

1. What is the diagnosis? Given the vagaries of current psychiatric knowledge, a clear unambiguous diagnosis is not always possible. A brief discussion of the two or three major possibilities (e.g., depression or dysthymia or both) or even a clear description of the major symptoms can be very useful even without a definitive diagnosis.

2. What are the possible treatments and what are the relative advantages and disadvantages of each? In treating anxiety, for example, the topics might include a brief discussion of the benzodiazepines, how they may be safer than prior tranquilizers such as barbiturates, and why Xanax is being recommended over Valium for this particular patient. Similarly, in choosing between Prozac, Zoloft, and Paxil to treat a mild depression with chronic rejection sensitivity, describing the essential similarities of the medications while noting the few differences (e.g., amount of sedation vs. activation, the interaction with other medications) would be appropriate.

3. What are the goals of the medication treatment? As already discussed, patients frequently have unrealistic expectations about medications, especially those recently released. Every new medication is described by its manufacturer (and duly reported by the press) as a breakthrough drug with either fewer side effects or greater efficacy or some unique biochemical profile compared with currently available agents. Of course, occasionally one of the claims is true, but more often they are grossly distorted. As with the children's game of telephone, the story gets less accurate with each telling, from pharmaceutical firm to newspaper to television to the patient's friend who saw it. Additionally, the capacity of a medication to cause a specific type of clinical response tells nothing about the likelihood of that response. As an example, the reports of personality transformations with serotonergic antidepressants such as Prozac are true, but they are uncommon, an observation that is rarely mentioned in the press. This becomes a source of great disappointment to those patients who feel better, but are not transformed.

Conversely, patients need to know that it is realistic to expect a medication to diminish or abolish panic attacks, or diminish the sleep, appetite, and energy symptoms of a major depressive episode.

4. What side effects are common with the particular medication being prescribed? Here too, patients differ in the amount of information they want. For some, knowing the possible, though unlikely, side effects, will heighten their anxiety and somatic preoccupation. Others will feel greater mastery knowing all the potential side effects.

    The type of patient who reads the *Physicians' Desk Reference* (PDR) is a particular challenge. The PDR is a reliable source of possible side effects (it lists virtually all side effects ever reported for any drug), but it does not easily distinguish between common and uncommon or between dangerous and distressing side effects. Risk/benefit ratios of any treatment —which are the basis of all good clinical psychopharmacological decisions—are not presented or discussed, as befits a marketing and medicolegal compendium. The problem is that the PDR is *not* a textbook of psychopharmacology, but is often used as one. For patients who do read the PDR, the discussion needs to emphasize the issue of rare versus common side effects and the purpose of the book.

5. How long should the patient stay on the medication? Are there long-term side effects? These questions arise more commonly later on in treatment and are valid and important concerns. In order to make the best decisions about a potential maintenance treatment, a discussion must review the risk/benefit ratio for continuing *and* for discontinuing the medications. The limitations of current knowledge (e.g., How long should a chronically depressed patient stay on an effective antidepressant? What are the chances of the same medication working if it is withdrawn and the person becomes depressed again?) should be acknowledged, not in the spirit of helplessness but in an honest assessment that allows for a properly collaborative decision.

MEDICATION COMPLIANCE: INTRA- AND INTERPERSONAL FACTORS

It is consistently observed that noncompliance with medication regimens occurs in 25 to 50 percent of psychiatric patients (Blackwell, 1976). Noncompliance can be minor, such as missing occasional doses or mistiming the medication—taking one pill in the morning and two in the evening instead of one pill three times daily. In the majority of these instances, the consequences are trivial. but noncompliance can also be significant, resulting in either missing enough doses to diminish treatment outcome, or taking too much medication with the risk of causing significant adverse effects. Therapists must be cognizant of these issues for two reasons. First, understanding factors related to compliance (and therefore, the ultimate success of the medication) helps in choosing an appropriate psychopharmacologist for any particular patient. Second, when patients are seen in a split treatment, the therapist is often the first to learn about the extent of noncompliance and the reasons for it. Some of these factors (see below) are rooted in irrational fears, beliefs, family interactions, or other psychological and psychosocial factors for which psychotherapeutic work may be fruitful. Thus, for those compliance problems rooted in the patient/psychopharmacologist interaction, the therapist may be able to help the patient interact in a more productive and satisfactory way with the physician.

Reasons for significant noncompliance are varied and often overly determined. Factors related to noncompliance may stem from patient, psychopharmacologist, or patient/psychopharmacologist interaction variables (Docherty and Fiester, 1985).

Patients may be noncompliant because of acute symptoms inherent in the disorder being treated or as a result of more long-term character traits. Acute disorder-related noncompliance is typically caused by paranoia, denial, or cognitive disorganization. For example, a patient with paranoid delusions may be noncompliant because of the conviction that the medications are poisonous or instruments of mind control, convictions that may vanish once the patient's paranoia diminishes. Denial of illness, seen frequently with mania or schizophrenia, makes treatment either meaningless or malevolent to the patient, and will also diminish compliance. Cognitive disorganization, in which awareness of time is lost or severely compromised, is a common symptom of depression, mania, psychotic disorders, attention deficit/hyperactivity disorder, or when drug/alcohol abuse complicates another disorder. This type of disorganization will prevent a patient from complying with even the simplest medication regimen.

Other patients have character pathology or psychological conflicts that affect compliance. These may include negative attitudes towards authority, fears of addiction (out of proportion to the realistic possibility), the assumption that taking medication implies "being crazy," or sensitivity about not being in control. Some patients need to act in the sick role for intrapersonal, interpersonal, or financial (secondary gain) reasons. In these cases, anything—such as treatment—that interferes with this role will be undermined by the patient and will be manifested by noncompliance.

With the increasing cost of newer medications, and an inconsistent health care system that provides financial assistance for medication costs only for some individuals, some patients discontinue psychotropic medication because they simply can't afford it. Often, patients do not tell either their therapists or psychopharmacologists, feeling ashamed of their lack of resources.

Compliance during a long-term maintenance treatment, such as for bipolar disorder, dysthymic disorder, recurrent major depression, or schizophrenia, requires increased attention to patient concerns. Many of the issues just noted—being controlled by a medication, stigma/shame about having a long-term psychiatric disorder, concerns about how others (including new lovers) will view the person, denial ("I've had no manic episodes for two years, maybe I no longer need a mood stabilizer")—often become more powerful over time. This may be especially true if the patient is doing well and the pain and consequences of the psychiatric disorder for which the medication was originally prescribed have faded with time.

A patient's sociocultural environment will also affect noncompliance through family and cultural attitudes towards medications. A patient whose family is deeply involved with a fundamentalist religion whose followers believe that psychiatric disorders are the work of the devil is at high risk to not take medication correctly, if at all. Similarly, cultural or ethnic factors within a family or a community may promote resistance to treatment of psychological problems in general, and specifically to the use of medications to treat them. Patients from these families will receive significant pressure to not take the prescribed medications. Patients from chaotic families have been demonstrated to comply less well than those from stable, supportive families (Docherty, 1988). Also, patients are sometimes profoundly influenced by uneducated opinions from friends, be they close or distant. All physicians have had the experience of a patient actively resisting taking a certain medication because a neighbor's brother's friend took a similar medication and had, say, a stroke. Naturally, resistances based on these kinds of distorted information may also mask more deepseated fears.

Another powerful cultural influence that may affect compliance is the general wariness/proscription against psychotropic medications for members of Alcoholics Anonymous or related organizations. Each local meeting has its own unique attitude toward the treatment of comorbid disorders often seen in those with alcohol abuse or dependence. It is worthwhile for patients with a mood disorder, anxiety disorder, or schizophrenia in addition to alcohol abuse to attend different meetings to see if one will be more accepting of appropriate pharmacotherapy for comorbid disorders. In some cities, there are groups specifically designed for these patients, who are sometimes referred to as "double trudgers."

The psychopharmacologist's approach to the patient can have an enormous impact on compliance and, therefore, outcome. In many ways, it is difficult to distinguish between physician-related factors on compliance and doctor/patient interactional factors (see below), since the physician's key to success in this area is being able to interact successfully with patients.

Some simple attributes of successful psychopharmacologists are the capacity to convey hope and optimism and an interest in the treatment. Interest in the treatment that will affect compliance might be shown, for instance, by an insistence on regular contact between patient and doctor. Patients whose physicians believe in the efficacy of their prescribed treatment have better compliance. In this way, effective physicians utilize positive placebo effects (all aspects of the treatment except those specifically related to the pharmacological properties of the drug) to maximize treatment outcome.

The doctor-patient relationship forms a key component of compliance (Docherty and Fiester, 1985). Patient and pharmacotherapist enter the consultation each with his own preconception. Yet they can and do influence each other within the first hour. Ultimately, some congruence of goals, expectations, and working relationship must be achieved for compliant and successful treatment to occur.

Aspects of the doctor/patient interaction that generally (but not always) foster compliance are:

1. Increased active participation by the patient. Patients who feel engaged in the treatment, and not like passive oral receptacles of the doctors' pills, are more likely to be compliant. Such participation may be fostered by discussing varied side effects among a class of medications and helping to pick the one(s) that would be most tolerable, or finding the easiest way to take the daily dose—all in the morning, for example, or three times daily. This gives the patient a greater sense of control in the treatment.

    Patient participation does not imply physician passivity. Excessive physician passivity diminishes compliance. What is needed is active collaboration between an engaged patient and an "expert provider" who can dispense knowledge, experience, and (it is hoped) wisdom as conjoint decisions are made.

2. Congruent expectations between patient and physician. In the first session, patient and physician must clarify treatment expectations—about what the treatment may or may not do, what information the patient may want or need, the structure of treatment (how often will they meet, for how long, costs), how long it will take for the medication to work, side effects, and so on.

A related concept is that of finding an explanatory model that is acceptable to the patient. Regardless of how the psychopharmacologist conceptualizes a disorder requiring medication, it is vital that the patient and doctor share some mutually acceptable explanation for the symptoms and for what the treatment might accomplish. At times, this may require the physician to focus on treating a symptom of the underlying disorder in order to engage the patient in the treatment. As an example, a patient may present with clear mania but demand treatment for the mania-related symptom of insomnia. In order to engage the patient in treatment, it would be appropriate initially to avoid the label of mania, targeting the treatment towards the insomnia using medications that treat the symptom *and* the underlying disorder.

3. Good communication between doctor and patient. As noted above, patient dissatisfaction with communication with the doctor can be extremely disruptive to treatment. General guidelines are that communication should be brief, clear, and comprehensible. Too often, physicians alternate between not giving enough information or giving it in technical language that is neither comprehensible nor helpful to a patient in distress. Additionally, medication instructions—how often to take the medication and at what time—must be communicated clearly, usually in writing, and using as simplified a regimen as is possible.

4. Affective tone. Not surprisingly, it is helpful for patient and psychopharmacologist to work in a context characterized by understanding and caring—the same traits that correlate with successful outcome in psychotherapy. Paranoid or suspicious patients, however, or those who had certain types of poor early parenting may experience excessive warmth as smothering and controlling and react negatively. Sheer volume of warmth and friendliness is less helpful than giving the appropriate amount for any individual patient.

Optimal affective tone may also change over time. A patient who is paranoid because of a psychosis may require a certain distance that then becomes unnecessary or even destructive once the paranoia recedes. Similar to psychotherapy, good psychopharmacology requires a repertoire of approaches that differ both between patients and with one patient whose needs change over the course of treatment.

Those aspects of treatment that foster compliance must not be seen as ends in themselves. They are necessary but not sufficient for providing optimal care. The wrong medication given in a warm, empathic manner to an actively involved patient in a collaborative effort is no more useful than is the right medication prescribed by a cold distancing psychopharmacologist to a patient who feels neglected—and who therefore doesn't take the pills as prescribed. Compliance is a necessary component of successful treatment but only if the right treatment is complied with.

TECHNICAL ASPECTS OF SPLIT TREATMENT

Choosing a Psychopharmacologist

In a community or group in which there is only one psychiatrist with psychopharmacological expertise, there are no options. But in many areas, a number of practitioners may be available. How might a therapist pick one or a few psychopharmacologists to work with in a split treatment model? Table 14–1 lists the important considerations for this decision. Some of these are relevant in every case—for instance, a specific competence in prescribing medications. Others may apply only in certain clinical situations.

Table 14–1
Considerations in Choosing a Psychopharmacologist

General clinical competence
Acceptance and respect for psychotherapy
Specific psychopharmacological competence
Comfort with the split treatment model
Capacity to communicate with the therapist
Capacity and willingness to educate patients
Personal style

Although the tasks for which a therapist engages the psychopharmacologist—making an accurate diagnosis, evaluating the patient for possible medication treatment, starting the medication and then monitoring it—are specific skills, it is generally preferable to work with someone whose skills extend beyond psychopharmacology. As noted in some of the cases presented above, the interactions and overlap between Axis I and Axis II disorders can be significant and difficult for the most skilled clinicians. Psychopharmacologists with no skill, interest, or experience in personality disorders may be very capable of prescribing medications correctly, but are at risk to be overly inclusive about whom to treat. They may, for instance, interpret all mood swings as bipolar disorder (ignoring both the mood liability of some depressive disorders as well as personality mood swings) or miss the often multiple sources of dysphoria in a patient with both a personality disorder and major depression. Classic cases of medication-responsive disorders will be diagnosed and treated correctly by even narrowly based practitioners. For the more difficult or sensitive patients, broad-based psychiatric skills will enhance the outcome of the consultation.

Additionally, some psychopharmacologists with no interest or acceptance of other treatment modalities may have disparaging feelings toward psychotherapy in general, or toward the specific type of therapy in which the patient is engaged. Inevitably, these feelings are communicated to the patient either overtly or covertly with predictable negative consequences.

Overall skill as a psychiatric clinician, however, does not immediately confer sophisticated knowledge of diagnosis and psychopharmacology. It is imperative that the pharmacotherapist you work with have specific competence in this area. A competent clinical psychopharmacologist need not know nor have experience with every medication in every class of treatment. Experience with ten antipsychotics, as opposed to five, will rarely, if ever, translate to useful clinical knowledge. A competent psychopharmacologist, though, will have at least *some* experience with more than one agent in each of the major medication classes.

In addition, the psychopharmacologist must feel comfortable and interested in prescribing medication. With medications increasingly utilized in treating psychiatric/psychological disorders and with fewer patients being referred to psychiatrists for intensive psychoanalytic psychotherapy, psychiatrists with little interest or skill in psychopharmacology are often asked to consult and prescribe medications. In this situation, even if medications are prescribed, it is frequently done in a haphazard, unthoughtful, and usually unsuccessful manner.

Arthur had a good response from the antidepressant, desipramine. As he ran out of medication two months after improving, he called Dr. A, his prescribing psychiatrist. Dr. A replied in irritation that Arthur need not call, that he would approve a refill if the pharmacy called. No provision was made for a follow-up. The next time Arthur ran out of medication, he simply stopped taking it. Three weeks later, he relapsed back into a depression. When his therapist asked why he had discontinued his medication, he replied that he didn't know how long he was supposed to take the antidepressant and that Dr. A had given him no instructions. Between his lack of information, his sense of being a bother to Dr. A, and his subsequent anger, he had simply stopped the medication.

After Susan moved to California from another state, she needed a psychiatrist to continue prescribing and monitoring her Prozac, which had very successfully treated her dysthymic disorder and recurrent major depressions. Susan's health insurance program required her to see one of the psychiatrists on its health panel. She chose Dr. M, a respected, somewhat senior psychiatrist in her geographic area. She told him of her needs and her lack of desire for psychotherapy in an initial meeting that lasted only fifteen minutes. Six months later, a second meeting which she thought was needed for an occasional checkup lasted only five minutes, during which time she keenly felt Dr. M's lack of interest. Further refills over the next year were handled through the pharmacy with neither Susan nor the doctor making any attempt to communicate with each other. During the following year, when she had some questions about the use of the medication during pregnancy, she sought private consultation outside her insurance program which she paid for out of pocket. Although seeing the private doctor was far more expensive for her, Susan felt that she could not trust Dr. M to take her concerns seriously. It was impossible for her to evaluate whether Dr. M was sufficiently knowledgeable to be of help; his lack of interest made his technical competence irrelevant. Without the development of a meaningful working alliance with him, she needed to seek care elsewhere.

An interested psychopharmacologist who is unsure of a specific technical point (e.g., how to treat the sexual side effects seen with SSRIs) can easily find the answer by informal discussion with colleagues, reading, or even calling the pharmaceutical firm. Without the interest in clinical psychopharmacology, however, the questions will remain unanswered and the outcome will be less satisfactory than it could have been.

Most psychopharmacologists are reasonably skilled at diagnosing and prescribing for most, if not all, major Axis I disorders, even if they have a specific clinical focus on one syndrome. There may be times, though, when a subspecialist in a specific disorder should be consulted. For instance, skill in treating severe anorexia nervosa or bulimia with medication involves not just a knowledge of the medications involved, but an awareness of the medical dangers of antidepressants when used to treat these specific disorders. As noted in chapter 6, treating patients with drug or alcohol abuse is particularly difficult and often requires specialized experience in this area.

Not all psychiatrists feel comfortable working in a split treatment model. They are uneasy about being part of a treatment in which they are not the primary therapists and therefore see the patient infrequently. If a psychiatrist with these concerns works in a split treatment model, boundaries become blurred, patients get confused, and therapeutic work is sabotaged.

> Dr. B, a psychiatrist who is both a psychoanalyst and a competent pharmacotherapist, often received referrals from therapists for psychopharmacological consultations. As he became more interested in psychoanalysis and less in medication treatment, he became more uneasy about his role as a pharmacotherapist to patients in therapy with others. He found himself feeling critical of the referring therapists, thinking frequently of how he would handle aspects of the treatment differently. After at least two different instances in which he accepted patients into therapy who had been initially referred to him for medication evaluation, Dr. B became aware that he had unconsciously sabotaged the previous therapies. At that point, he stopped accepting pharmacological consultations and prescribed only for patients who were seeing him in psychotherapy.

Not all psychiatrists are as self-aware as was Dr. B. A pharmacotherapist who is not comfortable with his role will undermine therapies repeatedly. If this happens with any regularity with a colleague, find another.

Although two professionals should be able to work together without having the same theoretical formulations, it is important that they share somewhat similar languages (or at least understand each other's languages!) in describing psychiatric problems. When communicating with each other, terms such as borderline, psychotic, or depression must refer to the same clinical phenomena. Otherwise, communication may be impaired or, ultimately, avoided, to the detriment of the patient's care.

Among the greatest failings of psychopharmacologists is their lack of attention to patient education. In choosing an appropriate pharmacotherapist for a patient, the match between the patient's anticipated need for information and the physician's capacity and skill to provide it should be considered.

Finally, there are times when the "match" of personal attributes between an individual patient and a psychopharmacologist can either enhance or interfere with successful treatment. These considerations are no different from those relevant to picking a psychotherapist. A dramatic, manipulative patient may work better with a pharmacotherapist who stays slightly disengaged. Conversely, a patient who needs more encouragement or nurturing might work more effectively with a more active practitioner. A schizoid patient may feel threatened by someone who is overly warm, while an obsessional patient may need a psychopharmacologist who has the patience for detailed explanations. As noted above, the quality of the therapeutic alliance between pharmacotherapist and patient will materially affect the therapeutic outcome.

Finding a Psychopharmacologist in Your Community or Group

Depending on the size of the psychiatric community, there will be a variable number of competent psychopharmacologists. Within HMOs or managed care groups, the choice of psychiatrists may be even more limited. In most communities or groups, however, there is typically more than one psychiatrist available for psychopharmacological consultation. The best initial approach to finding a psychopharmacologist in your area or group is the time-honored one of asking colleagues about their own experiences. Using the criteria listed above, an initial cursory assessment of the strengths and weaknesses of the available psychiatrists in your community or group can be made. If possible, it is helpful to identify at least two psychopharmacologists so that if one is unavailable because of vacation, you already have another known to you who will be able to see your patient. It is also helpful, if possible, to know at least one male and one female pharmacotherapist for those patients who would clearly work better with clinicians of one sex or the other.

Once you have the name of a potential practitioner with whom to work, there are two ways to evaluate whether this will be a successful therapeutic relationship. The simplest way is to refer a patient at an appropriate time and to see how it works out, from your point of view and that of your patient. Some therapists want to meet the psychopharmacologist in person, in order to evaluate the psychiatrist's personality, interest, and style of working. This can be very helpful, but is also time consuming. Many psychiatrists are disinclined to take the time to be "interviewed," especially if their practices are already relatively busy. In addition, the medical model, in which all psychiatrists have trained, virtually never uses the interviewing approach to find specialists for consultation purposes. Thus, a lack of desire to meet with a therapist first may have little to do with the psychopharmacologist's competence with your patient or his capacity to work well with you.

The Consultation Process

The Initial Consultation

The first step toward a psychopharmacological consultation is to discuss the possibility with the patient. As noted above, the suggestion may be met by a variety of reactions that have important transference implications. With some patients, these issues must be worked out before the actual consultation process can begin. With others, or in times of clinical crisis, the consultation can begin while its meanings are being explored. Even in those situations in which patients themselves suggest a consultation, the expectations of the pharmacotherapy should be at least probed, since the unrealistic fantasies noted above, if present (e.g., "a pill will solve all my problems"), should be elicited and discussed. Optimally, the consultation should be framed by the therapist as a question to be addressed: would medication aid in the patient's treatment, and if so, which medication? The contrasting approach—referring patients so they can get a prescription for Prozac, a decision made by a patient and/or therapist prior to the pharmacological consultation—both demeans the consultation process and hampers the open-ended thinking that characterizes the best consultations.

The timing of the consultation reflects the judgment of the therapist as well as the acceptance by the patient of medication as a potential therapeutic modality. Often, because of resistance caused by some of the factors noted above, it may take a patient many months to agree to a consultation that has been suggested.

Arthur was an artist in all senses of the word. Supported by his family, he had spent his life painting. After a recent marriage, he was made aware of his marked mood lability. Because his mood swings were often triggered by life events (such as a fight with his wife), he had al-

ways attributed them to his artistic nature. When his mood swings became problematic in his marriage, he entered therapy. Because of the
intensity of his mood swings and a strong family history of depression
(his father had had a severe depressive episode when Arthur was a
teenager, during which he killed himself), the therapist gently posed
the option of antidepressants. Arthur equally gently declined the option, fearing a dampening of his creativity and of being controlled by
a chemical. Nine months of effective psychotherapy was very helpful
in dealing with issues of unexpressed anger and grief about his father's death as well as how this experience related to some current
marital problems. The mood swings, however, continued. On a number of occasions, the therapist brought up the idea of antidepressants,
but Arthur's response was always the same, fearing the loss of his
artistic muse.

Finally, after a physician suggested the use of fluoxetine for a
chronic pain disorder, Arthur agreed to a medication trial for both the
pain and the mood swings. Given Arthur's profound wariness of antidepressants, the consulting pharmacotherapist started him on fluoxetine 2.5 mg daily (prescribed in the liquid form), increasing to 5 mg
daily after ten days. Within two weeks, Arthur noted a marked difference in his moodiness. For the first time in his adult life, he was able
to be upset without becoming paralyzed. His painting, rather than
being diminished by the medication, became bolder and Arthur became more productive, eventually becoming far more successful.
Once he was better, Arthur was able to acknowledge that a major
component of his medication reluctance was his fear that taking the
antidepressant would identify him with his psychiatrically ill father.
When the antidepressant was suggested for pain relief, it gave him a
rationale to pursue this line of treatment with less concern about its
meaning.

Once both therapist and patient agree to pursue a consultation, it is
wisest for the therapist to call the psychopharmacologist first. This ac-
complishes a number of goals: (1) if the therapist and psychopharmacologist haven't worked together before, it serves as an introduction;
(2) it establishes the availability of the pharmacotherapist (or if he is
unavailable, allows the therapist to restart the process with someone
else before the patient calls); and (3) it introduces the patient's name
and briefly describes the problem in question to the consultant. In my
experience, the level of personal attention the pharmacotherapist gives
the patient during the first telephone call increases if the groundwork
has been laid by the therapist beforehand. (This is equally important in

those clinical settings, such as managed care settings, in which patients have little choice in who treats them.) If the two professionals have not worked together previously, it can be helpful to clarify the consultation procedure during this call. How many visits will the consultation take? What are the fees? (If the patient's insurance will only pay for consultations with physicians on its clinician panel who accept a predetermined fee structure, it should be clarified whether the pharmacotherapist is on the panel.) How much information does the pharmacotherapist want beforehand? This information can then be given to the patient. All too frequently, patients who are referred for psychiatric consultation expect elaborate neurological testing and are disappointed when it is not done. Conversely, some patients expect to be interviewed for fifteen minutes and given medication. A realistic appreciation of the nature of a psychopharmacological consultation is vital for coordinated treatment and patient compliance.

There is no universal method of psychopharmacological consultation. In large part in response to financial pressures from third-party payors, patients are usually seen only once before a diagnostic decision and recommendation for treatment is made. For a patient who presents with a classic melancholic depression or a clear-cut panic disorder, this poses no problem. However, a more complicated patient, such as a 24-year-old man with borderline personality disorder who has been hospitalized twice and has been on multiple medications (the names of which are frequently forgotten) will usually require more visits and past information.

Unfortunately, there is very little magic in a psychopharmacological consultation. Within the interview, the psychopharmacologist will seek a careful delineation of symptoms and a sense of their timing with an additional emphasis on past psychiatric treatments and family and medical history. An interview that concentrates on eliciting symptoms may offend patients who are accustomed to the more psychodynamic examination of "why?" instead of the more symptom-based questions of "what?" Patients may get confused when the needed answer to the question "when did you start feeling depressed?" involves a time frame—"in May"—and not just "after my mother got sick." Timing and evolution of symptom clusters are vital pieces of diagnostic information. Life events and stressors, although important, are not *as* primary in a psychopharmacological consultation. Therefore, in the beginning of the first interview, some consultants explain that the interview will focus more on "what" rather than "why"; that for the purposes of the consultation—to clarify the nature of the problem, to decide whether medication might be helpful, and, if so, which medication—the "what" questions are vital.

The amount of medical information and number of lab tests needed in a consultation varies among psychopharmacologists and from patient to patient. It is impossible to state specifically in advance the extent and cost of the tests. A young healthy male with insomnia or depression requires only a minimal number of blood tests in order to exclude obvious abnormalities. An older depressed man with a history of heart disease may require consultation with an internist and an electrocardiogram and other sophisticated tests. The lab tests ensure the patient's physical health and rule out medical disorders that may either cause the psychiatric syndrome in question or interact with its treatment. Further details on these tests are presented in the previous chapters. It must be emphasized, though, that no test substitutes for a careful history. Except in unusual cases (e.g., the discovery of a brain tumor on a CT scan or of overt hyperthyroidism in a patient with anxiety), an accurate clinical history carries more weight than do the less easily interpretable lab tests.

If the consultation requires more than one session, the psychopharmacologist may call you after the first one to clarify certain clinical points that remain unclear after meeting with the patient. For instance, in evaluating a depressed patient it is often difficult, but important, to accurately date the course of symptoms: is the patient always depressed, as in dysthymic disorder, with superimposed depressive episodes, or does he have clear periods of normal mood? A depressed patient with the cognitive distortions of his disorder may perceive himself as having been depressed for years or a lifetime. The therapist who has seen the patient over months or years may have seen clear periods of normal mood. This distinction can have important implications in predicting response to antidepressants and evaluating the effect of treatment.

Once the consultant has finished his evaluation, he should communicate his thoughts both to the patient directly and to you via a telephone call. A consultation in which the referring therapist has not been given the conclusions of the consultant (assuming the therapist made the initial contact) has achieved only half its goal and should be considered incomplete. If this happens regularly with any particular consultant, bring it to his attention; if the pattern continues, find another pharmacotherapist for future collaborative work. If pharmacotherapy is appropriate, psychopharmacologists typically prescribe the medications at the end of the consultation and then inform the therapist, thereby saving the patient the expense of another visit. Written reports are sent by some, but not all consultants. They are time consuming and someone (usually the patient) ends up paying for it. When a written report is needed (e.g., for medicolegal reasons when working with a suicidal patient), let the consultant know. Similarly, it is sometimes recommended that the patient, therapist, and pharmacotherapist all meet together at the end of the consultation. Although this would aid in reducing the possibility of splitting and would enhance communication, it is usually difficult to arrange and expensive for the patient. If the two professionals are comfortable with the split treatment model, a three-way meeting is unnecessary.

Working in an Ongoing Split Treatment

If medication is prescribed, the psychopharmacologist will typically talk with the patient by telephone after three to ten days to evaluate side effects and possibly adjust the medication dose. One to four weeks after medication is begun, patient and pharmacotherapist usually meet to evaluate the potential therapeutic effect and to ask about side effects in a more detailed manner than is possible on the telephone. During times of active dose adjustment and clinical change, more contact, either by phone or in person, is needed. Once a patient is on a stable dose of medication, the frequency of contact decreases. Although telephone calls are often necessary to make minor dose adjustments or for patients to ask about unusual side effects, they cannot substitute for occasional face-to-face meetings in achieving a solid relationship between prescribing physician and patient. When virtually all the contact between patient and psychopharmacologist is by telephone, it can be easily assumed by the patient (and sometimes correctly!) that the physician is uninterested in the patient or the treatment, a feeling that is likely to have a negative effect on the outcome. Face-to-face meetings will enhance any placebo effect, foster compliance with the medication regimen, and decrease the possibilities of a negative transference with the pharmacotherapist. Together, these translate into a better treatment response.

Meetings between patient and pharmacotherapist typically last between fifteen and thirty minutes. The brevity of the meeting sharpens the boundaries between the psychotherapy sessions and the "med" visits. Seeing two mental health professionals for psychotherapy-length sessions, even if the stated goal of one of them is medication management, invites confusion and "parallel" therapies. With some extremely anxious patients, medication checkups may need to be forty-five minutes in order to answer all of the patient's questions and to allay any fears of the medication. In these cases, it is important that the extended "med" visits focus on the medication treatment.

Because the psychotherapist almost always sees the patient more frequently than the psychopharmacologist, questions pertaining to the medication ("Is the fatigue I feel due to the antidepressant?") are often directed to the therapist. The majority of these questions should be redirected to the pharmacotherapist. Except in the case of profoundly disturbed patients who are incapable of making the call, therapists should not call the psychopharmacologist to relay questions; the patient should call directly. This strengthens the alliance between physician and patient, promotes a more active stance on the patient's part in the treatment and diminishes the chance for a triangulation of the therapeutic relationship. If the patient has characterological issues with parental authority figures, this also allows for an interpersonal experience that, if successful, may be corrective or an important focus for psychotherapeutic treatment if problems arise.

For patients who are in maintenance treatment that may last many months or years, the amount of contact between patient and pharmacotherapist may vary from once a month to every six months. Similarly, it is difficult to suggest an appropriate frequency of contact between the therapist and psychopharmacologist over the course of a prolonged split treatment. What is needed is a balance between the extremes of two parallel treatments done in isolation versus overly enmeshed contact with the other professional. If contact is too infrequent, important observations and insights will not be shared, and the two professionals may push the treatment (and the patient) in opposite directions. Patients are also greatly relieved to know that the two professionals communicate with each other about them on an intermittent basis. With the pressure of time, however, and the sheer number of patients that many psychopharmacologists follow (which can be in excess of two hundred patients), regular contact between the two professionals is often difficult except at times when the patient is in a true crisis. A simple, effective option that is less time-consuming than actual conversations is via the magic of telephone answering machines (or voice mail) which allow observations, concerns, and questions to be raised and responses given without the need for formal discussions. If a more complex discussion (e.g., regarding potential hospitalization) is required, a direct conversation can be arranged.

Dr. H provided psychopharmacological treatment for Sarah, who was in long-term psychotherapy with Dr. N. Sarah's multiple difficulties included dysthymia with intermittent major depression, bulimia, intermittent drug abuse, mixed personality disorder with some borderline features, and significant marital discord. Not surprisingly, her course was stormy with times of functioning reasonably well interspersed with occasional crises of variable intensity. With both Dr. H and Dr. N having busy practices, they quickly evolved a system in which Dr. N would alert Dr. H to a new crisis with Sarah by leaving a message with a brief description of his clinical observations. He would also instruct the patient to call Dr. H. After the consultation, Dr. H would leave a brief return message for Dr. N., summarizing his findings and whatever medication changes he made. In this way, the two professionals were able to communicate frequently and efficiently with each other without excessive time burdens.

Too much contact between professionals absorbing too much time can result in subsequent resentment on the part of one or both professionals. It may also be a clue to seductive, manipulative pathology on the patient's part, promoting the mobilization and overengagement of "caretakers" around him as he waits passively to be rescued or cured.

Contact between the two professionals should always occur in the following circumstances:

1. When the patient's clinical condition changes acutely. The discussion should focus on the nature of the change and any stressors that might have precipitated it. A coordinated plan of action can then be agreed upon and implemented.
2. If the patient becomes significantly suicidal. Questions to be addressed include the possibility of hospitalization, frequency of therapeutic contact, and whether the patient has a lethal amount of medication at home if an overdose is attempted. At times, if a suicidal patient is not hospitalized, the therapist (who is likely to see the patient more frequently) can keep the pills in his office, dispensing a week (or less) of medication at a time to the patient. This would drastically decrease the risk in case of an impulsive overdose.
3. When a major change in diagnosis requires a medication shift. An example would be adding a mood stabilizer because of a conviction that the patient had bipolar disorder and not major depression as initially thought. Changing antidepressants because of side ef-

fects or minor dosage alterations do not need to be discussed every time.

4.   Whenever an important clinical question arises. For instance, trying to distinguish between a mild hypomania, especially if precipitated by antidepressants, and the emergence of true assertiveness is often difficult (as in the case of Roberta, described earlier in the chapter). Similarly, distinguishing between an exacerbation of depressed mood in a patient with both major depression and chronic self-esteem problems and depressive personality is easier with multiple observers.

Cynthia was in psychotherapy, dealing with her feelings of inadequacy and dependency on her mother. Additionally, her recurrent depressions were successfully treated by a pharmacotherapist with desipramine 150 mg daily. Following a threat by her mother to force her to move to her own apartment, Cynthia became frantic and suicidal. When she saw her pharmacotherapist, she asked to be hospitalized, describing hypersomnia and fatigue that had lasted for weeks. She did not mention the fight with her mother nor did she say that the hypersomnia occurred only on weekends when she was home all day with her mother. When the two treating professionals discussed the situation, the therapist clarified the acute and recent nature of the exacerbation as well as the variable course of the vegetative symptoms of depression. Because of this information, it was decided not to increase the antidepressant or to hospitalize the patient but to focus the work on her interactions with caregivers such as her mother and the psychopharmacologist.

5.   If there is any evidence that therapeutic splitting has occurred and is not diminishing through psychotherapeutic work. The clearest sign of the split is the patient devaluing the other professional— "he doesn't understand me the way you do" or "she doesn't help me at all"—often accompanied by a seductive overevaluation of the professional being addressed. In these situations, a personal knowledge of the other professional helps. If exploring transference implications of the split is not sufficient, it is often helpful for the two professionals to communicate.

Sometimes, two professionals may genuinely disagree as to the precipitant and appropriate intervention when a patient seems to be worse: Is the depressive exacerbation in a patient due to the emergence of early, painful memories being worked through or is it a seasonal mood disorder? It is confusing for patients to be given divergent explanations. At these times, the two clinicians need to confer and to make sure that even with disagreement, information can be presented to the patient in a way that does not undermine either treatment.

Psychiatric Medications

Note: Medications are listed alphabetically in the first column using both generic and trade names. When trade names are listed, however, the reader is instructed to look up the generic name or medication class for other trade names for the same product.

Name	Trade Name(s)	Medication Class[a]
Adapin: *see* Doxepin		
Akineton: *see* Biperiden		
Alprazolam	Xanax	BZP antianx/hyp
Amantadine	Symmetrel	Antipark, anti-s.e.
Ambien: *see* Zolpidem		
Amitriptyline	Elavil, Endep	Cyclic AD
Amobarbital	Amytal	Barb antianx/hyp
Amoxapine	Asendin	Cyclic AD
d-Amphetamine	Dexedrine	Stimulant
Amytal: *see* Amobarbital		
Anafranil: *see* Clomipramine		
Antabuse: *see* Disulfiram		
Artane: *see* Trihexyphenidyl		
Asendin: *see* Amoxapine		
Atarax: *see* Hydroxyzine		
Atenolol	Tenormin	Antianx, anti-s.e.
Ativan: *see* Lorazepam		
Aventyl: *see* Nortriptyline		
Benadryl: *see* Diphenhydramine		
Benztropine	Cogentin	Antipark
Biperiden	Akineton	Antipark
Bromocriptine	Parlodel	Cocaine abuse

[a]Abbreviations: AD = antidepressant; ADHD=attention deficit/hyperactivity disorder; Antianx = antianxiety; Antihist = antihistamine; Antipark = antiparkinsonian; Anti-s.e. = anti-side effect; Barb = barbiturate; BZP = Benzodiazepine; Hyp = hypnotic; Nonbarb = nonbarbiturate; OCD = obsessive compulsive disorder; PMS = premenstral syndrome; PTSD = post-traumatic stress disorder; SSRI = selective serotonin reuptake inhibitor.

Name	Trade Name(s)	Medication Class[a]
Buprenorphine	Buprenex	Opiate abuse
Buprenex: *see* Buprenorphine		
Bupropion	Wellbutrin	Cyclic AD
Buspar: *see* Buspirone		
Buspirone	Buspar	Antianx
Butabarbital	Butisol	Barb antianx/hyp
Butisol: *see* Butabarbital		
Calan: *see* Verapamil		
Carbamazepine	Tegretol	Mood stabilizer
Catapres: *see* Clonidine		
Chloral hydrate	Noctec	Hypnotic
Chlordiazepoxide	Librium	BZP antianx/hyp
Chlorpromazine	Thorazine	Antipsychotic
Clomipramine	Anfranil	Cyclic AD, OCD
Clonazepam	Klonopin	BZP antianx/hyp
Clonidine	Catapres	Antianx, Tourette's, ADHD
Clorazepate	Tranxene	BZP antianx
Clozapine	Clozaril	Antipsychotic
Clorazil: *see* Clozapine		
Cogentin: *see* Benztropine		
Cognex: *see* Tacrine		
Cylert: *see* Pemoline		
Cyproheptadine	Periactin	Anorexia nervosa, anti-sexual s.e.
Dalmane: *see* Flurazepam		
Danazol		PMS
Depakote: *see* Divalproex, Valproate		
Desipramine	Norpramin, Pertofrane	Cyclic AD
Desoxyn: *see* Methamphetamine		
Desyrel: *see* Trazodone		
Dexedrine: *see* d-Amphetamine		
Diazepam	Valium	BZP antianx/hyp
Diethylpropion		Stimulant
Dilantin: *see* Phenytoin		
Diphenhydramine	Benadryl	Antihist, antianx/hyp, antipark
Disulfiram	Antabuse	Alcohol abuse
Divalproex	Depakote	Mood stabilizer
Doral: *see* Quazepam		
Doriden: *see* Glutethimide		
Doxepin	Adapin, Sinequan	Cyclic AD
Droperidol	Inapsine	Antipsychotic

Name	Trade Name(s)	Medication Class[a]
Effexor: *see* Venlafaxine		
Elavil: *see* Amitriptyline		
Eldepryl: *see* Selegiline		
Endep: *see* Amitriptyline		
Eskalith-CR: *see* Lithium		
Estazolam	Prosom	BZP hyp
Ethchlorvynol	Placidyl	Nonbarb hypnotic
Ethinamate	Valmid	Nonbarb hypnotic
Etrafon (combination of amitriptyline and perphenazine)		
Evening primrose oil		PMS
Fenfluramine	Pondimin	Autism, OCD adjunct
Fluoxetine	Prozac	SSRI AD
Fluphenazine	Prolixin	Antipsychotic
Flurazepam	Dalmane	BZP hypnotic
Fluvoxamine	Luvox	SSRI AD, OCD
Glutethimide	Doriden	Nonbarb hypnotic
Guanfacine	Tenex	ADHD
Halazepam	Paxipam	BZP antianxiety
Halcion: *see* Triazolam		
Haldol: *see* Haloperidol		
Haloperidol	Haldol	Antipsychotic
Hydergine		Alzheimer's disease
Hydroxyzine	Atarax, Vistaril	Antihist, antianx/hyp
Imipramine	Tofranil	Cyclic AD
Inapsine: *see* Droperidol		
Inderal: *see* Propranolol		
Isoptin: *see* Verapamil		
Kemadrin: *see* Procyclidine		
Klonopin: *see* Clonazepam		
LAAM		Opiate abuse
Leuprolide	Lupron	PMS
Librium: *see* Chlordiazepoxide		
Limbitrol (combination of amitriptyline and chlordiazepoxide)		
Lithium	Eskalith, Lithonate, Lithotabs, Lithobid, Eskalith-CR, Cibalith-S	Mood stabilizer
Lithobid: *see* Lithium		
Lorazepam	Ativan	BZP antianx/hyp
Loxapine	Loxitane	Antipsychotic

Name	Trade Name(s)	Medication Class[a]
Loxitane: *see* Loxapine		
Ludiomil: *see* Maprotiline		
Luminal: *see* Phenobarbital		
Lupron: *see* Leuprolide		
Luvox: *see* Fluvoxamine		
Maprotiline	Ludiomil	Cyclic AD
Mebaral: *see* Mephobarbital		
Mellaril: *see* Thioridazine		
Mephobarbital	Mebaral	Barb antianx
Meprobamate	Miltown	Nonbarb antianx/hyp
Mesoridazine	Serentil	Antipsychotic
Methamphetamine	Desoxyn	Stimulant
Methylphenidate	Ritalin	Stimulant
Methyprylon	Noludar	Nonbarb hypnotic
Miltown: *see* Meprobamate		
Moban: *see* Molindone		
Molindone	Moban	Antipsychotic
Naltrexone	ReVia	Opiate addiction, alcohol abuse
Nardil: *see* Phenelzine		
Navane: *see* Thiothixene		
Nefazodone	Serzone	Novel AD
Nembutal: *see* Pentobarbital		
Noctec: *see* Chloral hydrate		
Noludar: *see* Methyprylon		
Norpramin: *see* Desipramine		
Nortriptyline	Aventyl, Pamelor	Cyclic AD
Orap: *see* Pimozide		
Oxazepam	Serax	BZP antianx/hyp
Pamelor: *see* Nortriptyline		
Parlodel: *see* Bromocriptine		
Parnate: *see* Tranylcypromine		
Paroxetine	Paxil	SSRI AD
Paxil: *see* Paroxetine		
Paxipam: *see* Halazepam		
Pemoline	Cylert	Stimulant
Pentobarbital	Nembutal	Barb antianx/hyp
Periactin: *see* Cyproheptadine		
Perphenazine	Trilafon	Antipsychotic
Pertofrane: *see* Desipramine		
Phendimetrazine		Stimulant
Phenelzine	Nardil	MAO inhibitor AD

Name	Trade Name(s)	Medication Class[a]
Phenergan: *see* Promethazine		
Phenobarbital	Luminal	Barb antianx
Phentermine		Stimulant
Pimozide	Orap	Tourette's syndrome
Placidyl: *see* Ethchlorvynol		
Pondimin: *see* Fenfluramine		
Procyclidine	Kemadrin	Antipark
Prolixin: *see* Fluphenazine		
Promethazine	Phenergan	Antihist antianx/hyp
Propranolol	Inderal	Antianx, anti-s.e.
Prosom: *see* Estazolam		
Protriptyline	Vivactil	Cyclic AD
Prozac: *see* Fluoxetine		
Pyridoxine/Vitamin B$_6$		PMS
Quazepam	Doral	BZD hyp
Restoril: *see* Temazepam		
ReVia: *see* Naltrexone		
Risperdal: *see* Risperidone		
Risperidone	Risperdal	Antipsychotic
Ritalin: *see* Methylphenidate		
Secobarbital	Seconal	Barb antianx/hyp
Seconal: *see* Secobarbital		
Selegiline	Eldepryl	MAO inhibitor AD
Serax: *see* Oxazepam		
Serentil: *see* Mesoridazine		
Sertraline	Zoloft	SSRI AD
Serzone: *see* Nefazodone		
Sinequan: *see* Doxepin		
Stelazine: *see* Trifluoperazine		
Surmontil: *see* Trimipramine		
Symmetrel: *see* Amantadine		
Tacrine	Cognex	Alzheimer's disease
Tegretol: *see* Carbamazepine		
Temazepam	Restoril	BZP antianx/hyp
Tenex: *see* Guanfacine		
Tenormin: *see* Atenolol		
Thioridazine	Mellaril	Antipsychotic
Thiothixene	Navane	Antipsychotic
Thorazine: *see* Chlorpromazine		
Tofranil: *see* Imipramine		
Tranxene: *see* Clorazepate		
Tranylcypromine	Parnate	MAO inhibitor AD

Name	Trade Name(s)	Medication Class[a]
Trazodone	Desyrel	Cyclic AD
Triavil (combination of amitriptyline and perhenazine)		
Triazolam	Halcion	BZP hypnotic
Trifluoperazine	Stelazine	Antipsychotic
Trifluopromazine	Vesprin	Antipsychotic
Trihexyphenidyl	Artane	Antipark
Trilafon: *see* Perphenazine		
Trimipramine	Surmontil	Cyclic AD
L-Tryptophan		Hypnotic
Valium: *see* Diazepam		
Valmid: *see* Ethinamate		
Valproate	Depakene, Depakote	Mood stabilizer
Venlafaxine	Effexor	Novel AD
Verapamil	Calan, Isoptin	Mood stabilizer
Vesprin: *see* Trifluopromazine		
Vistaril: *see* Hydroxyzine		
Vitamin E		Tardive dyskinesia
Vivactil: *see* Protriptyline		
Wellbutrin: *see* Bupropion		
Xanax: *see* Alprazolam		
Zoloft: *see* Sertraline		
Zolpidem	Ambien	Hypnotic

References

ABBEY, S. E., & GARFINKEL, P. E. (1991). Neurasthenia and chronic fatigue syndrome: The role of culture in the making of a diagnosis. *American Journal of Psychiatry, 148,* 1638–1646.

ADELMAN, S. (1985). Pills as transitional objects: A dynamic understanding of the use of medication in psychotherapy. *Psychiatry, 48,* 246–253.

AGRAS, W. S., ROSSITER, E. M., ARNOW, B., SCHNEIDER, J. A., TELCH, C. F., RAEBURN, S. D., BRUCE, B., PERL, M., & KORAN, L. M. (1992). Pharmacological and cognitive-behavioral treatment for bulimia nervosa: A controlled comparison. *American Journal of Psychiatry, 149,* 82–87.

AKISKAL, H. S., DJENDEREDJAN, A. H., ROSENTHAL, R. H., & KHANI, M. K. (1977). Cyclothymic disorder: Validating criteria for inclusion in the bipolar affective group. *American Journal of Psychiatry, 134,* 1227–1233.

AKISKAL, H. S., KHANI, M., & SCOTT-STRAUSS, A. (1979). Cyclothymic temperamental disorders. *Psychiatric Clinics of North America, 2,* 527–554.

AKISKAL, H. S., ROSENTHAL, T. L., HAYKAL, R. F., LEMMI, H., ROSENTHAL, R. H., & SCOTT-STRAUSS, A. (1980). Characterological depressions: Clinical and sleep EEG findings separating 'subaffective dysthymias' from 'character spectrum disorders.' *Archives of General Psychiatry, 37,* 777–783.

ALEXOPOULOS, G. S., MEYERS, B. S., YOUNG, R. C., MATTIS, S., & KAKUMA, T. (1993). The course of geriatric depression with "reversible dementia": A controlled study. *American Journal of Psychiatry, 150,* 1693–1699.

ALTSHULER, L. L., BURT, V. K., McMULLEN, M., & HENDRICK, V. (1995). Breastfeeding and sertraline: A 24-hour analysis. *Journal of Clinical Psychiatry, 56,* 243–245.

ALTSHULER, L. L., COHEN, L., SZUBA, M. P., BURT, V., GITLIN, M., & MINTZ, J. Pregnancy and psychiatric illness: Dilemmas and guidelines in pharmacologic management. *American Journal of Psychiatry,* in press.

ALTSHULER, L. L., HENDRICK, V., & PARRY, B. (1995). Pharmacological management of premenstrual disorder. *Harvard Review of Psychiatry, 2,* 233–245.

ALVIR, J. M. J., LIEBERMAN, J. A., SAFFERMAN, A. Z., SCHWIMMER, J. L., & SCHAAF, J. A. (1993). Clozapine-induced agranulocytosis. *New England Journal of Medicine, 329,* 162–167.

AMBELAS, A. (1987). Life events and mania: A special relationship. *British Journal of Psychiatry, 150,* 235–240.

AMERICAN ACADEMY OF PEDIATRICS COMMITTEE ON DRUGS. (1994). The transfer of drugs and other chemicals into human milk. *Pediatrics, 93,* 137–150.

AMERICAN PSYCHIATRIC ASSOCIATION. (1994a). *Diagnostic and statistical manual of mental disorders,* Fourth Edition. Washington, DC: American Psychiatric Association.

AMERICAN PSYCHIATRIC ASSOCIATION. (1994b). Practice guideline for the treatment of patients with bipolar disorder. *American Journal of Psychiatry, 151,* (Suppl), 1–36.

AMERICAN PSYCHIATRIC ASSOCIATION. (1993a). *Practice guidelines for eating disorders.* Washington, DC: American Psychiatric Association Press, *150,* 212–228.

AMERICAN PSYCHIATRIC ASSOCIATION. (1993b). Practice guideline for major depressive disorder in adults. *American Journal of Psychiatry, 150,* (Suppl), 1–26.

473

AMERICAN PSYCHIATRIC ASSOCIATION. (1990). *The practice of electroconvulsive therapy: Recommendations for treatment, training and privileging: A task force report.* Washington, DC: American Psychiatric Press.

ANDREASEN, N. C., ARNDT, S., ALLIGER, R., MILLER, D., & FLAUM, M. (1995). Symptoms of schizophrenia: Methods, meanings, and mechanisms. *Archives of General Psychiatry, 52,.* 341–351.

ANDREASEN, N. C., & CARPENTER, W. T. (1993). Diagnosis and classification of schizophrenia. *Schizophrenia Bulletin, 19,* 199–214.

ANGRIST, B., D'HOLLOSY, M., SANFILIPO, M., SATRIANO, J., DIAMOND, G., SIMBERKOFF, M., & WEINREB, H. (1992). Central nervous system stimulants as symptomatic treatments for AIDS-related neuropsychiatric impairment. *Journal of Clinical Psychopharmacology, 12,* 268–272.

ANGST, J. (1973). The course of monopolar depression and bipolar psychoses. *Psychiatrie, Neurologie et Neurochirurgie, 76,* 489–500.

ANGST, J., & HOCHSTRASSER, B. (1994). Recurrent brief depression: The Zurich Study. *Journal of Clinical Psychiatry, 55* (4, Suppl), 3–9.

ARANA, G. W., GOFF, D. C., BALDESSARINI, R. J., & KEEPERS, G. A. (1988). Efficacy of anticholinergic prophylaxis for neuroleptic-induced acute dystonia. *American Journal of Psychiatry, 145,* 993–996.

ARNDT, S., ANDREASEN, N. C., FLAUM, M., MILLER, D., & NOPOULOS, P. (1995). A longitudinal study of symptom dimensions in schizophrenia: Predictions and patterns of change. *Archives of General Psychiatry, 52,* 352–360.

ASCHER, J. A., COLE, G. O., COLIN, J-N., FEIGHNER, J. P., FERRIS, R. M., FIBIGER, H. C., GOLDEN, R. N., MARTIN, P., POTTER, W. Z., RICHELSON, E., & SULSER, F. (1995). Bupropion: A review of its mechanisms of antidepressant activity. *Journal of Clinical Psychiatry, 56,* 395–401.

AYD, F., & BLACKWELL, D. (EDS.). (1970). *Discoveries in biological psychiatry.* Philadelphia: Lippincott.

BACHRACH, L. L. (1992). What we know about homelessness among mentally ill persons: An analytical review and commentary. In H. R. Lamb, L. L. Bachrach, & F. I. Kass (Eds.), *Treating the homeless mentally ill.* Washington, DC: American Psychiatric Press, 13–40.

BAER, L., JENIKE, M. A., RICCIARDI, J. N., HOLLAND, A. D., SEYMOUR, R. J., MINICHIELLO, W. E., & BUTTOLPH, M. L. (1990). Standardized assessment of personality disorders in obsessive-compulsive disorder. *Archives of General Psychiatry, 47,* 826–830.

BAER, L., RAUCH, S. L., BALLANTINE, H. T., MARTUZA, R., COSGROVE, R., CASSEM, E., GIRIUNAS, I., MANZO, P. A., DIMINO, C., & JENIKE, M. A. (1995). Cingulotomy for intractable obsessive-compulsive disorder: Prospective long-term follow-up of 18 patients. *Archives of General Psychiatry, 52,* 384–392.

BALDESSARINI, R. J., COHEN, B. M., & TEICHER, M. H. (1988). Significance of neuroleptic dose and plasma level in the pharmacological treatment of psychoses. *Archives of General Psychiatry, 45,* 79–91.

BALLENGER, J. C. (1993). Panic disorder: Efficacy of current treatments. *Psychopharmacology Bulletin, 29,* 477–486.

BALLENGER, J. C., BURROWS, G. D., DuPONT, R. L., LESSER, I. M., NOYES, R., PECKNOLD, J. C., RIFKIN, A., & SWINSON, R. P. (1988). Alprazolam in panic disorder and agoraphobia: Results from a multicenter trial. 1. Efficacy in short-term treatment. *Archives of General Psychiatry, 45,* 413–422.

BANOV, M. D., ZARATE, C. A., TOHEN, M., SCIALABBA, D., WINES, J. D., KOLBRENER, M., KIM, J., & COLE, J. O. (1994). Clozapine therapy in refractory affective disorders: Polarity predicts response in long-term follow-up. *Journal of Clinical Psychiatry, 55,* 295–300.

BASOGLU, M., MARKS, I. M., & SENGUN, S. (1992). A prospective study of panic and anxiety in agoraphobia with panic disorder. *British Journal of Psychiatry, 160,* 57–64.

BAUER, M. S., CALABRESE, J., DUNNER, D. L., POST, R., WHYBROW, P. C., GYULAI, L., TAY, L. K., YOUNKIN, S. R., BYNUM, D., LAVORI, P., & PRICE, R. A. (1994). Multisite data reanalysis of the validity of rapid cycling as a course modifier for bipolar disorder in DSM-IV. *American Journal of Psychiatry, 151,* 506–515.

BAUER, M. S., & WHYBROW, P. C. (1990). Rapid cycling bipolar affective disorder. II: Treatment of refractory rapid cycling with high-dose levothyroxine: A preliminary study. *Archives of General Psychiatry, 47,* 435–440.

BAXTER, L. R. (1994). Positron emission tomography studies of cerebral glucose metabolism in obsessive compulsive disorder. *Journal of Clinical Psychiatry, 55* (10, Suppl), 54–59.

BAXTER, L. R., SCHWARTZ, J. M., BERGMAN, K. S., SZUBA, M. P., GUZE, B. H., MAZZIOTA, J. C., ALAZRAKI, A., SELIN, C. E., FERNG, H. K., MUNFORD, P., & PHELPS, M. E. (1992). Caudate glucose metabolic rate changes with both drug and behavior therapy for obsessive-compulsive disorder. *Archives of General Psychiatry, 49,* 681–689.

BEASLEY, C. M., MASICA, D. N., HEILIGENSTEIN, J. H., WHEADON, D. E., & ZERBE, R. L. (1993). Possible monoamine oxidase inhibitor–serotonin uptake inhibitor interaction: Fluoxetine clinical data and preclinical findings. *Journal of Clinical Psychopharmacology, 13,* 312–320.

BEERS, M. H., & OUSLANDER, J. G. (1989). Risk factors in geriatric drug prescribing: A practical guide to avoiding problems. *Drugs, 37,* 105–112.

BEIN, H. J. (1970). Biological research in the pharmaceutical industry with reserpine. In F. Ayd & B. Blackwell (Eds.), *Discoveries in biological psychiatry.* Philadelphia: Lippincott, 152–164.

BEITMAN, B. (1988). Combining pharmacotherapy and psychotherapy: Diagnostic considerations. In F. Flach (Ed.), *Psychobiology and psychopharmacology.* New York: Norton.

BELONGIA, E. A., HEDBERG, C. W., GLEICH, G. J., WHITE, K. E., MAYENO, A. N., LOEGERING, D. A., DUNNETTE, S. L., PIRIE, P. L., MACDONALD, K. L., & OSTERHOLM, M. T. (1990). An investigation of the cause of the eosinophilia myalgia syndrome associated with tryptophan use. *New England Journal of Medicine, 323,* 357–365.

BERNSTEIN, D. P., USEDA, D., & SIEVER, L. J. (1993). Paranoid personality disorder: Review of the literature and recommendations for DSM-IV. *Journal of Personality Disorders, 7,* 53–62.

BERNSTEIN, G. A., & PERWIEN, A. R. (1995). Anxiety disorders: *Child and Adolescent Psychiatric Clinics of North America, 4,* 305–322.

BIEDERMAN, J., FARAONE, S. V., SPENCER, T., WILENS, T., NORMAN, D., LAPEY, K. A., MICK, E., LEHMAN, B. K., & DOYLE, A. (1993). Patterns of psychiatric comorbidity, cognition, and psychosocial functioning in adults with deficit hyperactivity disorder. *American Journal of Psychiatry, 150,* 1792–1798.

BIEDERMAN, J., LERNER, Y., & BELMAKER, R. N. (1979). Combination of lithium carbonate and haloperidol in schizo-affective disorder: A controlled study. *Archives of General Psychiatry, 36,* 327–333.

BIEDERMAN, J., NEWCORN, J., & SPRICH, S. (1991). Comorbidity of attention deficit hyperactivity disorder with conduct, depressive, anxiety, and other disorders. *American Journal of Psychiatry, 148,* 564–577.

BIGELOW, G. E., & PRESTON, K. L. (1995). Opioids. In F. E. Bloom and D. J. Kupfer (Eds.), *Psychopharmacology: The fourth generation of progress.* New York: Raven Press, 1731–1744.

BIRMAHER, B., WATERMAN, G. S., RYAN, N., CULLY, M., BALACH, L., INGRAM, J., & BRODSKY, M. (1994). Fluoxetine for childhood anxiety disorders. *Journal of the American Academy of Child Adolescent Psychiatry, 33,* 993–999.

BLACK, D. W., NOYES, R., GOLDSTEIN, R. B., & BLUM, N. (1992). A family study of obsessive-compulsive disorder. *Archives of General Psychiatry, 49,* 362–368.

BLACK, D. W., WESNER, R., BOWERS, W., & GABEL, J. (1993). A comparison of fluvoxamine, cognitive therapy, and placebo in the treatment of panic disorder. *Archives of General Psychiatry, 50,* 44–50.

BLACK, D. W., WINOKUR, G., & NASRALLAH, A. (1986). ECT in unipolar and bipolar disorders: A naturalistic evaluation of 460 patients. *Convulsive Therapy, 2,* 231–237.

BLACKWELL, B. (1976). Treatment adherence. *British Journal of Psychiatry, 129,* 513–531.

BLAND, R. C., NEWMAN, S. C., & ORR, H. (1986). Recurrent and non-recurrent depression: A family study. *Archives of General Psychiatry, 43,* 1085–1089.

BLEHAR, M. C., & ROSENTHAL, N. E. (1989). Seasonal affective disorders and phototherapy. *Archives of General Psychiatry, 46,* 469–474.

BOHN, M. J. (1993). Alcoholism. *Psychiatric Clinics of North America, 16,* 679–692.

BOND, W. S. (1986). Psychiatric indications for clonidine: The neuropharmacologic and clinical basis. *Journal of Clinical Psychopharmacology, 6,* 81–87.

BOTTERON, K. N., & GELLER, B. (1995). Pharmacologic treatment of childhood and adolescent mania. *Child and Adolescent Psychiatric Clinics of North America, 4,* 283–304.

BOUCHARD, T. J., LYKKEN, D. T., MCGUE, M., SEGAL, N. L., & TELLEGAN, A. (1990). Sources of human psychological differences: The Minnesota Study of twins reared apart. *Science, 250,* 223–228.

BOWDEN, C. L., BRUGGER, A. M., SWANN, A. C., CALABRESE, J. R., JANICAK, P. G., PETTY, F., DILSAVER, S. C., DAVIS, J. M., RUSH, A. J., SMALL, J. G., GARZA-TREVINO, E. S., RISCH, S. C., GOODNICK, P. J., & MORRIS, D. D. (1994). Efficacy of divalproex vs lithium and placebo in the treatment of mania. *Journal of the American Medical Association, 271,* 918–924.

BOWRING, M. A., & KOVACS, M. (1992). Difficulties in diagnosing manic disorders among children and adolescents. *Journal of the American Academy of Child and Adolescent Psychiatry, 31,* 611–614.

BRAWMAN-MINTZER, O., LYDIARD, R. B., EMMANUEL, N., PAYEUR, R., JOHNSON, M., ROBERTS, J., JARRELL, M. P., & BALLENGER, J. C. (1993). Psychiatric comorbidity in patients with generalized anxiety disorder. *American Journal of Psychiatry, 150,* 1216–1218.

BREGMAN, J. D. (1995). Psychopharmacologic treatment of neuropsychiatric conditions in mental retardation. *Child and Adolescent Psychiatric Clinics of North America, 4,* 401–433.

BREIER, A., BUCHANAN, R. W., KIRKPATRICK, B., DAVIS, O. R., IRISH, D., SUMMERFELT, A., & CARPENTER, W. T. (1994). Effects of clozapine on positive and negative symptoms in outpatients with schizophrenia. *American Journal of Psychiatry, 151,* 20–26.

BREIER, A., CHARNEY, D. S., & HENINGER, G. R. (1984). Major depression in patients with agoraphobia and panic disorders. *Archives of General Psychiatry, 41,* 1129–1135.

BREWERTON, T. D., LYDIARD, R. B., HERZOG, D. B., BROTMAN, A. W., O'NEIL, P. M., & BALLENGER, J. C. (1995). Comorbidity of Axis I psychiatric disorders in bulimia nervosa. *Journal of Clinical Psychiatry, 56,* 77–80.

BROADHEAD, W. E., BLAZER, D. G., GEORGE, L. K., & TSE, C. K. (1990). Depression, disability days, and days lost from work in a prospective epidemiologic survey. *Journal of the American Medical Association, 264,* 2524–2528.

BROWN, S. A., INABA, R. K., GILLIN, J. C., SCHUCKIT, M. A., STEWART, M. A., & IRWIN, M. R. (1995). Alcoholism and affective disorder: Clinical course of depressive symptom. *American Journal of Psychiatry, 152,* 45–52.

BROWN, T. A., BARLOW, D. H., & LIEBOWITZ, M. R. (1994). The empirical basis of generalized anxiety disorder. *American Journal of Psychiatry, 151,* 1272–1280.

BUCHANAN, R. W., STRAUSS, M. E., KIRKPATRICK, B., HOLSTEIN, C., BREIER, A., & CARPENTER, W. T. (1994). Neuropsychological impairments in deficit vs non-deficit forms of schizophrenia. *Archives of General Psychiatry, 51,* 804–811.

BUNNEY, W. E., & DAVIS, J. M. (1965). Norepinephrine in depressive disorders: A review. *Archives of General Psychiatry, 13,* 483–494.

BYERLEY, B., & GILLIN, J. C. (1984). Diagnosis and management of insomnia. *Psychiatric Clinics of North America, 7,* 773–789.

CADE, J. F. J. (1949). Lithium salts in the treatment of psychotic excitement. *Medical Journal of Australia, 2,* 349–352.

CALABRESE, J. R., BOWDEN, C., & WOYSHVILLE, M. J. (1995). Lithium and the anticonvulsants in the treatment of bipolar disorder. In F. E. Bloom and D. S. Kupfer (Eds.), *Psychopharmacology: The fourth generation of progress.* New York: Raven Press, 1099–1111.

CALDWELL, C. B., & GOTTESMAN, I. I. (1990). Schizophrenics kill themselves too: A review of risk factors for suicide. *Schizophrenia Bulletin, 16,* 571–589.

CANTWELL, D. P. (1985). Hyperactive children have grown up: What have we learned about what happens to them? *Archives of General Psychiatry, 42,* 1026–1028.

CARLSON, G. A., & CANTWELL, D. P. (1980). Unmasking masked depression in children and adolescents. *American Journal of Psychiatry, 137,* 445–449.

CARPENTER, W. T. (1995). Serotonin-dopamine antagonists and treatment of negative symptoms. *Journal of Clinical Psychopharmacology, 15* (1, Suppl), 30S–35S.

CARPENTER, W. T., HANLON, T. E., HEINRICHS, D. W., SUMMERFELT, A. T., KIRKPATRICK, B., LEVINE, J., & BUCHANAN, R. W. (1990). Continuous versus targeted medications in schizophrenic outpatients: Outcome results. *American Journal of Psychiatry, 147,* 1138–1148.

CARPENTER, W. T., HEINRICHS, D. W., & WAGMAN, A. M. I. (1988). Deficit and non-deficit forms of schizophrenia: The concept. *American Journal of Psychiatry, 145,* 578–583.

CARROLL, K. M., ROUNSAVILLE, B. J., GORDON, L. T., NICH, C., JATLOW, P., BISIGHINI, R. M., & GAWIN, F. H. (1994). Psychotherapy and pharmacotherapy for ambulatory cocaine abusers. *Archives of General Psychiatry, 51,* 177–187.

CASEY, D. E. (1993). Neuroleptic-induced acute extrapyramidal syndromes and tardive dyskinesia. *Psychiatric Clinics of North America, 16,* 589–610.

CASEY, D. E. (1995). Tardive dyskinesia: Pathophysiology. In F. E. Bloom and D. J. Kupfer (Eds.), *Psychopharmacology: The fourth generation of progress.* New York: Raven Press, 1497–1502.

CASPAR, R. C., REDMOND, D. E., KATZ, M. M., SCHAFFER, C. B., DAVIS, J. M., & KOSLOW, S. H. (1985). Somatic symptoms in primary affective disorder. Presence and relationship to the classification of depression. *Archives of General Psychiatry, 42,* 1098–1104.

CAVALLARO, R., REGAZZETTI, M. G., COVELLI, G., & SMERALDI, E. (1993). Tolerance and withdrawal with zolpidem. *Lancet, 342,* 374–375.

CHAPPELL, P. B., LECKMAN, J. F., & RIDDLE, M. A. (1995). The pharmacologic treatment of tic disorders. *Child and Adolescent Psychiatric Clinics of North America, 4,* 197–216.

CHARNEY, D. S., BREMER, J. D., & REDMOND, D. E. (1995). Noradrenergic neural substrates for anxiety and fear: Clinical associations based on preclinical research. In

F. E. Bloom and D. J. Kupfer (Eds.), *Psychopharmacology: The fourth generation of progress.* NewYork: Raven Press, 387–395.

CHARNEY, D. S., DEUTCH, A. Y., KRYSTAL, J. H., SOUTHWICK, S. M., & DAVIS, M. (1993). Psychobiological mechanisms of posttraumatic stress disorder. *Archives of General Psychiatry, 50,* 294–305.

CHARNEY, D. S., HENINGER, G. R., & JATLOW, P. I. (1985). Increased anxiogenic effects of caffeine in panic disorders. *Archives of General Psychiatry, 42,* 233–243.

CHARNEY, D. S., WOODS, S. W., NAGY, L. M., SOUTHWICK, S. M., KRYSTAL, J. H., & HENINGER, G. R. (1990). Noradrenergic function in panic disorder. *Journal of Clinical Psychiatry, 51* (12, Suppl A), 5–11.

CHIARELLO, R. J., & COLE, J. O. (1987). The use of psychostimulants in general psychiatry: A reconsideration. *Archives of General Psychiatry, 44,* 286–295.

CHOU, J. C. Y. (1991). Recent advances in treatment of acute mania. *Journal of Clinical Psychopharmacology, 11,* 3–21.

CHRISTENSON, G. A., MACKENZIE, T. B., MITCHELL, J. E., & CALLIES, A. L. (1991). A placebo-controlled, double-blind crossover study of fluoxetine in trichotillomania. *American Journal of Psychiatry, 148,* 1566–1571.

CHRISTISON, G. W., KIRCH, D. G., & WYATT, R. J. (1991). When symptoms persist: Choosing among alternative somatic treatments for schizophrenia. *Schizophrenia Bulletin, 17,* 217–240.

CLEIN, P. D., & RIDDLE, M. A. (1995). Pharmacokinetics in children and adolescents. *Child and Adolescent Clinics of North America, 4,* 59–75.

COCCARO, E. F., & SIEVER, L. J. (1995). The neuropsychopharmacology of personality disorders. In F. E. Bloom and D. J. Kupfer (Eds.), *Psychopharmacology: The fourth generation of progress.* NewYork: Raven Press, 1567–1579.

COCHRAN, S. (1984). Preventing medical noncompliance in the outpatient treatment of bipolar affective disorders. *Journal of Consulting and Clinical Psychology, 52,* 873–878.

COFFEY, B. J., MIGUEL, E. C., SAVAGE, C. R., & RAUCH, S. L. (1994). Tourette's disorder and related problems: review and update. *Harvard Review of Psychiatry, 2,* 121–132.

COFFEY, C. E. (1994). The role of structural brain imaging in ECT. *Psychopharmacology Bulletin, 30,* 477–483.

COHEN, L. S., FRIEDMAN, J. M., JEFFERSON, J. W., JOHNSON, M., & WEINER, M. L. (1994). A reevaluation of risk of in utero exposure to lithium. *Journal of the American Medical Association, 271,* 146–150.

COLE, J. O., GOLDBERG, S. C., & KLERMAN, G. L. (1964). Phenothiazine treatment in acute schizophrenia. *Archives of General Psychiatry, 10,* 246–261.

CONSENSUS CONFERENCE. (1985). Electroconvulsive therapy. *Journal of the American Medical Association, 254,* 2103–2108.

CONSENSUS DEVELOPMENT PANEL. (1985). Mood disorders: Pharmacologic prevention of recurrences. *American Journal of Psychiatry, 142,*469–476.

CONTE, H., PLUTCHNIK, R., WILD, K., & KARASU, T. B. (1986). Combined psychotherapy and pharmacotherapy for depression: A systematic analysis of the evidence. *Archives of General Psychiatry, 43,* 471–479.

COOK, E. H., & LEVENTHAL, B. L. (1995). Autistic disorder and other pervasive developmental disorders. *Child and Adolescent Psychiatric Clinics of North America, 4,* 381–399.

COOPER, J. E., KENDALL, R. E., & KURLAND, B. J. (1972). *Psychiatric diagnosis in New York and London: Maudsley Monograph No. 20.* London: Oxford University Press.

COOPER, P. J., CAMPBELL, E. A., DAY, A., KENNERLY, H., & BOND, A. (1988). Nonpsychotic psychiatric disorder after childbirth: A prospective study of prevalence, incidence, course and nature. *British Journal of Psychiatry, 152,* 799–806.

COPLAN, J. D., WOLK, S. I. & KLEIN, D. F. (1995). Anxiety and the serotonin$_{1A}$ receptor. In F. E. Bloom and D. J. Kupfer (Eds.), *Psychopharmacology: The fourth generation of progress.* New York: Raven Press, 1301–1310.

CORYELL, W., ENDICOTT, J., & KELLER, M. (1992). Rapidly cycling affective disorder: Demographics, diagnosis, family history, and course. *Archives of General Psychiatry, 49,* 126–131.

CORYELL, W., KELLER, M., LAVORI, P., & ENDICOTT, J. (1990a). Affective syndromes, psychotic features, and prognosis: I. Depression. *Archives of General Psychiatry, 47,* 651–657.

CORYELL, W., KELLER, M., LAVORI, P., & ENDICOTT, J. (1990b). Affective syndromes, psychotic features, and prognosis: II. Mania. *Archives of General Psychiatry, 47,* 658–662.

COWDRY, R. W., & GARDNER, D. L. (1988). Pharmacotherapy of borderline personality disorder: Alprazolam, carbamazepine, trifluoperazine, and tranylcypromine. *Archives of General Psychiatry, 45,* 111–119.

COWLEY, D. S., & ARANA, G. W. (1990). The diagnostic utility of lactate sensitivity in panic disorder. *Archives of General Psychiatry, 47,* 277–284.

CREESE, I., BURT, D. R., & SNYDER, S. H. (1976). Dopamine receptor binding predicts clinical and pharmacological potencies of antischizophrenic drugs. *Science, 192,* 481–483.

CROW, T. J. (1980). Molecular pathology of schizophrenia: More than one disease process? *British Medical Journal, 280,* 66–68.

CROWE, R. R. (1974). An adoption study of antisocial personality. *Archives of General Psychiatry, 31,* 785–791.

CULLEN, M., MITCHELL, P., BRODATY, H., BOYCE, P., PARKER, G., HICKIE, I., & WILHELM, K. (1991). Carbamazepine for treatment-resistant melancholia. *Journal of Clinical Psychiatry, 52,* 472–476.

CUMMINGS, J. L. (1992). Depression and Parkinson's disease: A review. *American Journal of Psychiatry, 149,* 443–454.

DABIRI, L. M., PASTA, D., DARBY, J. K., & MOSBACHER, D. (1994). Effectiveness of vitamin E for treatment of long-term tardive dyskinesia. *American Journal of Psychiatry, 151,* 925–926.

DAHL, R. E. (1995). Child and adolescent sleep disorders. *Child and Adolescent Psychiatric Clinics of North America, 4,* 323–341.

DAVIDSON, J. (1992). Drug therapy of post-traumatic stress disorder. *British Journal of Psychiatry, 160,* 309–314.

DAVIDSON, J. (1989). Seizures and bupropion: A review. *Journal of Clinical Psychiatry, 50,* 256–261.

DAVIDSON, J. R. T., GILLER, E. L., ZISOOK, S., & OVERALL, J. E. (1988). An efficacy study of isocarboxazid and placebo in depression, and its relationship to depressive nosology. *Archives of General Psychiatry, 45,* 120–127.

DAVIDSON, J. R. T., HUGHES, D. C., GEORGE, L. K., & BLAZER, D. G. (1994). The boundary of social phobia: Exploring the threshold. *Archives of General Psychiatry, 51,* 975–983.

DAVIDSON, J., SWARTZ, M., STORCK, M., KRISHNAN, R. R., & HAMMETT, E. (1985). A diagnostic and family study of posttraumatic stress disorder. *American Journal of Psychiatry, 142,* 90–93.

DAVIDSON, J. R. T., TUPLER, L. A., & POTTS, N. L. S. (1994). Treatment of social phobia with benzodiazepines. *Journal of Clinical Psychiatry, 55* (6, Suppl), 28–32.

DAVIS, J. M., KOSLOW, S. H., GIBBONS, R. D., MAAS, J. W., BOWDEN, C. L., CASPER, R., HANIN, I., JAVAID, J., CHANG, S. S., & STOKES, P. E. (1988). Cerebrospinal fluid and urinary biogenic amines in depressed patients and healthy controls. *Archives of General Psychiatry, 45,* 705–717.

DAVIS, J. M., WANG, Z., & JANICAK, P. G. (1993). A quantitative analysis of clinical drug trials for the treatment of affective disorders. *Psychopharmacology Bulletin, 29,* 175–181.

DAVIS, K. L., KAHN, R. S., KO, G., & DAVIDSON, M. (1991). Dopamine in schizophrenia: A review and reconceptualization. *American Journal of Psychiatry, 148,* 1474–1486.

DELVA, N. J., & LETEMENDIA, F. J. (1982). Lithium treatment in schizophrenia and schizo-affective disorder. *British Journal of Psychiatry, 141,* 387–400.

DENIKER, P. (1970). Introduction of neuroleptic chemotherapy in psychiatry. In F. Ayd & B. Blackwell (Eds.), *Discoveries in biological psychiatry.* Philadelphia: Lippincott, 155–164.

DEVANE, C. L. (1994). Pharmacogenetics and drug metabolism of newer antidepressant agents. *Journal of Clinical Psychiatry, 55* (12, Suppl), 38–45.

DEVINSKY, O., & PACIA, S. V. (1994). Seizures during clozapine therapy. *Journal of Clinical Psychiatry, 55* (9, Suppl B), 153–156.

DIETCH, J. T., & JENNINGS, R. K. (1988). Aggressive dyscontrol in patients with benzodiazepines. *Journal of Clinical Psychiatry, 49,* 184–188.

DILSAVER, S. C., DEL MEDICO, V. J., QUADRI, A., & JAECKLE, R. S. (1990). Pharmacological responsiveness of winter depression. *Psychopharmacology Bulletin, 26,* 303–309.

DISTA. (1995). Data on file. Indianapolis, Indiana.

DOCHERTY, J. (1988). Managing compliance problems in psychopharmacology. In F. Flach (Ed.), *Psychobiology and psychopharmacology,* New York: Norton.

DOCHERTY, J., & FIESTER, S. (1985). The therapeutic alliance and compliance with psychopharmacology. In R. E. Hales & A. J. Frances (Eds.), *Annual review,* Vol. 4. Washington, DC: American Psychiatric Press, 607–632.

DOCHERTY, J., FIESTER, S., & SHEA, T. (1986). Syndrome diagnosis and personality disorders. In A. J. Frances & R. E. Hales (Eds.), *Annual review,* Vol. 5, Washington, DC: American Psychiatric Press, 315–355.

DOWNING, R., & RICKELS, K. (1987). Early treatment response in anxious outpatients treated with diazepam. *Acta Psychiatrica Scandinavia, 72,* 522–528.

DREIFUS, F., SANTILLI, N., & LANGER, D. (1987). Valproic acid hepatic fatalities: A retrospective review. *Neurology, 37,* 379–385.

DUBOVSKY, S. L., & THOMAS, M. (1995). Serotonergic mechanisms and current and future psychiatric practice. *Journal of Clinical Psychiatry, 56* (Suppl 2), 38–48.

DWORKIN, R. H., & CALIGOR, E. (1988). Psychiatric diagnosis and chronic pain: DSM-III-R and beyond. *Journal of Pain and Symptom Management, 3,* 87–98.

EATON, W. W., KESSLER, R. C., WITTCHEN, H. U., & MAGEE, W. J. (1994). Panic and panic disorder in the United States. *American Journal of Psychiatry, 151,* 413–420.

EISEN, J. L., & RASMUSSEN, S. A. (1993). Obsessive compulsive disorder with psychotic features. *Journal of Clinical Psychiatry, 54,* 373–379.

ELKIN, I., SHEA, M. T., WATKINS, J. T., IMBER, S. D., SOTSKY, S. M., COLLINS, J. F., GLASS, D. R., PILKONIS, P. A., LEBER, W. R., DOCHERTY, J. P., FIESTER, S. J., & PARLOFF, M. B. (1989). National Institute of Mental Health Treatment of Depression collaborative research program: General effectiveness of treatments. *Archives of General Psychiatry, 46,* 971–982.

EYSENCK, H. J., & EYSENCK, S. B. G. (1964). *Manual of the Eysenck Personality Inventory.* London: University of London Press.

FAEDDA, G. L., TONDO, L., BALDESSARINI, R. J., SUPPES, T., & TOHEN, M. (1993). Outcome after rapid vs gradual discontinuation of lithium treatment in bipolar disorders. *Archives of General Psychiatry, 50,* 448–455.

FAEDDA, G. L., TONDO, L., TEICHER, M. H., BALDESSARINI, R. J., GELBARD, H. A., & FLORIS, G. F. (1993). Seasonal mood disorders: Patterns of seasonal recurrence in mania and depression. *Archives of General Psychiatry, 50,* 17–23.

FAWCETT, J., KRAVITZ, H. M., ZAJECKA, J. M., & SCHAFF, M. R. (1991). CNS stimulant potentiation of monoamine oxidase inhibitors in treatment-refractory depression. *Journal of Clinical Psychopharmacology, 11,* 127–132.

FEIGHNER, J. P., BOYER, W. F., TYLER, D. L., & NEBORSKY, R. J. (1990). Adverse consequences of fluoxetine-MAOI combination therapy. *Journal of Clinical Psychiatry, 51,* 222–225.

FEIGHNER, J. P., HERBSTEIN, J., & DAMLOUJI, N. (1985). Combined MAOI, TCA, and direct stimulant therapy of treatment-resistant depression. *Journal of Clinical Psychiatry, 46:* 206–209.

FENTON, W. S., & McGLASHAN, T. H. (1991). Natural history of schizophrenia subtypes: I: Longitudinal study of paranoid, hebephrenic, and undifferentiated schizophrenia. *Archives of General Psychiatry, 48,* 969–977.

FENTON, W. S., WYATT, R. J., & McGLASHAN, T. H. (1994). Risk factors for spontaneous dyskinesia in schizophrenia. *Archives of General Psychiatry, 51,* 643–650.

FERNANDEZ, F., & LEVY, J. K. (1994). Psychopharmacology in HIV spectrum disorders. *Psychiatric Clinics of North America, 17,* 135–148.

FERNSTROM, M. A., KROWINSKI, R., & KUPFER, D. (1986). Chronic imipramine treatment and weight gain. *Psychiatric Research, 17,* 269–273.

FERRIS, R. M., & COOPER, B. R. (1993). Mechanism of antidepressant activity of bupropion. *Journal of Clinical Psychiatry Monograph, 11*(1), 2–14.

FESLER, F. A. (1991). Valproate in combat-related posttraumatic stress disorder. *Journal of Clinical Psychiatry, 52,* 361–364.

FINK, M. (1990). Is catatonia a primary indication for ECT? *Convulsive Therapy, 6,* 1–4.

FINK, M. (1994). Indications for the use of ECT. *Psychopharmacology Bulletin, 30,* 269–280.

FLEISCHHACKER, W. W., ROTH, S. D., & KANE, J. M. (1990). The pharmacologic treatment of neuroleptic-induced akathisia. *Journal of Clinical Psychopharmacology, 10,* 12–21.

FLUOXETINE BULIMIA NERVOSA COLLABORATIVE STUDY GROUP. (1992). Fluoxetine in the treatment of bulimia nervosa: A multicenter, placebo-controlled, double-blind trial. *Archives of General Psychiatry, 49,* 139–147.

FOA, E. S., & KOZAK, M. J. (1995). DSM-IV field trial: Obsessive-compulsive disorder. *American Journal of Psychiatry, 152,* 90–96.

FRANCES, R. J., & BORG, L. (1993). The treatment of anxiety in patients with alcoholism. *Journal of Clinical Psychiatry, 54* (5, Suppl), 37–43.

FRANK, E., KUPFER, D. J., PEREL, J. M., CORNES, C., MALLINGER, A. G., THASE, M. E., McEACHRAN, A. B., & GROCHOCINSKI, V. J. (1993). Comparison of full-dose versus half-dose pharmacotherapy in the maintenance of recurrent depression. *Journal of Affective Disorders, 27,* 139–145.

FRANK, J. B., KOSTEN, T. R., GILLER, E. L., & DAN, E. (1988). A randomized clinical trial of phenelzine and imipramine for post-traumatic stress disorder. *American Journal of Psychiatry, 145,* 1289–1291.

FRANKENBURG, F. R., & ZANARINI, M. C. (1993). Clozapine treatment of borderline patients: A preliminary study. *Comprehensive Psychiatry, 34,* 402–405.

FRANKENBURG, F. R., & ZANARINI, M. C. (1994). Uses of clozapine in nonschizophrenic patients. *Harvard Review of Psychiatry, 2,* 142–150.

FRAZIER, J. A., GORDON, C. T., McKENNA, K., LENANE, M. C., JIH, D., & RAPOPORT, J. L. (1994). An open trial of clozapine in 11 adolescents with childhood-onset schizophrenia. *Journal of the American Academy of Child and Adolescent Psychiatry, 33,* 658–663.

FYER, A. J. (1993). Heritability of social anxiety: A brief review. *Journal of Clinical Psychiatry, 54* (12, Suppl), 10–12.

GADOW, K. D., SVERD, J., SPRAFKIN, J., NOLAN, E. E., & EZOR, S. N. (1995). Efficacy of methylphenidate for attention-deficit hyperactivity disorder in children with tic disorder. *Archives of General Psychiatry, 52,* 444–455.

GARDOS, G., CASEY, D. E., COLE, J. O., PERENYI, A., KOCSIS, É., ARATO, M., SAMSON, J. A., & CONLEY, C. (1994). Ten-year outcome of tardive dyskinesia. *American Journal of Psychiatry, 151,* 836–841.

GARDOS, G., & COLE, J. O. (1995). The treatment of tardive dyskinesia. In F. E. Bloom and D. J. Kupfer (Eds.), *Psychopharmacotherapy: The fourth generation of progress.* New York: Raven Press, 1503–1511.

GARLAND, E. J., REMICK, R. A., & ZIS, A. P. (1988). Weight gain with antidepressants and lithium. *Journal of Clinical Psychopharmacology, 8,* 323–330.

GAWIN, F. H., & KLEBER, H. D. (1986). Pharmacological treatment of cocaine abuse. *Psychiatric Clinics of North America, 9,* 573–583.

GAWIN, F. H., KLEBER, H. D., BYCK, R., ROUNSAVILLE, B. J., KOSTEN, T. R., JATLOW, P. I., & MORGAN, C. (1989). Desipramine facilitation of initial cocaine abstinence. *Archives of General Psychiatry, 46,* 117–121.

GELENBERG, A. J., KANE, J. M., KELLER, M. B., LAVORI, P., ROSENBAUM, J. F., COLE, K., & LAVELLE, J. (1989). Comparison of standard and low serum levels of lithium for maintenance treatment of bipolar disorder. *New England Journal of Medicine, 321,* 1489–1493.

GELERNTER, C. S., UHDE, T. W., CIMBOLIC, P., ARNKOFF, D. B., VITTONE, B. J., TANCER, M. E., & BARTKO, J. J. (1991). Cognitive-behavioral and pharmacological treatments of social phobia: A controlled study. *Archives of General Psychiatry, 48,* 938–945.

GERLACH, J., & CASEY, D. E. (1994). Drug treatment of schizophrenia: Myths and realities. *Current Opinion in Psychiatry, 7,* 65–70.

GEORGOTAS, A., McCUE, R. E., HAPWORTH, W., FRIEDMAN, E., KIM, O. M., WELKOWITZ, J., CHANG, I., & COOPER, T. B. (1986). Comparative efficacy and safety of MAOIs versus TCAs in treating depression in the elderly. *Biological Psychiatry, 21,* 1155–1166.

GILBERT, P. L., HARRIS, M. J., McADAMS, & L. JESTE, D. V. (1995). Neuroleptic withdrawal in schizophrenic patients. *Archives of General Psychiatry, 52,* 173–188.

GILLIN, J. C., & BYERLEY, W. F. (1990). The diagnosis and management of insomnia. *New England Journal of Medicine, 322,* 239–247.

GILLIN, J. C., SPINWEBER, C. C., & JOHNSON, L. C. (1989). Rebound insomnia: A critical review. *Journal of Clinical Psychopharmacology, 9,* 161–172.

GITLIN, M. J. (1993a). Lithium-induced renal insufficiency. *Journal of Clinical Psychopharmacology, 13,* 276–279.

GITLIN, M. J. (1993b). Pharmacotherapy of personality disorders: Conceptual framework and clinical strategies. *Journal of Clinical Psychopharmacology, 13,* 343–353.

GITLIN, M. J. (1995a). Pharmacotherapy for personality disorders. *Psychiatric Clinics of North America: Annual of Drug Therapy, 2,* 151–185.

GITLIN, M. J. (1995b). Effects of depression and antidepressants on sexual functioning. *Bulletin of the Menninger Clinic, 5,* 232–248.

GITLIN, M., COCHRAN, S., & JAMISON, K. (1989). Maintenance lithium treatment: Side effects and compliance. *Journal of Clinical Psychiatry, 50,* 127–131.

GITLIN, M., & PASNAU, R. O. (1989). Psychiatric syndromes linked to reproductive function in women: A review of current knowledge. *American Journal of Psychiatry, 146,* 1413–1422.

GITLIN, M. J., WEINER, D. F., FAIRBANKS, L., HERSHMAN, J. M., & FRIEDFELD, N. (1987). Failure of T_3 to potentiate antidepressant response. *Journal of Affective Disorders, 13,* 267–272.

GITTELMAN-KLEIN, R., & KLEIN, D. F. (1971). Controlled imipramine treatment of school phobia. *Archives of General Psychiatry, 25*, 204–207.

GITTELMAN-KLEIN, R., LANDA, B., MATTES, J. A., & KLEIN, D. F. (1988). Methylphenidate and growth in hyperactive children: A controlled withdrawal study. *Archives of General Psychiatry, 45*, 1127–1130.

GITTELMAN-KLEIN, R., & MANNUZZA, S. (1988). Hyperactive boys almost grown up. III. Methylphenidate effects on ultimate height. *Archives of General Psychiatry, 45*, 1131–1134.

GLASSMAN, A. H., & PREUD'HOMME, X. A. (1993). Review of the cardiovascular effects of heterocyclic antidepressants. *Journal of Clinical Psychiatry, 54* (2, Suppl), 16–22.

GLAZER, W. M., MOORE, D. C., SCHOOLER, N. R., BRENNER, L. M., & MORGENSTERN, H. (1984). Tardive dyskinesia: A discontinuation study. *Archives of General Psychiatry, 41*, 623–627.

GOFF, D. C., BROTMAN, A. W., WAITES, M., & McCORMICK, S. (1990). Trial of fluoxetine added to neuroleptics for treatment-resistant schizophrenic patients. *American Journal of Psychiatry, 147*, 492–494.

GOLDBERG, S. C., KLERMAN, G. L., & COLE, J. O. (1965). Changes in schizophrenic psychopathology and ward behavior as a function of phenothiazine treatment. *British Journal of Psychiatry, 111*, 120–133.

GOLLUB, R. L., & HYMAN, S. E. (1995). G proteins and second messengers in psychiatry. *Harvard Review of Psychiatry, 3*, 41–44.

GOODMAN, W. K., McDOUGLE, C. J., BARR, L. C., ARONSON, S. C., & PRICE, L. H. (1993). Biological approaches to treatment-resistant obsessive compulsive disorder. *Journal of Clinical Psychiatry, 54* (6, Suppl), 16–26.

GOODNICK, P. J., & SANDOVAL, R. (1993). Psychotropic treatment of chronic fatigue syndrome and related disorders. *Journal of Clinical Psychiatry, 54*, 13–20.

GOODWIN, F., & JAMISON, K. (1990). *Manic-depressive illness.* Washington, DC: Oxford University Press.

GOODWIN, F. K., & JAMISON, K. (1984). The natural course of manic-depressive illness. In R. M. Post & J. C. Ballenger (Eds.), *Neurobiology of mood disorders.* Baltimore, MD: Williams & Wilkins, 20–37.

GORMAN, J. M., LIEBOWITZ, M., FYER, A., & STEIN, J. (1989). A neuroanatomical hypothesis for panic disorder. *American Journal of Psychiatry, 146*, 148–161.

GRABOWSKI, J., RHOADES, H., ELK, R., SCHMITZ, J., DAVIS, C., CRESON, D., & KIRBY, K. (1995). Fluoxetine is ineffective for treatment of cocaine dependence: Two placebo-controlled, double-blind trials. *Journal of Clinical Psychopharmacology, 15*, 163–174.

GREEN, M. F., NUECHTERLEIN, K. H., VENTURA, J., & MINTZ, J. (1990). The temporal relationship between depressive and psychotic symptoms in recent-onset schizophrenia. *American Journal of Psychiatry, 147*, 179–182.

GREEN, W. H. (1995). The treatment of attention-deficit hyperactivity disorder with nonstimulant medications. *Child and Adolescent Psychiatric Clinics of North America, 4*, 169–195.

GREENBLATT, D. J. (1991). Benzodiazepine hypnotics: Sorting the pharmacokinetic facts. *Journal of Clinical Psychiatry, 52* (9, Suppl), 4–10.

GREENBLATT, D. J., HARMATZ, J., ENGELHARDT, N., & SHADER, R. I. (1989). Pharmacokinetic determinants of dynamic differences among three benzodiazepines. *Archives of General Psychiatry, 46*, 326–332.

GREENBLATT, D. J., HARMATZ, J. S., & SHADER, R. I. (1993). Plasma alprazolam concentrations: Relation to efficacy and side effects in the treatment of panic disorder. *Archives of General Psychiatry, 50*, 715–722.

GREENHILL, L. (1995). Attention deficit hyperactivity disorder: The stimulants. *Child and Adolescent Clinics of North America, 4*, 123–168.

GREIST, J. H. (1994). Behavior therapy for obsessive compulsive disorder. *Journal of Clinical Psychiatry, 55* (10, Suppl), 60–68.

GREIST, J., CHOUINARD, G., DUBOFF, E., HALARIS, A., KIM, S. W., KORAN, L., LIEBOWITZ, M., LYDIARD, R. B., RASMUSSEN, S., WHITE, K., & SIKES, C. (1995a). Double-blind parallel comparison of three dosages of sertraline and placebo in outpatients with obsessive-compulsive disorder. *Archives of General Psychiatry, 52,* 289–295.

GREIST, J. H., JEFFERSON, J. W., KOBAK, K. A., KATZELNICK, D. J., & SERLIN, R. C. (1995b). Efficacy and tolerability of serotonin transport inhibitors in obsessive-compulsive disorder. *Archives of General Psychiatry, 52,* 53–60.

GRINSPOON, L., & BAKALAR, J. (1986). Psychedelics and arylcyclohexylamines. In A. J. Frances & R. E. Hales (Eds.), *Annual review,* Vol. 5. Washington DC: American Psychiatric Press, 212–225.

GROF, P., ANGST, J., & HAINES, T. (1973). The clinical course of depression: Practical issues. In J. Angst & J. Stuttgart (Eds.), *Classification and prediction of outcome of depression.* New York: F. K. Schattauer Verlag, 141–148.

GUNDERSON, J. G., & ELLIOTT, G. R. (1985). The interface between borderline personality disorder and affective disorder. *American Journal of Psychiatry, 142,* 277–288.

GUNDERSON, J. G., & PHILLIPS, K. A. (1995). Personality disorders. In H. I. Kaplan and B. J. Sadock (Eds.), *Comprehensive Textbook of Psychiatry,* Sixth Edition. Baltimore: Williams & Wilkins, 1425–1461.

GUNDERSON, J. G., & PHILLIPS, K. A. (1991). A current view of the interface between borderline personality disorder and depression. *American Journal of Psychiatry, 148,* 967–975.

GUZE, S. (1976). *Criminality and psychiatric disorders.* New York: Oxford University Press.

GWIRTSMAN, H. E. (1994). Dysthymia and chronic depressive states: Diagnostic and pharmacotherapeutic considerations. *Psychopharmacology Bulletin, 30,* 45–51.

GWIRTSMAN, H. E., GUZE, B. H., YAGER, J., & GAINSLEY, B. (1990). Fluoxetine treatment of anorexia nervosa: An open clinical trial. *Journal of Clinical Psychiatry, 51,* 378–382.

HAMILTON, M. S., & OPLER, L. A. (1992). Akathisia, suicidality, and fluoxetine. *Journal of Clinical Psychiatry, 53,* 401–406.

HARDING, C. M., BROOKS, G. W., ASHIKAGA, T., STRAUSS, J. S., & BRIER, A. (1987). The Vermont longitudinal study of persons with severe mental illness, I: Methodology, study sample, and overall status 32 years later. *American Journal of Psychiatry, 144,* 718–726.

HARRINGTON, R., FUDGE, H., RUTTER, M., PICKLES, A., & HILL, J. (1990). Adult outcomes of childhood and adolescent depression: I. Psychiatric status. *Archives of General Psychiatry, 47,* 465–473.

HARTMANN, E. (1977). L-Tryptophan: A rational hypnotic with clinical potential. *American Journal of Psychiatry, 134,* 366–370.

HASPEL, T. (1995). Beta-blockers and the treatment of aggression. *Harvard Review of Psychiatry, 2,* 274–281.

HAURI, P., & SATEIA, M. (1985). Nonpharmacological treatment of sleep disorders. In R. E. Hales & A. J. Frances (Eds.), *Annual review,* Vol. 4, Washington, DC: American Psychiatric Press, 361–378.

HAYKAL, R. F., & AKISKAL, H. S. (1990). Bupropion as a promising approach to rapid cycling bipolar II patients. *Journal of Clinical Psychiatry, 51,* 450–455.

HELLERSTEIN, D. J., YANOWITCH, P., ROSENTHAL, J., SAMSTAG, L. W., MAURER, M., KASCH, K., BURROWS, L., POSTER, M., CANTILLON, M., & WINSTON, A. (1993). A randomized double-blind study of fluoxetine versus placebo in the treatment of dysthymia. *American Journal of Psychiatry, 150,* 1169–1175.

HELZER, J. E., ROBINS, L. N., & McEVOY, L. (1987). Post-traumatic stress disorder in the general population: Findings of the epidemiologic catchment area survey. *New England Journal of Medicine, 317,* 1630–1634.

HERZ, M. I., GLAZER, W. M., MOSTERT, M. A., SHEARD, M. A., SZYMANSKI, H. V., HAFEZ, H., MIRZA, M., & VANA, J. (1991). Intermittent vs maintenance medication in schizophrenia. *Archives of General Psychiatry, 48,* 333–339.

HESTBECH, J., HANSEN, H. E., AMDISEN, A., & OLSEN, S. (1977). Chronic renal lesions following long-term treatment with lithium. *Kidney International, 12,* 205–213.

HIMMELHOCH, J. M., THASE, M. E., MALLINGER, A. G., & HOUCK, P. (1991). Tranylcypromine versus imipramine in anergic bipolar depression. *American Journal of Psychiatry, 148,* 910–916.

HIRSCHFELD, R. M. A., & HOLZER, C. E. (1994). Depressive personality disorder: Clinical implications. *Journal of Clinical Psychiatry, 55* (4, Suppl), 10–17.

HIRSCHFELD, R. M. A., KLERMAN, G. L., CLAYTON, P. J., KELLER, M. B., McDONALD-SCOTT, P., & LARKIN, B. H. (1983). Assessing personality: Effects of the depressive state on trait measurement. *American Journal of Psychiatry, 40,* 695–699.

HOGARTY, G. E., McEVOY, J. P., MUNETZ, M., DiBARRY, A. L., BARTONE, P., CATHER, R., COOLEY, S. J., ULRICH, R. F., CARTER, M., & MADONIA, M. J.: Environmental/Personal Indicators in the Course of Schizophrenia Research Group. (1988). Dose of fluphenazine, familial expressed emotion, and outcome in schizophrenia: Results of a two-year controlled study. *Archives of General Psychiatry, 45,* 797–805.

HOLLANDER, E., COHEN, L. J., & SIMEON, D. (1993). Body dysmorphic disorder. *Psychiatric Annals, 23,* 359–364.

HOLLISTER, L. E., MOTZENBECKER, F., & DEGAN, R. (1961). Withdrawal reactions from chlordiazepoxide (Librium). *Psychopharmacologia, 2,* 63–68.

HOLLISTER, L. E., MUELLER-OERLINGHAUSEN, B., RICKELS, K., & SHADER, R. I. (1993). Clinical uses of benzodiazepines. *Journal of Clinical Psychopharmacology, 13,* (Suppl 1), 1S–169S.

HOLLISTER, L. E., & YESAVAGE, J. (1984). Ergyloid mesylates for senile dementia: Unanswered questions. *Annals of Internal Medicine, 100,* 894–898.

HORNE, R. L., FERGUSON, J. M., POPE, H. G., HUDSON, J. I., LINEBERRY, C. G., ASCHER, J., & CATO, A. (1988). Treatment of bulimia with bupropion: A multicenter controlled trial. *Journal of Clinical Psychiatry, 49,* 262–266.

HORWATH, E., LISH, J. D., JOHNSON, J., HORNIG, C. D., & WEISSMAN, M. M. (1993). Agoraphobia without panic: Clinical reappraisal of an epidemiologic finding. *American Journal of Psychiatry, 150,* 1496–1501.

HOWLAND, R. H. (1991). Pharmacotherapy of dysthymia: A review. *Journal of Clinical Psychopharmacology, 11,* 83–92.

HUDSON, J. L., & POPE, H. G. (1990). Affective spectrum disorder: Does antidepressant response identify a family of disorders with a common pathophysiology? *American Journal of Psychiatry, 147,* 552–564.

HUNT, R. D., ARNSTEN, A. F. T., & ASBELL, M. D. (1995). An open trial of guanfacine in the treatment of attention-deficit hyperactivity disorder. *Journal of the American Academy of Child and Adolescent Psychiatry, 34,* 50–54.

HUTTUNEN, M. (1995). The evolution of the serotonin-dopamine antagonist concept. *Journal of Clinical Psychopharmacology, 15* (Suppl, 1), 4S–10S.

HYDE, T. M., & WEINBERGER, D. R. (1995). Tourette's syndrome: A model neuropsychiatric disorder. *Journal of the American Medical Association, 273,* 498–501.

HYMAN, S. E., & GOLLUB, R. L. (1994). More serotonin: Not as simple as it seems. *Harvard Review of Psychiatry, 2,* 222–224.

HYMAN, S. E., & NESTLER, E. J. (1993). *The molecular foundations of psychiatry.* Washington, DC: American Psychiatric Press.

INDERBITZIN, L. B., LEWINE, R. R. J., SCHELLER-GILKEY, G., SWOFFORD, C. D., EGAN, G. J., GLOERSEN, B. A., VIDANAGAMA, B. P., & WATERNAUX, C. (1994). A double-blind dose-reduction trial of fluphenazine decanoate for chronic, unstable schizophrenic patients. *American Journal of Psychiatry, 151,* 1753–1759.

INSEL, T., NINAN, P., ALOI, J., JIMERSON, D. C., SKOLNICK, P., & PAUL, S. M. (1984). A benzodiazepine-receptor mediated model of anxiety. Studies in non-human primates and clinical implications. *Archives of General Psychiatry, 41,* 741–750.

JACOBSEN, F. M. (1993). Low-dose valproate: A new treatment for cyclothymia, mild rapid cycling disorders, and premenstrual syndrome. *Journal of Clinical Psychiatry, 54,* 229–234.

JANICAK, P. G., DAVIS, J. M., GIBBONS, R. D., ERICKSEN, S., CHANG, S., & GALLAGHER, P. (1985). Efficacy of ECT: A meta-analysis. *American Journal of Psychiatry, 142,* 297–302.

JEFFERSON, J. W. (1995). Social phobia: A pharmacologic treatment overview. *Journal of Clinical Psychiatry, 56* (Suppl 5), 18–24.

JEFFERSON, J. W., GREIST, J. H., ACKERMAN, D. L., & CARROLL, J. A. (1987). *Lithium encyclopedia for clinical practice,* 2nd ed. Washington, DC: American Psychiatric Association Press.

JEFFERSON, J. W., GREIST, J. H., CLAGNAZ, P. J., EISCHENS, R. R., MARTEN, W. C., & EVENSON, M. A. (1982). Effect of strenuous exercise on serum lithium level in man. *American Journal of Psychiatry, 139,* 1593–1595.

JESTE, D. V., PAULSEN, J. S., & HARRIS, M. J. (1995). Late-onset schizophrenia and other related psychoses. In F. E. Bloom and D. J. Kupfer (Eds.), *Psychopharmacology: The fourth generation of progress.* New York: Raven Press, 1437–1446.

JOFFE, R., POST, R. M., ROY-BYRNE, P., & UHDE, T. W. (1985). Hematological effects of carbamazepine in patients with affective illness. *American Journal of Psychiatry, 142,* 1196–1199.

JOFFE, R. T., & SCHULLER, D. R. (1993). An open study of buspirone augmentation of serotonin reuptake inhibitors in refractory depression. *Journal of Clinical Psychiatry, 54,* 269–271.

JOFFE, R. T., SINGER, W., LEVITT, A. J., & MACDONALD, C. (1993). A placebo-controlled comparison of lithium and triiodothyronine augmentation of tricyclic antidepressants in unipolar refractory depression. *Archives of General Psychiatry, 50,* 387–393.

JOHANSON, C. E., & SCHUSTER, C. R. (1995). Cocaine. In F. E. Bloom and D. J. Kupfer (Eds.), *Psychopharmacology: The fourth generation of progress.* New York: Raven Press, 1685–1697.

JONES, K. L., LACRO, R. V., JOHNSON, K. A., & ADAMS, J. (1989). Pattern of malformations in the children of women treated with carbamazepine during pregnancy. *New England Journal of Medicine, 320,* 1661–1666.

JUDD, L., & HUEY, L. (1984). Lithium antagonizes ethanol intoxication in alcoholics. *American Journal of Psychiatry, 141,* 1517–1521.

JUDD, L. L., RAPAPORT, M. H., PAULUS, M. P., & BROWN, J. L. (1994). Subsyndromal symptomatic depression: A new mood disorder? *Journal of Clinical Psychiatry, 54* (4, Suppl), 18–28.

KAFANTARIS, V. (1995). Treatment of bipolar disorder in children and adolescents. *Journal of the American Academy of Child and Adolescent Psychiatry, 34,* 732–741.

KAFKA, M. P. (1994). Sertraline pharmacotherapy for paraphilias and paraphilia-related disorders: An open trial. *Annals of Clinical Psychiatry, 6,* 189–194.

KAHN, R. J., MCNAIR, D. M., LIPMAN, R. S., COVI, L., RICKELS, K., DOWNING, R., FISHER, J., & FRANKENTHALER, L. M. (1986). Imipramine and chlordiazepoxide in depressive and anxiety disorders. II. Efficacy in anxious outpatients. *Archives of General Psychiatry, 43,* 79–85.

KAHN, R. S., & DAVIS, K. L. (1995). New developments in dopamine and schizophrenia. In F. E. Bloom and D. J. Kupfer (Eds.), *Psychopharmacology: The fourth generation of progress.* New York: Raven Press, 1192–1203.

KALES, A., SOLDATOS, C. R., BIXTER, E. O., & KALES, J. D. (1983). Early morning insomnia with rapidly eliminated benzodiazepines. *Science, 220,* 95–97.

KALES, A., SOLDATOS, C. R., CALDWELL, A. B., KALES, J. D., HUMPHREY, F. J., CHARNEY, D. S., & SCHWEITZER, P. K. (1980). Somnabulism: Clinical characteristics and personality patterns. Archives of General Psychiatry, 37, 1406–1410.

KANE, J. (1995a). Clinical developments in the use of nonstandard neuroleptic antipsychotic agents: Interview. *Currents in Affective Illness, 14,* 16–20.

KANE, J. M. (1995b). Tardive dyskinesia: Epidemiologic and clinical presentation. In F. E. Bloom and D. J. Kupfer (Eds.), *Psychopharmacology: The fourth generation of progress.* New York: Raven Press, 1485–1495.

KANE, J., HONIGFELD, G., SINGER, J., MELTZER, H., & THE CLOZARIL COLLABORATIVE STUDY GROUP. (1988). Clozapine for the treatment-resistant schizophrenic. *Archives of General Psychiatry, 45,* 789–796.

KANE, J. M., & MARDER, S. R. (1993). Psychopharmacologic treatment of schizophrenia. *Schizophrenia Bulletin, 19,* 287–302.

KANE, J. M., QUITKIN, F. M., RIFKIN, A., RAMOS-LORENZI, J. R., NAYAK, D. D., & HOWARD, A. (1982). Lithium carbonate and imipramine in the prophylaxis of unipolar and bipolar II illness: A prospective placebo-controlled comparison. *Archives of General Psychiatry, 39,* 1065–1069.

KANE, J. M., WOERNER, M. G., POLLACK, S., SAFFERMAN, A. Z., & LIEBERMAN, J. A. (1993). Does clozapine cause tardive dyskinesia? *Journal of Clinical Psychiatry, 54,* 327–330.

KATZ, I. R. (1993). Drug treatment of depression in the frail elderly: Discussion of the NIH consensus development conference on the diagnosis and treatment of depression in late life. *Pharmacology Bulletin, 29,* 101–108.

KAVALE, K. A., & FORNESS, S. R. (1983). Hyperactivity and diet treatment: A meta-analysis of the Feingold hypothesis. *Journal of Learning Disabilities, 16,* 324–330.

KAYE, W. H., WELTZIN, T. E., HSU, L. K. G., & BULIK, C. M. (1991). An open trial of fluoxetine in patients with anorexia nervosa. *Journal of Clinical Psychiatry, 52,* 464–471.

KAYSER, A., ROBINSON, D. S., YINGLING, K., HOWARD, D. B., CORCELLA, J., & LAUX, D. (1988). The influence of panic attacks on response to phenelzine and amitriptyline in depressed outpatients. *Journal of Clinical Psychopharmacology, 8,* 246–253.

KECK, P. E., MCELROY, S. L., STRAKOWSKI, S. M., & WEST, S. A. (1994). Pharmacologic treatment of schizoaffective disorder. *Psychopharmacology, 114,* 529–538.

KECK, P. E., POPE, H. G., COHEN, B. M., MCELROY, S. G., & NIRENBERG, A. A. (1989). Risk factors for neuroleptic malignant syndrome: A case control study. *Archives of General Psychiatry, 46,* 914–918.

KECK, P. E., TAYLOR, V. E., TUGRUL, K. C., MCELROY, S. L., & BENNETT, J. A. (1993). Valproate treatment of panic disorder and lactate-induced panic attacks. *Biological Psychiatry, 33,* 542–546.

KEELER, M. H., TAYLOR, C. I., & MILLER, W. C. (1979). Are all recently detoxified alcoholics depressed? *American Journal of Psychiatry, 136,* 586–588.

KEEPERS, G. A., & CASEY, D. E. (1991). Use of neuroleptic-induced extrapyramidal symptoms to predict future vulnerability to side effects. *American Journal of Psychiatry, 148,* 85–89.

KELLER, M. B., LAVORI, P. W., KANE, J. M., GELENBERG, A. J., ROSENBAUM, J. F., WALZER, E. A., & BAKER, L. A. (1992). Subsyndromal symptoms in bipolar disorder: A comparison of standard and low serum levels of lithium. *Archives of General Psychiatry, 49,* 371–376.

KELLER, M., LAVORI, P. W., RICE, J., CORYELL, W., & HIRSCHFELD, R. M. A. (1986). The persistent risk of chronicity in recurrent episodes of non-bipolar major depressive disorder: A prospective follow-up. *Archives of General Psychiatry, 143,* 24–28.

KELLER, M. B., & SHAPIRO, R. W. (1982). "Double depression:" Superimposition of acute depressive episodes on chronic depressive disorders. *American Journal of Psychiatry, 139.* 438–442.

KELLER, M. B., SHAPIRO, R. W., LAVORI, P. W., & WOLFE, N. (1982). Recovery in major depressive disorder: Analysis with the life table and the regression models. *Archives of General Psychiatry, 39,* 905–910.

KENDLER, K. S. (1980). The nosologic validity of paranoia (simple delusional disorder): A review. *Archives of General Psychiatry, 37,* 699–706.

KENDLER, K. S., & DIEHL, S. R. (1993). The genetics of schizophrenia: A current, genetic-epidemiologic perspective. *Schizophrenia Bulletin, 19,* 261–285.

KENDLER, K. S., GRUENBERG, A. M., & KINNEY, D. K. (1994). Independent diagnoses of adoptees and relatives as defined by DSM-III in the provincial and national samples of the Danish adoption study of schizophrenia. *Archives of General Psychiatry, 51,* 456–468.

KENDLER, K. S., MCGUIRE, M., GRUENBERG, A. M., O'HARE, A., SPELLMAN, M., & WALSH, D. (1993a). The Roscommon family study: I. Methods, diagnosis of probands, and risk of schizophrenia in relatives. *Archives of General Psychiatry, 50,* 527–540.

KENDLER, K. S., MCGUIRE, M., GRUENBERG, A. M., O'HARE, A., SPELLMAN, M., & WALSH, D. (1993b). The Roscommon family study: III: Schizophrenia-related personality disorders in relatives. *Archives of General Psychiatry, 50,* 781–788.

KENDLER, K. S., MCGUIRE, M., GRUENBERG, A. M., & WALSH, D. (1994). Outcome and family study of the subtypes of schizophrenia in the west of Ireland. *American Journal of Psychiatry, 151,* 849–856.

KENDLER, K. S., NEALE, M. C., KESSLER, R. C., HEATH, A. C., & EAVES, L. J. (1992). Generalized anxiety disorder in women: A population-based twin study. *Archives of General Psychiatry, 49,* 267–272.

KENNEDY, S. H., PIRAN, N., WARSH, J. J., PRENDERGAST, P., MAINPRIZE, E., WHYNOT, C., & GARFINKEL, P. E. (1988). A trial of isocarboxazid in the treatment of bulimia nervosa. *Journal of Clinical Psychopharmacology, 8,* 391–396.

KESSLER, D. A. (1989). The regulation of investigational drugs. *New England Journal of Medicine, 321,* 281–288.

KESSLER, R. C., MCGONAGLE, K. A., ZHAO, S., NELSON, C. B., HUGHES, M., ESHLEMAN, S., WITTCHEN, H. U., & KENDLER, K. S. (1994). Lifetime and 12-month prevalence of DSM-III-R psychiatric disorders in the United States. *Archives of General Psychiatry, 51,* 8–19.

KESSLER, R. C., SONNEGA, A., BROMET, E., HUGHES, M., & NELSON, C. B. (1995). Posttraumatic stress disorder in the national comorbidity survey. *Archives of General Psychiatry, 52,* 1048–1060.

KETTER, T. A., GEORGE, M. S., RING, H. A., PAZZAGLIA, P., MARANGELL, L., KIMBRELL, T. A., & POST, R. M. (1994). Primary mood disorders: Structural and resting functional studies. *Psychiatric Annals, 24,* 637–642.

KETY, S. S., WENDER, P. H., JACOBSEN, B., INGRAHAM, L. J., JANSSON, L., FABER, B., & KINNEY, D. K. (1994). Mental illness in the biological and adoptive relatives of schizophrenic adoptees: Replication of the Copenhagen study in the rest of Denmark. *Archives of General Psychiatry, 51,* 442–455.

KIMMEL, S. E., CALABRESE, J. R., WOYSHVILLE, M. J., & MELTZER, H. Y. (1994). Clozapine in treatment-refractory mood disorders. *Journal of Clinical Psychiatry, 55* (9, Suppl B), 91–93.

KINON, B. J., KANE, J. M., JOHNS, C., PEROVICH, R., ISMI, M., KOREEN, A., & WEIDEN, P. (1993). Treatment of neuroleptic-resistant schizophrenic relapse. *Psychopharmacology Bulletin, 29,* 309–314.

KLEIN, D. F. (1993a). False suffocation alarms, spontaneous panics, and related conditions: An integrated hypothesis. *Archives of General Psychiatry, 50,* 306–317.

KLEIN, D. F. (1993b). Clinical psychopharmacologic practice: The need for developing a research base. *Archives of General Psychiatry, 50,* 491–494.

KLEIN, D. F. (1964). Delineation of two drug-responsive anxiety syndromes. *Psychopharmacologia, 5,* 397–408.

KLEIN, D. F., GITTELMAN, R., QUITKIN, F., & RIFKIN, A. (1980). *Diagnosis and drug treatment of psychiatric disorders: Adults and children,* 2nd ed. Baltimore, MD: Williams & Wilkins.

KLEIN, E., COLIN, V., STOLK, J., & LENOX, R. H. (1994). Alprazolam withdrawal in patients with panic disorder and generalized anxiety disorder: Vulnerability and effect of carbamazepine. *American Journal of Psychiatry, 151,* 1760–1766.

KLERMAN, G. L. (1991). Ideological conflicts in integrating pharmacotherapy and psychotherapy. In B. D. Beitman & G. L. Klerman (Eds.), *Integrating pharmacotherapy and psychotherapy.* Washington, DC: American Psychiatric Press, 3–19.

KNAPP, M. J., KNOPMAN, D. S., SALOMON, P. R., PENDLEBURY, W. W., DAVIS, C. S., GRACON, S. I., & THE TACRINE STUDY GROUP. (1994). A 30-week randomized, controlled trial of high-dose tacrine in patients with Alzheimer's disease. *Journal of the American Medical Association, 271,* 985–991.

KNIGHTS, A., & HIRSCH, S. R. (1981). "Revealed depression" and drug treatment for schizophrenia. *Archives of General Psychiatry, 38,* 806–811.

KOSLOW, S. H., MAAS, J. W., BOWDEN, C. L., DAVIS, J. M., HANIN, I., & JAVAID, J. (1983). CSF and urinary biogenic amines and metabolites in depression and mania: A controlled, univariate analysis. *Archives of General Psychiatry, 40,* 999–1010.

KOSTEN, T. R., & McCANCE-KATZ, E. (1995). New pharmacotherapies. In J. M. Oldham & M. B. Riba (Eds.), *Review of Psychiatry,* Vol. 14. Washington, DC: American Psychiatric Press, 105–126.

KOVACS, M., AKISKAL, H. S., GATSONIS, C., & PARRONE, P. L. (1994). Childhood-onset dysthymic disorder: Clinical features and prospective naturalistic outcome. *Archives of General Psychiatry, 51,* 365–374.

KRAMER, M. S., VOGEL, W. H., diJOHNSON, C., DEWEY, D. A., SHEVES, P., CAVICCHIA, C., LITLE, P., SCHMIDT, R., & KIMES, I. (1989). Antidepressants in "depressed" schizophrenic inpatients: A controlled trial. *Archives of General Psychiatry, 46,* 922–928.

KRAMER, P. (1993). *Listening to Prozac.* New York: Viking Press.

KRANZLER, H. R., BURLESON, J. A., DEL BOCA, F. K., BABOR, T. F., KORNER, P., BROWN, J., & BOHN, M. J. (1994). Buspirone treatment of anxious alcoholics: A placebo-controlled trial. *Archives of General Psychiatry, 51,* 720–731.

KRANZLER, H. R., BURLESON, J. A., KORNER, P., DEL BOCA, F. K., BOHN, M. J., BROWN, J., & LIEBOWITZ, N. (1995). Placebo-controlled trial of fluoxetine as an adjunct to relapse prevention in alcoholics. *American Journal of Psychiatry, 152,* 391–397.

KRANZLER, H. R., & ORROK, B. (1989). The pharmacotherapy of alcoholism. In A. Tasman, R. E. Hales, & A. J. Frances (Eds.), *Review of psychiatry,* Vol. 8. Washington, DC: American Psychiatric Press.

KRAUPL-TAYLOR, F. (1989). The damnation of benzodiazepines. *British Journal of Psychiatry, 154,* 697–704.

KROESSLER, D. (1985). Relative efficacy rates for therapies of delusional depression. *Convulsive Therapy, 1,* 173–182.

KRUPP, L. B., MENDELSON, W. B., & FRIEDMAN, R. (1991). An overview of chronic fatigue syndrome. *Journal of Clinical Psychiatry, 52,* 403–410.

KUKOPULOS, A., MINNAI, G., & MULLER-OERLINGHAUSEN, B. (1985). The influence of mania and depression on the pharmacokinetics of lithium: A longitudinal single-case study. *Journal of Affective Disorders, 8,* 159–166.

KUPFER, D. J., FRANK, E., PEREL, J. M., CORNES, C., MALLINGER, A. G., THASE, M. E., MCEACHRAN, A. B., & GROCHOCINSKI, V. J. (1992). Five-year outcome for maintenance therapies in recurrent depression. *Archives of General Psychiatry, 49,* 769–773.

KYE, C., & RYAN, N. (1995). Pharmacologic treatment of child and adolescent depression. *Child and Adolescent Psychiatric Clinics of North America, 4,* 261–281.

LADER, M. (1988). B-receptor antagonists in neuropsychiatry: An update. *Journal of Clinical Psychiatry, 49,* 213–223.

LAHEY, B. B., APPLEGATE, B., MCBURNETT, K., BIEDERMAN, J., GREENHILL, L., HYND, G. W., BARKLEY, R. A., NEWCORN, J., JENSEN, P., RICHTERS, J., GARFINKEL, B., KERDYK, L., FRICK, P. J., OLLENDICK, T., PEREZ, D., HART, E. L., WALDMAN, I., & SHAFFER, D. (1994). DSM-IV field trials for attention deficit hyperactivity - disorder in children and adolescents. *American Journal of Psychiatry, 151,* 1673–1685.

LAMMER, E. J., SEVER, L. E., & OAKLEY, G. P. (1987). Teratogen Update: Valproic acid. *Teratology, 35,* 465–473.

LAPENSEE, M. A. (1992a). A review of schizoaffective disorder: I: Current concepts. *Canadian Journal of Psychiatry, 37,* 335–346.

LAPENSEE, M. A. (1992b). A review of schizoaffective disorder: II: Somatic treatment. *Canadian Journal of Psychiatry, 37,* 347–349.

LEJOYEUX, M., & ADES, J. (1993). Evaluation of lithium treatment in alcoholism. *Alcohol & Alcoholism, 28,* 273–279.

LE MOAL, M. (1995). Mesocorticolimbic dopaminergic neurons: Functional and regulatory roles. In F. E. Bloom and D. J. Kupfer (Eds.), *Psychopharmacology: The fourth generation of progress.* New York: Raven Press, 283–294.

LEONARD, H. L., SWEDO, S. E., LENANE, M. C., RETTEW, D. C., HAMBURGER, S. D., BARTKO, J. J., & RAPOPORT, J. L. (1993). A 2- to 7-year follow-up study of 54 obsessive-compulsive children and adolescents. *Archives of General Psychiatry, 50,* 429–439.

LERER, B., SHAPIRA, B., CALEV, A., TUBI, N., DREXLER, H., KINDLER, S., LIDSKY, D., & SCHWARTZ, J. E. (1995). Antidepressant and cognitive effects of twice- versus three-times-weekly ECT. *American Journal of Psychiatry, 152,* 564–570.

LESSER, I. M., RUBIN, R. T., PECKNOLD, J. C., RIFKIN, A., SWINSON, R. P., LYDIARD, R. B., BURROWS, G. D., NOYES, R., & DUPONT, R. L. (1988). Secondary depression in panic disorder and agoraphobia. 1. Frequency, severity, and response to treatment. *Archives of General Psychiatry, 45,* 437–443.

LEVITT, A. J., JOFFE, R. T., ENNIS, J., MACDONALD, K., & KUTCHER, S. P. (1990). The prevalence of cyclothymia in borderline personality disorder. *Journal of Clinical Psychiatry, 51,* 335–339.

LEVITT, A. J., JOFFE, R. T., MOUL, D. E., LAM, R. W., TEICHER, M. H., LEBEGUE, B., MURRAY, M. G., OREN, D. A., SCHWARTZ, P., BUCHANAN, A., GLOD, C. A., & BROWN, J. (1993). Side effects of light therapy in seasonal affective disorder. *American Journal of Psychiatry, 150,* 650–652.

LEVITT, J. J., & TSUANG, M. T. (1988). The heterogeneity of schizoaffective disorders: Implications for treatment. *American Journal of Psychiatry, 145,* 926–936.

LEWINE, R. R. J. (1988). Gender and Schizophrenia. In M. T. Tsuang & J. C. Simpson (Eds.), *Handbook of Schizophrenia: Volume 3. Nosology, epidemiology, and genetics of schizophrenia.* Amsterdam: Elsevier, 379–397.

LIEBERMAN, J. A., BROWN, A. S., & GORMAN, J. M. (1994). Biological markers: Schizophrenia. In J. M. Oldham and M. B. Riba (Eds.), *Review of Psychiatry*, Vol. 13. Washington, DC: American Psychiatric Press, 133–170.

LIEBERMAN, J. A., SAFFERMAN, A. Z., POLLACK, S., SZYMANSKI, S., JOHNS, C., HOWARD, A., KRONIG, M., BROOKSTEIN, P., & KANE, J. M. (1994). Clinical effects of clozapine in chronic schizophrenia: Response to treatment and predictors of outcome. *American Journal of Psychiatry, 151,* 1744–1752.

LIEBOWITZ, M. (1992). Diagnostic issues in anxiety disorders. In A. Tasman and M. B. Riba (Eds.), *Review of Psychiatry*, Vol. 11. Washington, DC: American Psychiatric Press, 247–259.

LIEBOWITZ, M. R., GORMAN, J. M., FYER, A. J., & KLEIN, D. F. (1985). Social phobia: Review of a neglected anxiety disorder. *Archives of General Psychiatry, 42,* 729–736.

LIEBOWITZ, M. R., KLEIN, D. F., QUITKIN, F. M., STEWART, J. W., & McGRATH, P. J. (1984). Clinical implications of diagnostic subtypes of depression. In R. M. Post & J. C. Ballenger (Eds.), *Neurobiology of mood disorders.* Baltimore, MD: Williams & Wilkins, 107–120.

LIEBOWITZ, M. R., QUITKIN, F. M., STEWART, J. W., McGRATH, P. J., HARRISON, W. M., MARKOWITZ, J. S., RABKIN, J. G., TRICANO, E., GOETZ, D. M., & KLEIN, D. F. (1988). Antidepressant specificity in atypical depression. *Archives of General Psychiatry, 45,* 129–137.

LIEBOWITZ, M. R., SCHNEIER, F., CAMPEAS, R., HOLLANDER, E., HATTERER, J., FYER, A., GORMAN, J., PAPP, L., DAVIES, S., GULLY, R., & KLEIN, D. F. (1992). Phenelzine vs atenolol in social phobia: A placebo-controlled comparison. *Archives of General Psychiatry, 49,* 290–300.

LINGJAERDE, O. (1991). Benzodiazepines in the treatment of schizophrenia: An updated survey. *Acta Psychiatria Scandinavia, 84,* 453–459.

LIPPER, S., DAVIDSON, J. R. T., GRADY, T. A., EDINGER, T. D., HAMMETT, E. B., MAHORNEY, S. L., & CAVENAR, J. O. (1986). Preliminary study of carbamazepine in post-traumatic stress disorder. *Psychosomatics, 27,* 849–854.

LORANGER, A. W. (1984). Sex differences in age at onset of schizophrenia. *Archives of General Psychiatry, 41,* 157–161.

LUCKI, I., & RICKELS, K. (1986). The behavioral effects of benzodiazepines following long-term use. *Psychopharmacology Bulletin, 22,* 424–433.

LUCKI, I., RICKELS, K., & GELLER, A. M. (1985). Psychomotor performance following the long-term use of benzodiazepines. *Psychopharmacology Bulletin, 21,* 93–96.

LYDIARD, R. B., LESSER, I. M., BALLENGER, J. C., RUBIN, R. T., LARAIA, M., & DuPONT, R. (1992). A fixed-dose study of alprazolam 2 mg, alprazolam 6 mg, and placebo in panic disorder. *Journal of Clinical Psychopharmacology, 12,* 96–103.

MAAS, J. W., KOSLOW, S. H., KATZ, M. M., GIBBONS, R. C., BOWDEN, C. L., ROBINS, E., & DAVIS, J. M. (1984). Pretreatment neurotransmitter metabolite levels and response to tricyclic antidepressant drugs. *American Journal of Psychiatry, 141,* 1159–1171.

MAES, M., & MELTZER, H. Y. (1995). The serotonin hypothesis of major depression. In F. E. Bloom and D. J. Kupfer (Eds.), *Psychopharmacology: The fourth generation of progress,* New York: Raven Press, 933–944.

MAJ, M. (1988). Lithium prophylaxis of schizoaffective disorders: A prospective study. *Journal of Affective Disorders, 14,* 129–135.

MANJI, H. K., POTTER, W. Z., & LENOX, R. H. (1995). Signal transduction pathways: Molecular targets for lithium's actions. *Archives of General Psychiatry, 52,* 531–543.

MANN, J. J. (1991). The history and current status of selegiline (1-deprenyl) in clinical practice. *Currents in Affective Illness, 10,* 5–13.

MANN, J. J., AARONS, S. F., WILNER, P. J., KEILP, J. G., SWEENEY, J. A., PEARLSTEIN, T., FRANCES, A. J., KOCSIS, J. H., & BROWN, R. P. (1989). A controlled study of the antidepressant efficacy and side effects of (-)-deprenyl. *Archives of General Psychiatry, 46,* 45–50.

MANN, J. J., & KAPUR, S. (1991). The emergence of suicidal ideation and behavior during antidepressant pharmacotherapy. *Archives of General Psychiatry, 48,* 1027–1033.

MANN, J. J., & KAPUR, S. (1994). Elucidation of biochemical basis of the antidepressant action of electroconvulsive therapy by human studies. *Psychopharmacology Bulletin, 30,* 445–453.

MANNUZZA, S., KLEIN, R. G., BESSLER, A., MALLOY, P., & LaPADULA, M. (1993). Adult outcome of hyperactive boys: Educational achievement, occupational rank, and psychiatric status. *Archives of General Psychiatry, 50,* 565–576.

MANOS, N., GKIOUZEPAS, J., & LOGOTHETIS, J. (1981). The need for continuous use of antiparkinsonian medication with chronic schizophrenic patients receiving long-term neuroleptic therapy. *American Journal of Psychiatry, 138,* 184–188.

MANSCHRECK, T. (1992). Delusional disorders: Clinical concepts and diagnostic strategies. *Psychiatric Annals, 22,* 241–251.

MARCH, J. S., ERHARDT, D., JOHNSTON, H., & CONNERS, C. K. (1995). Pharmacotherapy for attention-deficit hyperactivity disorder. In J. W. Jefferson and J. H. Greist (Eds.), *Psychiatric Clinics of North America: Annual of Drug Therapy, 2,* 187–213.

MARCH, J. S., LEONARD, H. L., & SWEDO, S. E. (1995). Pharmacotherapy of obsessive-compulsive disorder. *Child and Adolescent Psychiatric Clinics of North America, 4,* 217–236.

MARDER, S. R., & MEIBACH, R. C. (1994). Risperidone in the treatment of schizophrenia. *American Journal of Psychiatry, 151,* 825–835.

MARDER, S., VAN PUTTEN, T., MINTZ, J., LEBELL, J., McKENZIE, J., & MAY, P. R. A. (1987). Low and conventional dose maintenance therapy with fluphenazine decanoate: Two year outcome. *Archives of General Psychiatry, 44,* 518–521.

MARDER, S., VAN PUTTEN, T., MINTZ, J., McKENZIE, J., LEBELL, M., FALTICO, G., & MAY, P. R. A. (1984). Costs and benefits of two doses of fluphenazine. *Archives of General Psychiatry, 41,* 1025–1029.

MARGRAF, J., EHLERS, A., & ROTH, W. T. (1988). Mitral valve prolapse and panic disorder: A review of their relationship. *Psychosomatic Medicine, 50,* 93–113.

MARKS, I. M. (1986). Genetics of fear and anxiety disorders. *British Journal of Psychiatry, 149,* 406–418.

MASAND, P., PICKETT, P., & MURRAY, G. B. (1991). Psychostimulants for secondary depression in medical illness. *Psychosomatics, 32,* 203–208.

MATTES, J. (1990). Comparative effectiveness of carbamazepine and propranolol for rage outbursts. *Journal of Neuropsychiatry and Clinical Neuroscience, 2,* 159–164.

MATTHEWS, K. A., WING, R. R., KULLER, L. H., MEILAHN, E. N., KELSEY, S. F., COSTELLO, E. J., & CAGGIULA, A. W. (1990). Influences of natural menopause on psychological characteristics and symptoms of middle-aged healthy women. *Journal of Consulting and Clinical Psychology, 58,* 345–351.

MAVISSAKALIAN, M., & PEREL, J. M. (1995). Imipramine treatment of panic disorder with agoraphobia: Dose ranging and plasma level-response relationships. *American Journal of Psychiatry, 152,* 673–682.

MAX, M. B., LYNCH, S. A., MUIR, J., SHOAF, S. E., SMOLLER, B., & DUBNER, R. (1992). Effects of desipramine, amitriptyline, and fluoxetine on pain in diabetic neuropathy. *New England Journal of Medicine, 326,* 1250–1256.

McClellan, J., & Werry, J. (1994). Practice parameters for the assessment and treatment of children and adolescents with schizophrenia. *Journal of the American Academy of Child and Adolescent Psychiatry, 33,* 616–635.

McDougle, C. J., Goodman, W. K., Leckman, J. F., Lee, N. C., Heninger, G. R., & Price, L. H. (1994). Haloperidol addition in fluvoxamine-refractory obsessive-compulsive disorder: A double-blind, placebo-controlled study in patients with and without tics. *Archives of General Psychiatry, 51,* 302–308.

McElroy, S. L., Keck, P. E., Pope, H. G., & Hudson, J. I. (1992a). Valproate in the treatment of bipolar disorder: Literature review and clinical guidelines. *Journal of Clinical Psychopharmacology, 12* (1, Suppl), 42S–52S.

McElroy, S. L., Keck, P. E., Pope, H. G., Hudson, J. I., Faedda, G. L., & Swann, A. C. (1992b). Clinical and research implications of the diagnosis of dysphoric or mixed mania or hypomania. *American Journal of Psychiatry, 149,* 1633–1644.

McElroy, S. L., Phillips, K. A., & Keck, P. E. (1994). Obsessive compulsive spectrum disorder. *Journal of Clinical Psychiatry, 55* (10, Suppl), 33–51.

McFarland, B. H. (1994). Cost-effectiveness considerations for managed care systems: Treating depression in primary care. *American Journal of Medicine, 97* (suppl 6A), 47S–58S.

McGlashan, T. H. (1988). A selective review of recent North American long-term follow-up studies of schizophrenia. *Schizophrenia Bulletin, 14,* 515–542.

McGlashan, T. H., & Carpenter, W. T. (1976). Post-psychotic depression in schizophrenia. *Archives of General Psychiatry, 33,* 231–239.

McGlashan, T. H., & Fenton, W. S. (1992). The positive-negative distinction in schizophrenia: Review of natural history validators. *Archives of General Psychiatry, 49,* 63–72.

McGrath, P. J., Stewart, J. W., Nunes, E. V., Ocepek-Welikson, K., Rabkin, J. G., Quitkin, F. M., & Klein, D. F. (1993). A double-blind crossover trial of imipramine and phenelzine for outpatients with treatment-refractory depression. *American Journal of Psychiatry, 150,* 118–123.

McGuffin, P., & Thapar, A. (1992). The genetics of personality disorder. *British Journal of Psychiatry, 160,* 20–23.

McKenna, K., Gordon, C. T., Lenane, M., Kaysen, D., Fahey, K., & Rapoport, J.L. (1994). Looking for childhood-onset schizophrenia: The first 71 cases screened. *Journal of the American Academy of Child and Adolescent Psychiatry, 33,* 636–644.

Mellinger, G. D., Balter, M. B., & Uhlenhuth, E. H. (1985). Insomnia and its treatment: Prevalence and correlates. *Archives of General Psychiatry, 42,* 225–232.

Meltzer, H. (1995). Atypical antipsychotic drugs. In F. E. Bloom and D. J. Kupfer (Eds.), *Psychopharmacology: The fourth generation of progress.* New York: Raven Press, 1277–1286.

Meltzer, H. Y., Cola, P., Way, L., Thompson, P. A., Bastani, B., Davies, M. A., & Snitz, B. (1993). Cost effectiveness of clozapine in neuroleptic-resistant schizophrenia. *American Journal of Psychiatry, 150,* 1630–1638.

Mendelson, W. B. (1993). Insomnia and related sleep disorders. *Psychiatric Clinics of North America, 16,* 841–851.

Mendelson, W. (1985). Pharmacological treatment of insomnia. In R. E. Hales & A.J. Frances (Eds.), *Annual review,* Vol. 4. Washington, DC: American Psychiatric Press, 379–394.

Metzger, E. D., & Friedman, R. S. (1994). Treatment-related depression. *Psychiatric Annals, 24,* 540–544.

Meyer, R. E. (1992). New Pharmacotherapies for cocaine dependence . . . revisited. *Archives of General Psychiatry, 49,* 900–904.

Miles, P. (1977). Conditions predisposing to suicide: A review. *Journal of Nervous and Mental Diseases, 164,* 231–246.

MILLER, H. L., DELGADO, P. L., SALOMON, R. M., LICINO, J., BARR, L. C., & CHARNEY, D. S. (1992). Acute tryptophan depletion: A method of studying antidepressant action. *Journal of Clinical Psychiatry, 53* (10, Suppl), 28–35.

MILLER, L. J. (1994). Use of electroconvulsive therapy during pregnancy. *Hospital and Community Psychiatry, 45,* 444–450.

MITCHELL, J. E., PYLE, R. L., ECKERT, E. D., HATSUKAMI, D., POMEROY, C., & ZIMMERMAN, R. (1990). A comparison study of antidepressants and structured intensive group psychotherapy in the treatment of bulimia nervosa. *Archives of General Psychiatry, 47,* 149–157.

MITCHELL, J. E., PYLE, R. L., ECKERT, E. D., HATSUKAMI, D., POMEROY, C., & ZIMMERMAN, R. (1989). Response to alternative antidepressants in imipramine nonresponders with bulimia nervosa. *Journal of Clinical Psychopharmacology, 9,* 291–293.

MONTGOMERY, S. A. (1993). Venlafaxine: A new dimension in antidepressant pharmacotherapy. *Journal of Clinical Psychiatry, 54,* 119–126.

MORIN, C. M., CULBERT, J. P., & SCHWARTZ, S. M. (1994). Nonpharmacological interventions for insomnia: A meta-analysis of treatment efficacy. *American Journal of Psychiatry, 151,* 1172–1180.

MUKHERJEE, S., SACKHEIM, H. A., & SCHNUR, D. B. (1994). Electroconvulsive therapy of acute manic episodes: A review of 50 years' experience. *American Journal of Psychiatry, 151,* 169–176.

MUNJACK, D. J., CROCKER, B., CABE, D., BROWN, R., USIGLI, R., ZULUETA, A., MCMANUS, M., MCDOWELL, D., PALMER, R., & LEONARD, M. (1989). Alprazolam, propranolol, and placebo in the treatment of panic disorder and agoraphobia with panic attacks. *Journal of Clinical Psychiatry, 9,* 22–27.

NATIONAL ADVISORY MENTAL HEALTH COUNCIL. (1993). Health care reform for Americans with severe mental illnesses: Report of the national advisory mental health council. *American Journal of Psychiatry, 150,* 1447–1465.

NIH CONSENSUS DEVELOPMENT CONFERENCE. (1993). Diagnosis and treatment of depression in late life: The NIH consensus development conference statement. *Psychopharmacology Bulletin, 29,* 87–100.

NELSON, J. C., JATLOW, P. I., & QUINLAN, D. M. (1984). Subjective complaints during desipramine treatment: Relative importance of plasma drug concentrations and the severity of depression. *Archives of General Psychiatry, 41,* 55–59.

NELSON, J. C., MAZURE, C. M., BOWERS, M. B., & JATLOW, P. I. (1991). A preliminary, open study of the combination of fluoxetine and desipramine for rapid treatment of major depression. *Archives of General Psychiatry, 48,* 303–307.

NESTLER, E. J., FITZGERALD, L. W., & SELF, D. W. (1995). Neurobiology. In J. M. Oldham and M. B. Riba (Eds.), *Review of Psychiatry,* Vol. 14. Washington, DC: American Psychiatric Press, 51–81.

NOFZINGER, E. A., BUYSSE, D. J., REYNOLDS, C. F., & KUPFER, D. J. (1993). Sleep disorders related to another mental disorder (nonsubstance/primary): A DSM-IV literature review. *Journal of Clinical Psychiatry, 54,* 244–255.

NOYES, R. (1985). Beta-adrenergic blocking drugs in anxiety and stress. *Psychiatric Clinics of North America, 8,* 119–132.

NOYES, R., GARVEY, M. J., COOK, B. L., & SAMUELSON, L. (1989). Problems with tricyclic antidepressant use in patients with panic disorder or agoraphobias: Results of a naturalistic follow-up study. *Journal of Clinical Psychiatry, 50,* 163–169.

NUNES, E. V., MCGRATH, P. J., QUITKIN, F. M., STEWART, J. P., HARRISON, W., TRICAMO, E., & OCEPEK-WELIKSON, K. (1993). Imipramine treatment of alcoholism with comorbid depression. *American Journal of Psychiatry, 150,* 963–965.

NURNBERG, H. G., & PRUDIC, J. (1984). Guidelines for treatment of psychosis during pregnancy. *Hospital & Community Psychiatry, 35,* 67–71.

O'BRIEN, C. P., ECKARD, I. M. J., & LINNOILA, M. I. (1995). Pharmacotherapy of alcoholism. In F. E. Bloom and D. J. Kupfer (Eds.), *Psychopharmacology: The fourth generation of progress*, New York: Raven Press, 1745–1755.

OLAJIDE, D., & LADER, M. (1987). A comparison of buspirone, diazepam, and placebo in patients with chronic anxiety states. *Journal of Clinical Psychiatry, 7*, 148–152.

O'MALLEY, S. S., JAFFE, A. J., CHANG, G., SCHOTTENFELD, R. S., MEYER, R. E., & ROUNSAVILLE, B. (1992). Naltrexone and coping skills therapy for alcohol dependence: A controlled study. *Archives of General Psychiatry, 49*, 881–887.

ONSTAD, S., SKRE, I., TORGERSEN, S., & KRINGLEN, E. (1991). Twin concordance for DSM-III-R schizophrenia. *Acta Psychiatria Scandinavia, 83*, 395–401.

OTTO, M. W., POLLACK, M. H., SACHS, G. S., REITER, S. R., MELTZER-BRODY, S., & ROSENBAUM, J. F. (1993). Discontinuation of benzodiazepine treatment: Efficacy of cognitive-behavioral therapy for patients with panic disorder. *American Journal of Psychiatry, 150*, 1485–1490.

PAPP, L. A., KLEIN, D. F., & GORMAN, J. M. (1993). Carbon dioxide hypersensitivity, hyperventilation, and panic disorder. *American Journal of Psychiatry, 150*, 1149–1157.

PARSONS, B., QUITKIN, F. M., MCGRATH, P. J., STEWART, J. W., TRICAMO, E., OCEPEK-WELIKSON, K., HARRISON, W., RABKIN, J. G., WAGER, S. G., & NUNES, E. (1989). Phenelzine, imipramine, and placebo in borderline patients meeting criteria for atypical depression. *Psychopharmacology Bulletin, 25*, 524–534.

PATTEN, S. B., & LOVE, E. J. (1993). Can drugs cause depression? A review of the evidence. *Journal of Psychiatry and Neuroscience, 18*, 92–102.

PAUL, S. (1995). GABA and glycine. In F. E. Bloom and D. J. Kupfer (Eds.), *Psychopharmacology: The fourth generation of progress*. New York: Raven Press, 87–94.

PAULS, D. L., ALSOBROOK, J. P., GOODMAN, W., RASMUSSEN, S., & LECKMAN, J. F. (1995). A family study of obsessive-compulsive disorder. *American Journal of Psychiatry, 152*, 76–84.

PELLOCK, J. M., & WILLMORE, L. J. (1991). A rational guide to routine blood monitoring in patients receiving antiepileptic drugs. *Neurology, 41*, 961–964.

PERKINS, D. O., STERN, R. A., GOLDEN, R. N., MURPHY, C., NAFTOLOWITZ, D., & EVANS, D. W. (1994). Mood disorders in HIV infection: Prevalence and risk factors in a nonepicenter of the AIDS epidemic. *American Journal of Psychiatry, 151*, 233–236.

PERRY, P. J., ZEILMANN, C., & ARNDT, S. (1994). Tricyclic antidepressant concentrations in plasma: An estimate of their sensitivity and specificity as a predictor of response. *Journal of Clinical Psychopharmacology, 14*, 230–240.

PFOHL, B., & ANDREASEN, N. C. (1986). Schizophrenia: Diagnosis and classification. In A. J. Frances & R. E. Hales (Eds.), *Annual review*, Vol. 5. Washington, DC: American Psychiatric Press, 7–24.

PHILIPP, M., & FICKINGER, M. (1993). Psychotropic drugs in the management of chronic pain syndromes. *Pharmacopsychiatry, 26*, 221–234.

PHILLIPS, K. A., MCELROY, S. L., KECK, P. E., HUDSON, J. I., & POPE, H. G. (1994). A comparison of delusional and nondelusional body dysmorphic disorder in 100 cases. *Psychopharmacology Bulletin, 30*, 179–186.

PHILLIPS, K. A., MCELROY, S. L., KECK, P. E., POPE, H. G., & HUDSON, J. I. (1993). Body dysmorphic disorder: 30 cases of imagined ugliness. *American Journal of Psychiatry, 150*, 302–308.

Physicians' Desk Reference. (1995). Montvale, N.J.: Medical Economics Co.

PIGGOTT, T. A., L'HEUREUX, F., DUBBERT, B., BERNSTEIN, S., & MURPHY, D. L. (1994). Obsessive-compulsive disorder: Comorbid conditions. *Journal of Clinical Psychiatry, 55* (10, Suppl), 15–27.

PISCIOTTA, A. V. (1982). Carbamazepine: Hematologic toxicity. In D. M. Woodbury, J. K. Penry, & C. Pippenger (Eds.), *Antiepileptic drugs*. New York: Raven Press, 309–341.

PLASKY, P. (1991). Antidepressant usage in schizophrenia. *Schizophrenia Bulletin, 17,* 649–657.

PLENGE, P., & MELLERUP, E. T. (1986). Lithium and the kidney: Is one daily dose better than two? *Comprehensive Psychiatry, 27,* 336–342.

PLOTKIN, D. A., GERSON, S. C., & JARVIK, L. F. (1987). Antidepressant drug treatment in the elderly. In H. Y. Meltzer (Ed.), *Psychopharmacology: The third generation of progress*. New York: Raven Press, 1149–1158.

POHL, R., BERCHOU, R., & RAINEY, J. M. (1982). Tricyclic antidepressants and monoamine oxidase inhibitors in the treatment of agoraphobia. *Journal of Clinical Psychopharmacology, 2,* 399–407.

POHL, R., YERAGANI, V. K., BALON, R., & LYCAKI, A. (1988). The jitteriness syndrome in panic disorder patients treated with antidepressants. *Journal of Clinical Psychiatry, 49,* 100–104.

POLLACK, M. H., & OTTO, M. W. (1994). Long-term pharmacologic treatment of panic disorder. *Psychiatric Annals, 24,* 291–298.

POLLACK, M. H., OTTO, M. W., ROSENBAUM, J. F., SACHS, G. S., O'NEIL, C., ASHER, R., & MELTZER-BRODY, S. (1990). Longitudinal course of panic disorder: Findings from the Massachusetts General Hospital naturalistic study. *Journal of Clinical Psychiatry, 51* (12, Suppl A), 12–16.

POPE, H. G., & KATZ, D. L. (1994). Psychiatric and medical side effects of anabolic-androgenic steroid use: A controlled study of 160 athletes. *Archives of General Psychiatry, 51,* 375–382.

POPE, H. G., & LIPINSKI, J. F. (1978). Diagnosis of schizophrenia and manic-depressive illness: A reassessment of the specificity of "schizophrenic symptoms" in the light of current research. *Archives of General Psychiatry, 35,* 811–828.

POPE, H. G., McELROY, S. L., KECK, P. E., & HUDSON, J. I. (1991). Valproate in the treatment of acute mania: A placebo-controlled study. *Archives of General Psychiatry, 48,* 62–68.

POPPER, C. W. (1993). Psychopharmacologic treatment of anxiety disorders in adolescents and children. *Journal of Clinical Psychiatry, 54* (5, Suppl), 52–63.

POST, R. M., LEVERICH, G. S., ALTSHULER, L., & MIKALAUSKAS, K. (1992). Lithium-discontinuation-induced refractoriness: Preliminary observations. *American Journal of Psychiatry, 149,* 1727–1729.

POST, R. M., LEVERICH, G. S., ROSOFF, A. S., & ALTSHULER, L. L. (1990). Carbamazepine prophylaxis in refractory affective disorders: A focus on long-term follow-up. *Journal of Clinical Psychiatry, 10,* 318–327.

POST, R. M., RUBINOW, D. R., & BALLENGER, J. C. (1984). Conditioning, sensitization and kindling: Implications for the course of affective illness. In R. M. Post & J. C. Ballenger (Eds.), *Neurobiology of mood disorders*. Baltimore, MD: Williams & Wilkins, 432–466.

POST, R. M., & UHDE, T. W. (1987). Clinical approaches to treatment resistant bipolar illness. In R. E. Hales & A. J. Frances (Eds.), *Annual review,* Vol. 6. Washington, DC: American Psychiatric Press, 125–150.

POST, R. M., UHDE, T. W., BALLENGER, J. C., CHATTERJI, D. C., GREENE, R. F., & BUNNEY, W. E. (1983). Carbamazepine and its -10, -11-epoxide metabolite in plasma and CSF. Relationship to antidepressant response. *Archives of General Psychiatry, 40,* 673–676.

POST, R. M., UHDE, T. W., PUTNAM, F. W., BALLENGER, J. C., & BERRETTINI, W. H. (1982). Kindling and carbamazepine in affective illness. *Journal of Nervous and Mental Disease, 170,* 717–731.

POST, R. M., & WEISS, S. R. B. (1995). The neurobiology of treatment-resistant mood disorders. In F. E. Bloom and D. J. Kupfer (Eds.), *Psychopharmacology: The fourth generation of progress*. New York: Raven Press, 1155–1170.

POST, R. M., WEISS, S. R. B., & CHUANG, D. M. (1992). Mechanisms of action of anticonvulsants in affective disorders: Comparisons with lithium. *Journal of Clinical Psychopharmacology, 12*, 23S–25S.

PRESKORN, S. H., ALDERMAN, J., CHUNG, M., HARRISON, W., MESSIG, M., & HARRIS, S. (1994). Pharmacokinetics of desipramine coadministered with sertraline or fluoxetine. *Journal of Clinical Psychopharmacology, 14*, 90–98.

PRICE, L. H. (1990). Pharmacological strategies in refractory depression. In A. Tasman, S. Golfinger, and C. Kaufmann (Eds.), *Review of Psychiatry*, Volume 9. Washington, DC: American Psychiatric Press, 116–131.

PRICE, L. H., GODDARD, A. W., BARR, L. C., & GOODMAN, W. K. (1995). Pharmacological challenges in anxiety disorders. In F. E. Bloom and D. J. Kupfer (Eds.), *Psychopharmacology: The fourth generation of progress*. New York: Raven Press, 1311–1323.

PRIEN, R. P., & KOCSIS, J. H. (1995). Long-term treatment of mood disorders. In F. E. Bloom and D. J. Kupfer (Eds.), *Psychopharmacology: The fourth generation of progress*. New York: Raven Press, 1067–1079.

PRIEN, R. F., & KUPFER, D. J. (1986). Continuation drug therapy for major depressive episodes: How long should it be maintained? *American Journal of Psychiatry, 143*, 18–23.

PRIEN, R. F., & POTTER, W. Z. (1990). NIMH workshop report on treatment of bipolar disorder. *Psychopharmacology Bulletin, 26*, 409–427.

PRUDIC, J., DEVANAND, D. P., SACKEIM, H. A., DECINA, P., & KERR, B. (1989). Relative response of endogenous and non-endogenous symptoms to electroconvulsive therapy. *Journal of Affective Disorders, 16*, 59–64.

PRUDIC, J., SACKEIM, H. A., & DEVANAND, D. P. (1990). Medication resistance and clinical response to electroconvulsive therapy. *Psychiatry Research, 31*, 287–296.

PUIG-ANTICH, J., PEREL, J. M., LUPATKIN, W., CHAMBERS, W. J., TABRIZI, M. A., KING, J., GOETZ, R., DAVIES, M., & STILLER, R. L. (1987). Imipramine in prepubertal major depressive disorders. *Archives of General Psychiatry, 44*, 81–89.

QUITKIN, F. M., RABKIN, J. G., ROSS, D., & MCGRATH, P. J. (1984). Duration of antidepressant drug treatment: What is an adequate trial? *Archives of General Psychiatry, 41*, 238–245.

RABKIN, J. G., QUITKIN, F. M., MCGRATH, P., HARRISON, W., & TRICAMO, E. (1985). Adverse reactions to monoamine oxidase inhibitors. Part II. Treatment correlates and clinical management. *Journal of Clinical Psychopharmacology, 5*, 2–9.

RABKIN, J. G., RABKIN, R., HARRISON, W., & WAGNER, G. (1994). Effect of imipramine on mood and enumerative measures of immune status in depressed patients with HIV illness. *American Journal of Psychiatry, 151*, 516–523.

RAFT, D., DAVIDSON, J., MATTOX, A., MUELLER, R., & WASIK, J. (1979). Double-blind evaluation of phenelzine, amitriptyline and placebo in depression associated with pain. In A. Singer (Ed.), *Monoamine oxidase: Structure, function and altered functions*. New York: Academic Press, 507–516.

RAO, U., RYAN, N. D., BIRMAHER, B., DAHL, R. E., WILLIAMSON, D. E., KAUFMAN, J., RAO, R., & NELSON, B. (1995). Unipolar depression in adolescents: Clinical outcome in adulthood. *Journal of the American Academy of Child and Adolescent Psychiatry, 34*, 566–578.

RAPOPORT, J. L., BUCHSBAUM, M. S., WEINGARTNER, H., ZAHN, T. P., LUDLOW, C., & MIKKELSEN, E. J. (1980). Dextroamphetamine: Its cognitive and behavioral effects in normal and hyperactive boys and normal men. *Archives of General Psychiatry, 37*, 933–943.

RASKIND, M. (1995). Alzheimer's disease: Treatment of neurocognitive behavioral abnormalities. In F. E. Bloom and D. J. Kupfer (Eds.), *Psychopharmacology: The fourth generation of progress.* New York: Raven Press, 1427–1435.

RASMUSSEN, S. A. (1994). Obsessive compulsive spectrum disorders. *Journal of Clinical Psychiatry, 55,* 89–91.

RASMUSSEN, S. A., AND EISEN, J. L. (1992). The epidemiology and clinical features of obsessive compulsive disorder. *Psychiatric Clinics of North America, 15,* 743–758.

RASMUSSEN, S. A., & TSUANO, M. T. (1986). Clinical characteristics and family history in DSM-III obsessive-compulsive disorder. *American Journal of Psychiatry, 143,* 317–322.

RAUCH, S. L., & RENSHAW, P. F. (1995). Clinical neuroimaging in psychiatry. *Harvard Review of Psychiatry, 2,* 297–312.

RAZANI, J., WHITE, K. L., WHITE, J., SIMPSON, G., SLOANE, R. B., REBAL, R., & PALMER, R. (1983). The safety and efficacy of combined amitriptyline and tranylcypromine antidepressant treatment: A controlled trial. *Archives of General Psychiatry, 40,* 657–661.

REGIER, D. A., FARMER, M. E., RAE, D. S., LOCKE, B. Z., KEITH, S. J., JUDD, L. L., & GOODWIN, F. K. (1990). Comorbidity of mental disorders with alcohol and other drug abuse. *Journal of the American Medical Association, 264,* 2511–2518.

REGIER, D. A., NARROW, W. E., RAE, D. S., MANDERSCHEID, R. W., LOCKE, B. Z., & GOODWIN, F. K. (1993). The de facto mental and addictive disorders service system: Epidemiologic catchment area prospective 1-year prevalence rates of disorders and services. *Archives of General Psychiatry, 50,* 85–94.

REICH, J. H. (1989). Familiarity of DSM-III dramatic and anxious personality clusters. *Journal of Nervous and Mental Disease, 177,* 96–100.

REICH, J., NOYES, R., & TROUGHTON, E. (1987). Dependent personality disorder associated with phobic avoidance in patients with panic disorder. *American Journal of Psychiatry, 144,* 323–326.

REICH, J., NOYES, R., & YATES, W. (1989). Alprazolam treatment of avoidant personality traits in social phobic patients. *Journal of Clinical Psychiatry, 50,* 91–95.

RENNER, J. A., & CIRAULO, D. (1994). Substance abuse and depression. *Psychiatric Annals, 24,* 532–539.

RICCIARDI, J. N., BAER, L., JENIKE, M. A., FISCHER, S. C., SHOLTZ, D., & BUTTOLPH, M. L. (1992). *American Journal of Psychiatry, 149,* 829–831.

RICE, E. H., SOMBROTTO, L. B., MARKOWITZ, J. C., & LEON, A. C. (1994). Cardiovascular morbidity in high-risk patients during ECT. *American Journal of Psychiatry, 151,* 1637–1641.

RICE, J., REICH, T., ANDREASEN, N. C., ENDICOTT, J., VAN EERDEWEGH, M., FISHMAN, R., HIRSCHFELD, R. M. A., & KLERMAN, G. L. (1987). The familial transmission of bipolar illness. *Archives of General Psychiatry, 44,* 441–447.

RICHELSON, E. (1984). Neuroleptic affinities for human brain receptors and their use in predicting adverse effects. *Journal of Clinical Psychiatry, 45,* 331–336.

RICKELS, K., AMSTERDAM, J. D., CLARY, C., PUZZUOLI, G., & SCHWEIZER, E. (1991). Buspirone in major depression: A controlled study. *Journal of Clinical Psychiatry, 52,* 34–38.

RICKELS, K., CASE, W. G., & DOWNING, R. W. (1982). Issues in long-term treatment with diazepam. *Psychopharmacology, 18,* 38–41.

RICKELS, K., CASE, W. G., DOWNING, R. W., & FRIEDMAN, R. (1986). One year follow-up of anxious patients treated with diazepam. *Journal of Clinical Psychopharmacology, 6,* 32–36.

RICKELS, K., CASE, W. G., DOWNING, R. W., & WINOKUR, A. (1983). Long-term diazepam therapy and clinical outcome. *Journal of the American Medical Association, 250,* 767–771.

RICKELS, K., CASE, W. G., SCHWEIZER, E., GARCIA-ESPANA, F., & FRIDMAN, R. (1991). Long-term benzodiazepine users 3 years after participation in a discontinuation program. *American Journal of Psychiatry, 148,* 757–761.

RICKELS, K., CHUNG, H. R., CSANALOSI, I. B., HUROWITZ, A. M., LONDON, J., WISEMAN, K., KAPLAN, M., & AMSTERDAM, J. D. (1987). Alprazolam, diazepam, imipramine, and placebo in outpatients with major depression. *Archives of General Psychiatry, 44,* 862–866.

RICKELS, K., DOWNING, R., SCHWEIZER, E., & HASSMAN, H. (1993). Antidepressants for the treatment of generalized anxiety disorder: A placebo-controlled comparison of imipramine, trazadone, and diazepam. *Archives of General Psychiatry, 50,* 884–895.

RICKELS, K., FOX, I. L., GREENBLATT, D. J., SANDLER, K. R., & SCHLESS, A. (1988). Clorazepate and lorazepam: Clinical improvement and rebound anxiety. *American Journal of Psychiatry, 145,* 312–317.

RICKELS, K., & SCHWEIZER, E. (1990). The clinical course and long-term management of generalized anxiety disorder. *Journal of Clinical Psychopharmacology, 10,* 101S–110S.

RICKELS, K., SCHWEIZER, E., CASE, W. G., & GARCIA-ESPANA, F. (1988). Benzodiazepine dependence, withdrawal severity, and clinical outcome: Effects of personality. *Psychopharmacology Bulletin, 24,* 415–420.

RICKELS, K., SCHWEIZER, E., CASE, W. G., & GREENBLATT, D. J. (1990). Long-term therapeutic use of benzodiazepines: I: Effects of abrupt discontinuation. *Archives of General Psychiatry, 47,* 899–907.

RICKELS, K., SCHWEIZER, E., WEISS, S., & ZAVODNICK, S. (1993). Maintenance drug treatment for panic disorder: II: Short- and long-term outcome after drug taper. *Archives of General Psychiatry, 50,* 61–68.

ROBBINS, T. W., & EVERITT, B. J. (1995). Central norepinephrine neurons and behavior. In F. E. Bloom and D. J. Kupfer (Eds.), *Psychopharmacology: The fourth generation of progress.* New York: Raven Press, 363–372.

ROBINS, E. (1986). Completed suicide. In A. Roy (Ed.), *Suicide,* Baltimore, MD: Williams & Wilkins, 123–133.

ROBINS, L. (1987). The epidemiology of antisocial personality. In R. Michels & J. Cavenar (Eds.), *Psychiatry,* Philadelphia: Lippincott, 231–244.

ROBINS, L., HELZER, J., WEISSMAN, M., ORVASCHEL, H., GRUENBERG, E., BURKE, J. D., & REGIER, D. A. (1984). Lifetime prevalence of specific psychiatric disorders in three sites. *Archives of General Psychiatry, 41,* 949–958.

ROBINSON, D. S., & KURTZ, N. M. (1987). Monoamine oxidase inhibiting drugs: Pharmacologic and therapeutic issues. In H. Y. Meltzer (Ed.), *Psychopharmacology: The third generation of progress,* New York: Raven Press, 1297–1304.

ROFFWARG, H., & ERMAN, M. (1985). Evaluation and diagnosis of the sleep disorders: Implications for psychiatry and other clinical specialties. In R. E. Hales & A. J. Frances (Eds.), *Annual review,* Vol. 4, Washington, DC: American Psychiatric Press, 294–328.

ROGERS, J. H., WIDIGER, T. A., & KRUPP, A. (1995). Aspects of depression associated with borderline personality disorder. *American Journal of Psychiatry, 152,* 268–270.

ROOSE, S. P., GLASSMAN, A. H., ATTIA, E., & WOODRING, S. (1994). Comparative efficacy of selective serotonin reuptake inhibitors and tricyclics in the treatment of melancholia. *American Journal of Psychiatry, 151,* 1735–1739.

ROSEBUSH, P. I., HILDEBRAND, A. M., FURLONG, B. G., & MAZUREK, M. F. (1990). Catatonic syndrome in a general psychiatric inpatient population: Frequency, clinical presentation, and response to lorazepam. *Journal of Clinical Psychiatry, 51,* 357–362.

ROSEBUSH, P. I., STEWART, T. D., & GELENBERG, A. J. (1989). 20 neuroleptic challenges after neuroleptic malignant syndrome in 15 patients. *Journal of Clinical Psychiatry, 50,* 295–298.

ROSENBAUM, J. F., BIEDERMAN, J., GERSTEN, M., HIRSHFELD, D. R., MEMINGER, S. R., HERMAN, J. B., KAGAN, J., REZNICK, J. S., & SNIDMAN, N. (1988). Behavioral inhibition in children of parents with panic disorder and agoraphobia. *Archives of General Psychiatry, 45,* 463–470.

ROSENBAUM, J. F., BIEDERMAN, J., HIRSHFELD, D. R., BOLDUC, E. A., FARAONE, S. T., KAGAN, J., SNIDMAN, N., & REZNICK, J. S. (1991). Further evidence of an association between behavioral inhibition and anxiety disorders: Results from a family study of children from a non-clinical sample. *Journal of Psychiatric Research, 25,* 49–65.

ROSENBERG, P. B., AHMED, I., & HURWITZ, S. (1991). Methylphenidate in depressed medically ill patients. *Journal of Clinical Psychiatry, 52,* 263–267.

ROSENSTEIN, D. L., NELSON, J., & JACOBS, S. C. (1993). Seizures associated with antidepressants: A review. *Journal of Clinical Psychiatry, 54,* 289–299.

ROSS, H. E., GLASER, F. B., & GERMANSON, T. (1988). The prevalence of psychiatric disorders in patients with alcohol and other drug problems. *Archives of General Psychiatry, 45,* 1023–1031.

ROTH, B. L. (1994). Multiple serotonin receptors: Clinical and experimental aspects. *Annals of Clinical Psychiatry, 6,* 67–78.

ROTH, B. L., & MELTZER, H. Y. (1995). The role of serotonin in schizophrenia. In F. E. Bloom and D. J. Kupfer (Eds.), *Psychopharmacology: The fourth generation of progress.* New York: Raven Press, 1215–1227.

ROTHSCHILD, A. J. (1992). Disinhibition, amnestic reactions, and other adverse reactions secondary to triazolam: A review of the literature. *Journal of Clinical Psychiatry, 53* (12, Suppl), 69–79.

ROY, A. (1990). Relationship between depression and suicidal behavior in schizophrenia. In L. E. deLisi (Ed.), *Depression in schizophrenia.* Washington, DC: American Psychiatric Press, 39–58.

ROY, A. (1986). Suicide in schizophrenia. In A. Roy (Ed.), *Suicide,* Baltimore, MD: Williams & Wilkins, 97–112.

ROY-BYRNE, P. P., SULLIVAN, M. D., COWLEY, D. S., & RIES, R. K. (1993). Adjunctive treatment of benzodiazepine discontinuation syndromes: A review. *Journal of Psychiatric Research, 27* (1, Suppl), 143–153.

RUDORFER, M. V. (1992). Monoamine oxidase inhibitors: Reversible and irreversible. *Psychopharmacology Bulletin, 28,* 45–57.

RUPP, A., & KEITH, S. J. (1993). The costs of schizophrenia. *Psychiatric Clinics of North America, 16,* 413–423.

RYAN, N. D., PUIG-ANTICH, J., AMBROSINI, P., RABINOVICH, H., ROBINSON, D., NELSON, B., IYENGAR, S., & TWOMAY, J. (1987). The clinical picture of major depression in children and adolescents. *Archives of General Psychiatry, 44,* 854–861.

SACHDEV, P., & LONERAGAN, C. (1991). The present status of akathisia. *Journal of Nervous and Mental Disease, 179,* 381–391.

SACHS, G. S., LAFER, B., STOLL, A. L., BANOV, M., THIBAULT, A. B., TOHEN, M., & ROSENBAUM, J. F. (1994a). A double-blind trial of bupropion versus desipramine for bipolar depression. *Journal of Clinical Psychiatry, 55,* 391–393.

SACHS, G. S., LAFER, B., TRUMAN, C. J., NOETH, M., & THIBAULT, A. B. (1994b). Lithium monotherapy: Miracle, myth and misunderstanding. *Psychiatric Annals, 24,* 299–306.

SACKEIM, H. A. (1992). The cognitive effects of electroconvulsive therapy. In W. H. Moos, E. R. Gamzu, and L. J. Thal (Eds.), *Cognitive disorders: Pathophysiology and treatment.* New York: Marcel Dekker, 183–228.

SACKEIM, H. A. (1994). Central issues regarding the mechanisms of action of electroconvulsive therapy: Directions for future research. *Psychopharmacology Bulletin, 30*, 281–308.

SACKEIM, H. A., DEVANAND, D. P., & NOBLER, M. S. (1995). Electroconvulsive therapy. In F. E. Bloom and D. J. Kupfer (Eds.), *Psychopharmacology: The fourth generation of progress.* New York: Raven Press, 1123–1141.

SACKEIM, H. A., PRUDIC, J., DEVANAND, D. P., KIERSKY, J. E., FITZSIMMONS, L., MOODY, B. J., MCELHINEY, M. C., COLEMAN, E. A., & SETTEMBRINO, J. M. (1993). Effects of stimulus intensity and electrode placement on the efficacy and cognitive effects of electroconvulsive therapy. *New England Journal of Medicine, 328*, 839–846.

SACKEIM, H. A., PRUDIC, J., DEVANAND, D. P., DECINA, P., KERR, B., & MALITZ, S. (1990). The impact of medication resistance and continuation pharmacotherapy on relapse following response to electroconvulsive therapy in major depression. *Journal of Clinical Psychopharmacology, 10*, 96–104.

SACKS, O. (1983). *Awakenings.* New York: Dutton.

SAKKAS, P., DAVIS, J. M., JANICAK, P. G., & WANG, Z. (1991). Drug treatment of the neuroleptic malignant syndrome. *Psychopharmacology Bulletin, 27*, 381–384.

SALIN-PASCUAL, R. J., ROEHRS, T. A., MERLOTTI, L. A., ZORICK, F., & ROTH, T. (1992). Long-term study of the sleep of insomnia patients with sleep state misperception and other insomnia patients. *American Journal of Psychiatry, 149*, 904–908.

SALZMAN, C. (1995). Interview: Update on selected topics pertaining to geriatric psychopharmacology. *Currents in Affective Disorder, 14*, 5–13.

SALZMAN, C. (1993). Benzodiazepine treatment of panic and agoraphobic symptoms: Use, dependence, toxicity, abuse. *Journal of Psychiatric Research, 27* (1, Suppl), 97–110.

SALZMAN, C., WOLFSON, A. N., SCHATZBERG, A., LOOPER, J., HENKE, R., ALBANESE, M., SCHWARTZ, J., & MIYAWAKI, E. (1995). Effect of fluoxetine on anger in symptomatic volunteers with borderline personality disorder. *Journal of Clinical Psychopharmacology, 15*, 23–29.

SATEL, S. L., & NELSON, J. C. (1989). Stimulants in the treatment of depression: A critical overview. *Journal of Clinical Psychiatry, 50*, 241–249.

SCHARF, M. B., FLETCHER, K., & GRAHAM, J. P. (1988). Comparative amnestic effects of benzodiazepine hypnotic agents. *Journal of Clinical Psychiatry, 49*, 134–137.

SCHATZBERG, A. F., & ROTHSCHILD, A. J. (1992). Psychotic (delusional) major depression: Should it be included as a distinct syndrome in DSM-IV? *American Journal of Psychiatry, 149*, 733–745.

SCHATZBERG, A. F., & SCHILDKRAUT, J. J. (1995). Recent studies on norepinephrine systems in mood disorders. In F. E. Bloom and D. J. Kupfer (Eds.), *Psychopharmacology: The fourth generation of progress,* New York: Raven Press, 911–920.

SCHMIDT, P. J., & RUBINOW, D. R. (1991). Menopause-related affective disorders: A justification for further study. *American Journal of Psychiatry, 148*, 844–852.

SCHNEIDER, L. S., OLIN, J. T., & PAWLUCZYK, S. (1993). A double-blind crossover pilot study of 1-deprenyl (selegiline) combined with cholinesterase inhibitor in Alzheimer's disease. *American Journal of Psychiatry, 150*, 321–323.

SCHNEIER, F. R., JOHNSON, J., HORNIG, C., LIEBOWITZ, M. R., & WEISSMAN, M. M. (1992). Social phobia: Comorbidity and morbidity in an epidemiologic sample. *Archives of General Psychiatry, 49*, 282–288.

SCHNEIER, F. R., SAOUD, J. B., CAMPEAS, R., FALLON, B. A., HOLLANDER, E., COPLAN, J., & LIEBOWITZ, M. R. (1993). Buspirone in social phobia. *Journal of Clinical Psychopharmacology, 13*, 251–256.

SCHNEIER, F. R., SPITZER, R. L., GIBBON, M., FYER, A. J., & LIEBOWITZ, M. R. (1991). The relationship of social phobia subtypes and avoidant personality disorder. *Comprehensive Psychiatry, 32*, 496–502.

SCHOU, M. (1986). Lithium treatment: A refresher course. *British Journal of Psychiatry, 149,* 541–547.

SCHOU, M. (1988). Effects of long-term lithium treatment on kidney function: An overview. *Journal of Psychiatric Research, 22,* 287–296.

SCHUCKIT, M. A. (1986). Genetic and clinical implications of alcoholism and affective disorder. *American Journal of Psychiatry, 143,* 140–147.

SCHUCKIT, M. A. (1983). Alcoholism and other psychiatric disorders. *Hospital and Community Psychiatry, 34,* 1022–1026.

SCHUCKIT, M. A., & HESSELBROCK, V. (1994). Alcohol dependence and anxiety disorders: What is the relationship? *American Journal of Psychiatry, 151,* 1723–1734.

SCHWARTZ, H. I. (1992). An empirical review of the impact of triplicate prescription of benzodiazepines. *Hospital and Community Psychiatry, 43,* 382–385.

SCHWEIZER, E., & RICKELS, K. (1994). New and emerging clinical uses for buspirone. *Journal of Clinical Psychiatry Monograph, 12,* 46–54.

SCHWEIZER, E., RICKELS, K., AMSTERDAM, J. D., FOX, I., PUZZUOLI, G., & WEISE, C. (1990). What constitutes an adequate antidepressant trial for fluoxetine? *Journal of Clinical Psychiatry, 51,* 8–11.

SCHWEIZER, E., RICKELS, K., CASE, W. G., & GREENBLATT, D. J. (1991). Carbamazepine treatment in patients discontinuing long-term benzodiazepine therapy: Effects on withdrawal severity and outcome. *Archives of General Psychiatry, 48,* 448–452.

SCHWEIZER, E., RICKELS, K., CASE, W. G., & GREENBLATT, D. J. (1990). Long-term therapeutic use of benzodiazepines: II: Effects of gradual taper. *Archives of General Psychiatry, 47,* 908–915.

SCHWEIZER, E., RICKELS, K., & UHLENHUTH, E. H. (1995). Issues in the long-term treatment of anxiety disorders. In F. E. Bloom and D. J. Kupfer (Eds.), *Psychopharmacology: The fourth generation of progress.* New York: Raven Press, 1349–1359.

SCHWEIZER, E., RICKELS, K., WEISS, S., & ZAVODNICK, S. (1993). Maintenance drug treatment of panic disorder: I: Results of a prospective, placebo-controlled comparison of alprazolam and imipramine. *Archives of General Psychiatry, 50,* 51–60.

SCOTT, A. I., & WHALLEY, L. J. (1993). The onset and rate of the antidepressant effect of electroconvulsive therapy. *British Journal of Psychiatry, 162,* 725–732.

SECUNDA, S., KATZ, M., SWANN, A., KOSLOW, S., MAAS, J., CHUANG, S., & CROUGHAN, J. (1985). Mania: Diagnosis, state measurement and prediction of response. *Journal of Affective Disorders, 8,* 113–121.

SEEMAN, P. (1992). Dopamine receptor sequences. *Neuropsychopharmacology, 7,* 261–284.

SERNYAK, M. J., & WOODS, S. W. (1993). Chronic neuroleptic use in manic-depressive illness. *Psychopharmacology Bulletin, 29,* 375–381.

SHADER, R. I., & GREENBLATT, D. J. (1993). Use of benzodiazepines in anxiety disorders. *New England Journal of Medicine, 328,* 1398–1405.

SHAW, E. D., MANN, J. J., STOKES, P. E., & MANEVITZ, A. Z. A. (1986). Effects of lithium carbonate on associative productivity and idiosyncrasy in bipolar outpatients. *American Journal of Psychiatry, 143,* 1166–1169.

SHEA, M. T., GLASS, D. R., PILKONIS, P. A., WATKINS, J., & DOCHERTY, J. P. (1987). Frequency and implications of personality disorders in a sample of depressed outpatients. *Journal of Personality Disorders, 1,* 27–42.

SHEAR, K. (1986). Pathophysiology of panic: A review of pharmacologic provocative tests and naturalistic monitoring data. *Journal of Clinical Psychiatry, 47* (Suppl), 18–26.

SHEEHAN, D. V., BALLENGER, J., & JACOBSEN, G. (1980). Treatment of endogenous anxiety with phobic, hysterical and hypochondriacal symptoms. *Archives of General Psychiatry, 37,* 51–59.

SIEVER, L. J., & DAVIS, K. L. (1991). A psychobiological perspective on the personality disorders. *American Journal of Psychiatry, 148,* 1647–1658.

SIEVER, L. J., KALUS, O. F., & KEEFE, R. S. E. (1993). The boundaries of schizophrenia. *Psychiatric Clinics of North America, 16,* 217–244.

SIEVER, L. J., STEINBERG, B. J., TRESTMAN, R. L., & INTRATOR, J. (1994). Personality disorders. In J. M. Oldham and M. B. Riba (Eds.), *Review of Psychiatry,* Vol. 13. Washington, DC: American Psychiatric Press, 253–290.

SILOVE, D., & MANICAVASAGER, V. (1993). Adults who feared school: Is early separation anxiety specific to the pathogenesis of panic disorder? *Acta Psychiatrica Scandinavia, 88,* 385–390.

SIRIS, S. G. (1991). Diagnosis of secondary depression in schizophrenia: Implications for DSM-IV. *Schizophrenia Bulletin, 17,* 75–98.

SIRIS, S. G., BERMANZOHN, P. C., MASON, S. E., & SHUWALL, M. A. (1994). Maintenance imipramine therapy for secondary depression in schizophrenia: A controlled trial. *Archives of General Psychiatry, 51,* 109–115.

SIRIS, S. G., MORGAN, V., FAGERSTROM, R., RIFKIN, A., & COOPER, T. B. (1987). Adjunctive imipramine in the treatment of postpsychotic depression: A controlled trial. *Archives of General Psychiatry, 42,* 533–539.

SITLAND-MARKEN, P. A., RICKMAN, L. A., WELLS, B. G., & MABIE, W. C. (1989). Pharmacologic management of acute mania in pregnancy. *Journal of Clinical Psychopharmacology, 9,* 78–87.

SKRE, I., ONSTAD, S., TORGERSEN, S., LYGREN, S., & KRINGLEN, E. (1993). A twin study of DSM-III-R anxiety disorders. *Acta Psychiatrica Scandinavia, 88,* 85–92.

SKY, A. J., & GROSSBERG, G. T. (1994). The use of psychotropic medication in the management of problem behaviors in the patient with Alzheimer's disease. *Medical Clinics of North America, 78,* 811–822.

SNYDER, S. H. (1988). *The new biology of mood.* New York: Roerig/Pfizer.

SOLOFF, P. H. (1989). Psychopharmacologic therapies in borderline personality disorder. In A. Tasman, R. E. Hales, and A. J. Frances, (Eds.), *Review of Psychiatry,* Volume 8. Washington, DC: American Psychiatric Press, 65–83.

SOLOFF, P. H., CORNELIUS, J., GEORGE, A., NATHAN, R. S., PEREL, J. M., & ULRICH, R. F. (1993). Efficacy of phenelzine and haloperidol in borderline personality disorder. *Archives of General Psychiatry, 50,* 377–385.

SOLOFF, P. H., GEORGE, A., NATHAN, R. S., SCHULZ, P. M., CORNELIUS, J. R., HERRING, J., & PEREL, J. M. (1989). Amitriptyline versus haloperidol in borderlines: Final outcomes and predictors of response. *Journal of Clinical Psychiatry, 9,* 238–246.

SOLOFF, P. H., GEORGE, A., NATHAN, R. S., SCHULZ, P. M., & PEREL, J. M. (1986). Paradoxical effects of amitriptyline on borderline patients. *American Journal of Psychiatry, 143,* 1603–1605.

SOUTHWICK, S. M., YEHUDA, R., & GILLER, E. L. (1993). Personality disorders in treatment-seeking combat veterans with posttraumatic stress disorder. *American Journal of Psychiatry, 150,* 1020–1023.

SOUZA, F. G. M., & GOODWIN, G. M. (1991). Lithium treatment and prophylaxis in unipolar depression: A meta-analysis. *British Journal of Psychiatry, 158,* 666–675.

SPENCER, T., BIEDERMAN, J., & WILENS, T. (1994). Tricyclic antidepressant treatment of children with ADHD and tic disorders. *Journal of the Academy of Child and Adolescent Psychiatry, 33,* 1203–1204.

SPENCER, T., BIEDERMAN, J., WILENS, T., & FARAONE, S. V. (1994). Is attention-deficit hyperactivity disorder in adults a valid disorder? *Harvard Review of Psychiatry, 1,* 326–335.

SPENCER, T., WILENS, T., BIEDERMAN, J., FARAONE, S. V., ABLON, S., & LAPEY, K. (1995). A double-blind, crossover comparison of methylphenidate and placebo in adults with childhood-onset attention-deficit hyperactivity disorder. *Archives of General Psychiatry, 52,* 434–443.

SPIKER, D. G., PEREL, J. M., HANIN, I., DEALY, R. S., GRIFFIN, S. J., SOLOFF, P. H., & COFSKY-WEISS, J. (1986). The pharmacological treatment of delusional depression: Part II. *Journal of Clinical Psychopharmacology, 6,* 339–342.

SPITZER, R. L., ENDICOTT, J., & ROBINS, E. (1978). The research diagnostic criteria: Rationale and reliability. *Archives of General Psychiatry, 35,* 773–782.

SQUIRE, L. (1985). The question of long-term effects. In *Electroconvulsive Therapy,* NIH Consensus Development Conference, NIH, Bethesda, Md.

STARKMAN, M., ZELNICK, T., TESSE, R., & CAMERON, O. G. (1985). Anxiety in patients with pheochromocytomas. *Archives of Internal Medicine, 145,* 248–252.

STEINER, M., HASKETT, R., & OSMUN, J. (1980). Treatment of premenstrual tension with lithium carbonate. *Acta Psychiatrica Scandinavia, 61,* 96–102.

STEINER, M., STEINBERG, S., STEWART, D., CARTER, D., BERGER, C., REID, R., GROVER, D., & STREINER, D. (1995). Fluoxetine in the treatment of premenstrual dysphoria. *New England Journal of Medicine, 332,* 1529–1534.

STEINGARD, R. J., DEMASO, D. R., GOLDMAN, S. J., SHORROCK, K. L., & BUCCI, J. P. (1995). Current perspectives on the pharmacotherapy of depressive disorders in children and adolescents. *Harvard Review of Psychiatry, 2,* 313–326.

STEINGARD, S., ALLEN, M., & SCHOOLER, N. R. (1994). A study of the pharmacologic treatment of medication-compliant schizophrenics who relapse. *Journal of Clinical Psychiatry, 55,* 470–472.

STERNBACH, H. (1991). The serotonin syndrome. *American Journal of Psychiatry, 148,* 705–713.

STEWART, D. E., KLOMPENHOUWER, J. L., KENDALL, R. E., & VAN HULST, A. M. (1991). Prophylactic lithium in puerperal psychosis: The experience of three centers. *British Journal of Psychiatry, 158,* 393–397.

STOEWE, J. K., KRUESI, M. J. P., & CELIO, D. F. (1995). Psychopharmacology of aggressive states and features of conduct disorder. *Child and Adolescent Psychiatric Clinics of North America, 4,* 359–379.

STOLL, A. L., BANOV, M., KOLBRENER, M., MAYER, P. V., TOHEN, M., STRAKOWSKI, S. M., CASTILLO, J., SUPPES, T., & COHEN, B. M. (1994). Neurologic factors predict a favorable valproate response in bipolar and schizoaffective disorders. *Journal of Clinical Psychopharmacology, 14,* 311–313.

STRAKOWSKI, S. M. (1994). Diagnostic validity of schizophreniform disorder. *American Journal of Psychiatry, 151,* 815–824.

STRAUSS, J. S., & CARPENTER, W. T. (1974). The prediction of outcome in schizophrenia. II. Relationships between predictor and outcome variables: A report from the WHO International Pilot Study of Schizophrenia. *Archives of General Psychiatry, 31,* 37–42.

STROBER, M., & CARLSON, G. (1982). Bipolar illness in adolescents: Clinical, genetic and pharmacologic predictors in a three-to-four year prospective follow-up. *Archives of General Psychiatry, 39,* 549–555.

STROBER, M., & KATZ, J. (1986). Depression in the eating disorders: A review and analysis of descriptive, family and biological findings. In D. M. Garner & P. E. Garfinkel (Eds.), *Diagnostic issues in anorexia nervosa and bulimia nervosa,* New York: Brunner/Mazel, 80–111.

STROBER, M., MORRELL, W., LAMPERT, C., & BURROUGHS, J. (1990). Relapse following discontinuation of lithium maintenance therapy in adolescents with bipolar I illness: A naturalistic study. *American Journal of Psychiatry, 147,* 457–461.

STUPPAECK, C. H., PYCHA, R., MILLER, C., WHITWORTH, A. B., OBERBAUER, H., & FLEISCHACKER, W. W. (1992). Carbamazepine versus oxazepam in the treat ment of alcohol withdrawal: A double-blind study. *Alcohol & Alcoholism, 27,* 153–158.

SUNDERLAND, T., COHEN, R. M., MOLCHAN, S., LAWLOR, B. A., MELLOW, A., NEW-HOUSE, P. A., TARIOT, P. N., MUELLER, E. A., & MURPHY, D. L. (1994). High-dose selegiline in treatment-resistant older depressive patients. *Archives of General Psychiatry, 51,* 607–615.

SUPPES, T., BALDESSARINI, R. J., FAEDDA, G. L., & TOHEN, M. (1991). Risk of recurrence following discontinuation of lithium treatment in bipolar disorder. *Archives of General Psychiatry, 48,* 1082–1088.

SUSSMAN, N. (1994). The uses of buspirone in psychiatry. *Journal of Clinical Psychiatry Monograph, 12,* 3–19.

SUTHERLAND, S. M., & DAVIDSON, J. R. (1994). Pharmacotherapy for post-traumatic stress disorder. *Psychiatric Clinics of North America, 17,* 409–423.

SUTKER, P. B., ALLAIN, A. N., & WINSTEAD, D. K. (1993). Psychopathology and psychiatric diagnoses of World War II Pacific theater prisoner of war survivors and combat veterans. *American Journal of Psychiatry, 150,* 240–245.

SZYMANSKI, L. S., RUBIN, I. L., & TARJAN, G. (1989). Mental retardation. In A. Tasman, R. E. Hales, & A. J. Frances (Eds.), *Review of Psychiatry,* Vol. 8, Washington DC: American Psychiatric Press, 217–241.

TAMMINGA, C. A., THAKER, G. K., MORAN, M., KAKIGI, T., & GAO, X. M. (1994). Clozapine in tardive dyskinesia: Observations from human and animal model studies. *Journal of Clinical Psychiatry, 55* (Suppl B), 102–106.

TAYLOR, J. L. & TINKLENBERG, J. R. (1987). Cognitive impairment and benzodiazepines. In H. Y. Meltzer (Ed.), *Psychopharmacology: The third generation of progress,* New York: Raven Press, 1448–1454.

TEICHER, M. H., GLOD, C., & COLE, J. O. (1990). Emergence of intense suicidal preoccupation during fluoxetine treatment. *American Journal of Psychiatry, 147,* 207–210.

TERMAN, M., TERMAN, J. S., QUITKIN, F. M., McGRATH, P. J., STEWART, J. W., & RAFFERTY, B. (1989). Light therapy for seasonal affective disorder: A review of efficacy. *Neuropsychopharmacology, 2,* 1–22.

THASE, M. E., KUPFER, D. J., FRANK, E., & JARRETT, D. B. (1989). Treatment of imipramine-resistant recurrent depression: II. An open clinical trial of lithium augmentation. *Journal of Clinical Psychiatry, 50,* 413–417.

THIENHAUS, O. J., MARGLETTA, S., & BENNETT, J. A. (1990). A study of the clinical efficacy of maintenance ECT. *Journal of Clinical Psychiatry, 51,* 141–144.

THOMPSON, J. L., MORAN, M. G., & NIES, A. S. (1983). Psychotropic drug use in the elderly. *New England Journal of Medicine, 308,* 134–138.

THOMPSON, J. W., & BLAINE, J. D. (1987). Use of ECT in the United States in 1975 and 1980. *American Journal of Psychiatry, 144,* 557–562.

THOMPSON, J. W., WEINER, R. D., & MYERS, C. P. (1994). Use of ECT in the United States in 1975, 1980, and 1986. *American Journal of Psychiatry, 151,* 1657–1661.

TOLLEFSON, G. D., RAMPEY, A. H., BEASLEY, C. M., ENAS, G. G., & POTVIN, J. H. (1994a). Absence of a relationship between adverse events and suicidality during pharmacotherapy for depression. *Journal of Clinical Psychopharmacology, 14,* 163–169.

TOLLEFSON, G. D., RAMPEY, A. H., POTVIN, J. H., JENIKE, M. A., RUSH, A. J., DOMINGUEZ, R. A., KORAN, L. M., SHEAR, M. K., GOODMAN, W., & GENDUSO, L. A. (1994b). A multicenter investigation of fixed-dose fluoxetine in the treatment of obsessive-compulsive disorder. *Archives of General Psychiatry, 51,* 559–567.

TORGERSEN, S. (1979). The nature and origin of common phobic fears. *British Journal of Psychiatry, 134,* 343–351.

TOWBIN, K. E. (1995). Evaluation, establishing the treatment alliance, and informed consent. *Child and Adolescent Psychiatric Clinics of North America, 4,* 1–14.

TYRER, P., CASEY, P., & FERGUSON, B. (1991). Personality disorder in perspective. *British Journal of Psychiatry, 159,* 463–471.

UHDE, T. W., STEIN, M. B., VITTONE, F. J., SIEVER, L. J., BOULENGER, J. P., KLEIN, E., & MELLMAN, T. A. (1989). Behavioral and physiologic effects of short-term and long-term administration of clonidine in panic disorder. *Archives of General Psychiatry, 46,* 170–177.

UHDE, T., VITTONE, B., & POST, R. (1984). Glucose tolerance tests in panic disorder. *American Journal of Psychiatry, 141,* 1461–1463.

UHLENHUTH, E. H., BALTER, M. B., MELLINGER, G. D., CISIN, I. H., & CLINTHORNE, J. (1983). Symptom checklist syndromes in the general population: Correlations with psychotherapeutic drug use. *Archives of General Psychiatry, 40,* 1167–1173.

VALLEJO, J., OLIVARES, J., MARCOS, T., BULBENA, A., & MENCHON, J. M. (1992). Clomipramine versus phenelzine in obsessive-compulsive disorder. *British Journal of Psychiatry, 161,* 665–670.

VAN DER KOLK, B. A., DREYFUSS, D., MICHAELS, M., SHERA, D., BERKOWITZ, R., FISLER, R., & SAXE, G. (1994). Fluoxetine in posttraumatic stress disorder. *Journal of Clinical Psychiatry, 55,* 517–522.

VAN KAMMEN, D., BUNNEY, W. E., DOCHERTY, J. P., MARDER, S. R., EBERT, M. H., ROSENBLATT, J. E., & RAYNER, J. N. (1982). d-Amphetamine-induced heterogeneous changes in psychotic behavior in schizophrenia. *American Journal of Psychiatry, 139,* 991–997.

VAN PUTTEN, T., & MARDER, S. (1987). Behavioral toxicity of antipsychotic drugs. *Journal of Clinical Psychiatry, 48* (Suppl.), 13–19.

VAN PUTTEN, T., & MAY, P. R. A. (1978). Subjective response as a predictor of outcome in pharmacotherapy. The consumer has a point. *Archives of General Psychiatry, 35,* 477–480.

VESTEGAARD, P. (1983). Clinically important side effects of long-term lithium treatment: A review. *Acta Psychiatrica Scandinavia, 67* (Suppl. 305), 11–33.

VESTEGAARD, P., AMDISEN, A., & SCHOU, M. (1980). Clinically significant side effects of lithium treatment: A survey of 237 patients in long-term treatment. *Acta Psychiatrica Scandinavia, 62,* 193–200.

VOLPICELLI, J. R., ALTERMAN, A. I., HAYASHIDA, M., & O'BRIEN, C. P. (1992). Naltrexone in the treatment of alcohol dependence. *Archives of General Psychiatry, 49,* 876–880.

VOLPICELLI, J. R., WATSON, N. T., KING, A. C., SHERMAN, C. E., & O'BRIEN, C. P. (1995). Effect of naltrexone on alcohol "high" in alcoholics. *American Journal of Psychiatry, 152,* 613–615.

WALLACE, A. E., KOFOED, L. L., & WEST, A. N. (1995). Double-blind, placebo-controlled trial of methylphenidate in older, depressed, medically ill patients. *American Journal of Psychiatry, 152,* 929–931.

WALSH, B. T., & DEVLIN, M. (1995). Psychopharmacology of anorexia nervosa, bulimia nervosa, and binge eating. In F. E. Bloom and D. J. Kupfer (Eds.), *Psychopharmacology: The fourth generation of progress.* New York: Raven Press, 1581–1589.

WALSH, B., GLADIS, M., ROOSE, S., STEWART, J. W., STETNER, F., & GLASSMAN, A. H. (1988). Phenelzine vs. placebo in 50 patients with bulimia. *Archives of General Psychiatry, 45,* 471–475.

WALSH, B. T., HADIGAN, C. M., DEVLIN, M. J., GLADIS, M., & ROOSE, S. P. (1991). Long-term outcome of antidepressant treatment for bulimia nervosa. *American Journal of Psychiatry, 148,* 1206–1212.

WALSH, J. K., & ENGELHARDT, C. L. (1992). Trends in the pharmacologic treatment of insomnia. *Journal of Clinical Psychiatry, 53* (12, Suppl), 10–17.

WALSH, S. L., PRESTON, K. L., SULLIVAN, J. T., FROMME, R., & BIGELOW, G. E. (1994). Fluoxetine alters the effects of intravenous cocaine in humans. *Journal of Clinical Psychopharmacology, 14,* 396–407.

WATSON, C. P. E. (1994). Antidepressant drugs as adjuvant analgesics. *Journal of Pain and Symptom Management, 9,* 392–405.

WEHR, T. A., & GOODWIN, F. K. (1987). Can antidepressants cause mania and worsen the course of affective illness? *American Journal of Psychiatry, 144,* 1403–1411.

WEINBERGER, D. (1987). Implications of normal brain development for the pathogenesis of schizophrenia. *Archives of General Psychiatry, 44,* 660–669.

WEINER, R. D., ROGERS, A. J., DAVIDSON, J. R., & SQUIRE, L. R. (1986). Effects of stimulus parameters on cognitive side effects. *Annals of New York Academy of Science, 462,* 315–325.

WEINTRAUB, M., SINGH, S., BYRNE, L., MAHARAJ, K., & GUTTMACHER, L. (1991). Consequences of the 1989 New York State triplicate benzodiazepine prescription regulations. *Journal of the American Medical Association, 266,* 2392–2397.

WEISSMAN, M. M. (1993). Family genetic studies of panic disorder. *Journal of Psychiatric Research, 27* (1, Suppl), 69–78.

WEISSMAN, M. M., WICKRAMARANTE, P., MERIKANGAS, K. R., LECKMAN, J. F., PRUSOFF, B. A., CARUSO, K. A., KIDD, K. K., & GAMMON, G. D. (1984). Onset of major depression in early adulthood. Increased familial loading and specificity. *Archives of General Psychiatry, 41,* 1136–1143.

WELLS, K. B., BURNAM, M. A., ROGERS, W., HAYS, R., & CAMP, P. (1992). The course of depression in adult outpatients: Results from the medical outcomes study. *Archives of General Psychiatry, 49,* 788–794.

WENDER, P. H., & REIMHERR, F. W. (1990). Bupropion treatment of attention-deficit hyperactivity disorder in adults. *American Journal of Psychiatry, 147,* 1018–1020.

WENDER, P., REIMHERR, F. W., & WOOD, D. R. (1981). Attention deficit disorder ("Minimal brain dysfunction") in adults: A replication study of diagnosis and drug treatments. *Archives of General Psychiatry, 38,* 449–456.

WENDER, P. H., REIMHERR, R. W., WOOD, D., & WARD, M. (1985). A controlled study of methylphenidate in the treatment of attention deficit disorder, residual type, in adults. *American Journal of Psychiatry, 142,* 547–552.

WENDER, P., WOOD, D., & REIMHERR, F. (1985). Pharmacological treatment of attention deficit disorder, residual type (ADD, RT, "minimal brain dysfunctions," "hyperactivity") in adults. *Psychopharmacological Bulletin, 21,* 222–231.

WIDIGER, T. A., & ROGERS, J. H. (1989). Prevalence and comorbidity of personality disorders. *Psychiatric Annals, 19,* 132–136.

WILENS, T. E., BIEDERMAN, J., & SPENCER, T. (1994). Clonidine for sleep disturbances associated with attention-deficit hyperactivity disorder. *Journal of the American Academy of Child and Adolescent Psychiatry, 33,* 424–426.

WILENS, T. E., BIEDERMAN, J., SPENCER, T. J., & PRINCE, J. (1995). Pharmacotherapy of adult attention deficit/hyperactivity disorder: A review. *Journal of Clinical Psychopharmacology, 15,* 270–279.

WILENS, T. E., SPENCER, T., BIEDERMAN, J., WOZNIAK, J., & CONNOR, D. (1995). Combined pharmacotherapy: An emerging trend in pediatric psychopharmacology. *Journal of the American Academy of Child and Adolescent Psychiatry, 34,* 110–112.

WINGARD, C. (1961). Is there any legitimate medical use for the compounds of lithium? *Journal of the American Medical Association, 75,* 340.

WINKER, A. (1994). Tacrine for Alzheimer's disease: Which patient, what dose? *Journal of the American Medical Association, 271,* 1023–1024.

WISNER, K. L., PEREL, J. M., & FOGLIA, J. P. (1995). Serum clomipramine and metabolite levels in four nursing mother-infant pairs. *Journal of Clinical Psychiatry, 56,* 17–20.

WISNER, K. L., & WHEELER, S. B. (1994). Prevention of recurrent postpartum major depression. *Hospital and Community Psychiatry, 45,* 1191–1196.

WITHERS, N. W., PULVIRENTI, L., KOOB, G. F., & GILLIN, J. C. (1995). Cocaine abuse and dependence. *Journal of Clinical Psychopharmacology, 15,* 63–78.

WITTCHEN, H. U., & ESSAU, C. A. (1993). Epidemiology of panic disorder: Progress and unresolved issues. *Journal of Psychiatric Research, 27* (1, Suppl), 47–68.

WITTCHEN, H. U., ZHAO, S., KESSLER, R. C., & EATON, W. W. (1994). DSM-III-R generalized anxiety disorder in the national comorbidity survey. *Archives of General Psychiatry, 51,* 355–364.

WOLKOWITZ, O. M., & PICKAR, D. (1991). Benzodiazepines in the treatment of schizophrenia: A review and reappraisal. *American Journal of Psychiatry, 148,* 714–726.

WOLRAICH, M. L., LUNDGREN, S. D., STUMBO, P. J., STEGINK, L. D., APPELBAUM, M. I., & KIRITSY, M. C. (1994)5. Effects of diets high in sucrose or aspartame on the behavior and cognitive performance of children. *New England Journal of Medicine, 330,* 301–307.

WOODMAN, C. L., & NOYES, R. (1994). Panic disorder: Treatment with valproate. *Journal of Clinical Psychiatry, 55,* 134–136.

WOODS, J. H., KATZ, J. L., & WINGER, G. (1995). Abuse and therapeutic use of benzodiazepines and benzodiazepine-like drugs. In F. E. Bloom and D. J. Kupfer (Eds.), *Psychopharmacology: The fourth generation of progress.* New York: Raven Press, 1777–1791.

WOODS, S. W., NAGY, L. M., KOLESZAR, A. S., KRYSTAL, J. H., HENINGER, G. R., & CHARNEY, D. S. (1992). Controlled trial of alprazolam supplementation during imipramine treatment of panic disorder. *Journal of Clinical Psychopharmacology, 12,* 32–38.

WOZNIAK, J., BIEDERMAN, J., KIELY, K., ABLON, J. S., FARAONE, S. V., MUNDY, E., & MENNIN, D. (1995). Mania-like symptoms suggestive of childhood onset bipolar disorder in clinically referred children. *Journal of American Academy of Child and Adolescent Psychiatry, 34,* 867–876.

WRAGG, R. E., & JESTE, D. V. (1989). Overview of depression and psychosis in Alzheimer's disease. *American Journal of Psychiatry, 146,* 577–587.

WYATT, R. J., KIRCH, D. G., & EGAN, M. F. (1995). Schizophrenia: neurochemical, viral and immunological studies. In H. I. Kaplan and B. J. Sadock (Eds.), *Comprehensive textbook of psychiatry.* Baltimore: Williams & Wilkins, 927–942.

WYETH-AYERST. Effexor package insert, 1994.

YASSA, R., & JESTE, D. V. (1992). Gender differences in tardive dyskinesia: A critical review of the literature. *Schizophrenia Bulletin, 18,* 701–715.

ZARIN, D. A., PINCUS, H. A., & McINTYRE, J. S. (1993). Practice guidelines. *American Journal of Psychiatry, 150,* 175–177.

ZIMMERMAN, M. (1990). Is DSM-IV needed at all? *Archives of General Psychiatry, 47,* 974–976.

ZINBARG, R. E., BARLOW, D. H., LIEBOWITZ, M., STREET, L., BROADHEAD, E., KATON, W., ROY-BYRNE, P., LEPINE, J. P., TEHERANI, M., RICHARDS, J., BRANTLEY, P. J., & KRAEMER, H. (1994). The DSM-IV field trial for mixed anxiety-depression. *American Journal of Psychiatry, 151,* 1153–1162.

ZISOOK, S., & SHUCHTER, S. R. (1993). Uncomplicated bereavement. *Journal of Clinical Psychiatry, 54,* 365–372.

ZOHAR, J., KAPLAN, Z., & BENJAMIN, J. (1993). Clomipramine treatment of obsessive compulsive symptomatology in schizophrenic patients. *Journal of Clinical Psychiatry, 54,* 385–388.

ZORNBERG, G. L., & POPE, H. G. (1993). Treatment of depression in bipolar disorder: New directions for research. *Journal of Clinical Psychopharmacology, 13,* 397–408.

ZORUMSKI, C. F., & ISENBERG, K.E . (1991). Insights into the structure and function of GABA-benzodiazepine receptors: Ion channels and psychiatry. *American Journal of Psychiatry, 148,* 162–173.

Index